AF594151

Bork
Bräuninger

Skin Diseases in Clinical Practice

Skin Diseases in Clinical Practice

2nd Edition

by

Konrad Bork, M. D.
Professor of Dermatology
University Hospital, Mainz, Germany

Wolfgang Bräuninger, M. D.
University Hospital, Mainz, Germany

Translated from the Original German Text by

Karl H. Müller, M. D.,
Ramsey Markus, M. D.,
The Medical College of Wisconsin,
Milwaukee, Wisconsin

and

Virginia Müller,
Tübingen, Germany

W. B. SAUNDERS COMPANY
A Division of Harcourt Brace and Company
Philadelphia London Toronto Montreal Sydney Tokyo

W. B. SAUNDERS COMPANY
A Division of Harcourt Brace & Company

The Curtis Center
Independence Square West
Philadelphia, PA 19106

Library of Congress Cataloging-in-Publication Data

Skin Diseases in Clinical Practice, 2nd Edition/Bork, Bräuninger

p. cm.

Includes bibliographical references and Index.

ISBN 0-7216-7480-1

1. skin diseases   2. dermatology

Translator's Note

Recommendations for therapy throughout this book are based on the experience of the authors and their colleagues in the Dermatology Clinic of the University Hospital, Mainz. Whenever possible, the names of German therapeutic preparations have been replaced in this English edition by equivalent U.S. product names.
Some German products have no exact U.S. equivalent or must be compounded, and these are designated by appropriate notes in the text, particularly in the final chapter on therapy. The treatment methods described are not necessarily those that would be recommended by the translators.

Skin Diseases in Clinical Practice   ISBN 0-7216-7480-1

English edition published by W. B. Saunders Company, 1998.

Printed in Germany
Last digit is the print number: 9 8 7 6 5 4 3 2 1

Preface to the Second Edition

The first edition of this book was accepted very favorably, and we have now prepared a new edition with a text that was revised and enlarged significantly. Again, it was our goal with this new edition to achieve the greatest usefulness for the practicing physician. To this end, the most characteristic illustrations were included, descriptions of the signs and symptoms one needs to know to arrive at the correct diagnosis are presented, and in particular, the appropriate therapeutic measures are provided. Several chapters were revised, such as the chapter on AIDS. A number of new clinical syndromes that are seen with increasing frequency by the practicing physician were included. Special emphasis was given to up-to-date advice on therapeutic measures. The last chapter was also brought up to date with a summary of practical recommendations for treatment. Only those therapeutic measures were included that have been found effective by the authors. This selection, of course, represents an evaluation of the different therapeutic measures. "Older" treatment methods that may still be in use are not included.

In the German edition, the diseases were presented in alphabetical order, but this could not be done in the American edition without reorganizing both the text and the color plates.

We thank Drs. S. Hellwig and C. Raulin, Karlsruhe, for their kind loan of Figure 288.

K. Bork, W. Bräuninger

Contents

I. Common General Skin Diseases

Acne . . . 3
A. Acne Vulgaris . . . 3
B. Acne Conglobata . . . 5
Age-Related Skin Changes . . . 7
A. Senile Atrophy of the Skin . . . 7
B. Changes in the Senile Skin due to Prolonged Exposure to Sunlight . . . 7
a) Pseudoscars, Senile Comedones and Senile Cysts . . . 7
b) Senile Purpura . . . 7
c) Chronic Actinic Cheilitis (Chronic Light-Induced Inflammation of the Lips) . . 9
d) Chondrodermatitis Helicis . . . 9
Aphthae . . . 11
Self-Induced Skin Lesions . . . 13
Side Effects of Drugs . . . 17
A. Macular Exanthemas . . . 17
B. Fixed Drug Eruptions . . . 19
C. Toxic Epidermal Necrolysis . . . 19
D. Light-Provoked Drug Reactions . . . 19
E. Urticaria and Angioedema . . . 19
F. Purpura, Cutaneous Hemorrhages . . . 21
G. Cortisone-Induced Skin Changes . . . 21
H. Acneiform Eruptions . . . 21
I. Skin Changes at the Site of Injections . . . 21
Vesiculobullous Diseases . . . 23
A. Pemphigus Vulgaris . . . 23
B. Bullous Pemphigoid . . . 23
C. Dermatitis Herpetiformis . . . 25
D. Epidermolysis Bullosa Hereditaria . . . 25
Decubitus Ulcer . . . 27
Vascular Disorders . . . 29
A. Obstructive Arterial Diseases . . . 29
B. Venous Disorders, Ulcus Cruris (Leg Ulcers) . . . 29
C. Other Common Vascular Disorders . . . 33
a) Acrocyanosis . . . 33
b) Livedo Reticularis . . . 35
c) Raynaud's Disease/Raynaud's Phenomenon . . . 35
Eczematous Diseases . . . 37
A. Acute Allergic Contact Dermatitis . . . 37
B. Chronic Allergic Contact Eczema . . . 39
C. Chronic, Non-Allergic Contact Eczema (Toxic Degenerative Eczema, Cumulative Toxic Contact Dermatitis) . . . 39
D. Atopic Dermatitis (Atopic Eczema; Disseminated Neurodermitis) . . . 41
E. Vesicular Palmoplantar Eczema (Pompholyx) . . . 45
F. Chronic, Hyperkeratotic Eczema of the Palms and the Soles . . . 47
G. Diaper Dermatitis, Diaper Rash . . . 47
H. Stasis Eczema, Stasis Dermatitis . . . 49
I. Seborrheic Dermatitis . . . 49
J. Bacterial Ear Eczema . . . 51
K. Nummular Eczema . . . 51
Frostbite . . . 55
Erysipelas . . . 57
Erythema Chronicum Migrans and Other Skin Disorders Transmitted by Ticks . . . 59
A. Erythema Chronicum Migrans . . . 59

B. Acrodermatitis Chronica Atrophicans 59
C. Lymphocytoma 59
Erythema Multiforme 61
Erythema Nodosum 63
Chilblains, Perniosis 65
Granuloma Annulare, Necrobiosis Lipoidica 67
A. Granuloma Annulare 67
B. Necrobiosis Lipoidica 67
Diseases of the Hair 69
A. Alopecia Areata 69
B. Diffuse Alopecia 71
C. Trichotillomania 71
D. External Damage to the Hair 71
Herpes Simplex 73
Hyperhidrosis and Sequelae 77
A. Hyperhidrosis 77
B. Trichomycosis Palmellina (Trichomycosis Axillaris) 77
C. Pitted Keratolysis (Keratoma Plantare Sulcatum) 77
Insect Bites 79
A. Mosquito Bites 79
B. Wasp and Bee Stings 79
C. Flea Bites 81
D. Bedbug Bites 81
E. Trombidiosis 81
Intertrigo, Erythrasma 83
A. Intertrigo 83
B. Erythrasma 83
Pruritus 85
A. Generalized Pruritus 85
B. Localized Pruritus 85
Lice 89
A. Pediculosis Capitis 89
B. Pediculosis Corporis 89
C. Pediculosis Pubis 91
Lichen Planus 93
Sun Reactions 95
A. Sunburn (Dermatitis Solaris) 95
B. Phototoxic Reactions 95
C. Photoallergic Reactions 97
D. Persistent Light Reaction, Actinic Reticuloid 97
E. Porphyria Cutanea Tarda 97
Inflammations of the Lips 99
A. Lip-Licking Cheilitis 99
B. Perlèche, Angular Cheilitis 99
C. Chronic Actinic Cheilitis, Chronic Light-Induced Inflammation of the Lips 99
D. Thrush Cheilitis, Candidiasis of the Lips 99
Lupus Erythematosus 101
A. Systemic Lupus Erythematosus 101
B. Discoid Lupus Erythematosus 101
Lymphedema 103
Miliaria 105
Diseases of the Nails 107
A. Ingrown Nail (Unguis Incarnatus) 107
B. Bacterial Paronychia 107
Pigmentation Disorders 109
A. Vitiligo 109
B. Pityriasis Alba 109
C. Universal Hyperpigmentation 109

D. Ephelides, Freckles . . . 111
E. Solar Lentigines (Sun-Induced Freckles) . . . 111
F. Melasma, Chloasma . . . 111
Fungal Diseases . . . 113
A. Diseases due to Dermatophytes . . . 113
    a) Tinea Capitis . . . 113
    b) Tinea Corporis . . . 113
    c) Tinea Pedis . . . 115
    d) Tinea Unguium, Onychomycosis . . . 115
B. Skin Diseases Caused by Yeasts (Candidiasis) . . . 117
    a) Candidal Infection of the Skin (Thrush) . . . 117
    b) Candidiasis of the Mucosa, Candidiasis of the Genital Area . . . 117
    c) Candidal Paronychia . . . 119
C. Pityriasis Versicolor . . . 119
Pityriasis Rosea . . . 123
Prurigo, Prurigo Nodularis . . . 125
Psoriasis . . . 127
Pyodermas . . . 131
A. Folliculitis, Follicular Pustules . . . 131
B. Furuncle and Furunculosis . . . 131
C. Carbuncle . . . 133
D. Sweat Gland Abscesses . . . 133
E. Impetigo Contagiosa . . . 133
F. Staphylococcal Scalded Skin Syndrome . . . 135
Radiation Damage to the Skin . . . 137
A. Acute Radiation Dermatitis . . . 137
B. Chronic Radiation Dermatitis . . . 137
Rosacea and Rosacea-Like Dermatitis . . . 139
A. Rosacea . . . 139
B. Perioral Rosacea-Like Dermatitis (Steroid Rosacea) . . . 139
Scabies . . . 141
Stomatitis, Inflammation of the Oral Mucosa . . . 143
Tattoos . . . 145
Thrombophlebitis . . . 147
Dry Skin, Ichthyosis . . . 149
A. Dry Skin . . . 149
B. Ichthyosis, Fish Skin . . . 149
Vacation Dermatoses . . . 151
A. Creeping Eruption . . . 151
B. Bacterial Ulcers . . . 151
C. Sand Flea Bites . . . 151
D. Furunculoid Myiasis Caused by Human Botflies . . . 151
Urticaria and Angioedema (Quincke's Edema) . . . 153
A. Urticaria . . . 153
B. Angioedema (Histamine-Mediated) . . . 155
C. Hereditary and Acquired Angioedemas Caused by C1-Inhibitor Deficiency . . . 155
Chemical Burns . . . 157
Burns, Scalding . . . 159
Herpes Zoster, Shingles . . . 161
Alterations of the Tongue . . . 163
A. Geographic Tongue, Exfoliatio Areata Linguae . . . 163
B. Fissured Tongue, Lingua Plicata . . . 163
C. Black Hairy Tongue, Lingua Villosa Nigra . . . 163
D. Median Rhomboid Glossitis . . . 165
E. Increased Coating of the Tongue . . . 165

II. Sexually Transmitted Diseases and Non-Venereal Genital Diseases

AIDS, HIV Infection 169
Gonorrhea 173
Syphilis 175
Non-Venereal Genital Diseases 179
A. Balanitis 179
B. Vulvovaginitis 179
C. Kraurosis Penis, Kraurosis Vulvae 179
D. Phimosis 181
E. Heterotopic Sebaceous Glands 181
F. Pearly Penile Papules (Hirsuties Papillaris Penis) 181

III. Benign Tumors

Atheromas, Retention Cysts, Pilar Cysts 185
Fibromas 187
A. Fibroma Molle (Skin Tags) 187
B. Histiocytoma, Dermatofibroma 187
Hemangiomas 189
A. Capillary Hemangioma (Strawberry Hemangioma) 189
B. Nevus Flammeus, Port-Wine Stain 189
a) Median Nevus Flammeus 191
b) Lateral Nevus Flammeus 191
C. Senile Angiomas 193
D. Venous Angioma of the Lips (Venous Lake) 193
E. Spider Nevi (Nevus Araneus, Eppinger Stars) 193
Keloids 195
Lipomas, Lipomatosis 197
A. Solitary or Multiple Lipomas 197
B. Benign, Symmetric Lipomatosis (Madelung's Syndrome) 197
Milia 199
Molluscum Contagiosum 201
Pigmented Nevi 203
A. Common Acquired Nevomelanocytic Nevus 203
B. Sutton's Nevus, Halo Nevomelanocytic Nevus 203
C. Congenital Nevomelanocytic Nevus 203
D. Spindle Cell Nevomelanocytic Nevus, Spitz Nevus 205
E. Nevus Spilus 205
F. Blue Nevus 205
Pyogenic Granuloma 207
Calluses 209
A. Clavi 209
B. Lip Calluses 209
C. Lip Callus of the Nursing Infant 209
D. Fiddler's Neck 209
E. Occupational Callus 211
F. Plantar Callus 211
G. Prayer Callus 211
H. Masticatory Welt 211
Seborrheic Keratoses 213
Infectious Warts 215
A. Common Warts (Verrucae vulgares) 215
B. Plantar Warts 217
C. Flat Warts 217
D. Condylomata Acuminata 217
Xanthoma, Xanthelasma 221
A. Eruptive Xanthoma 221
B. Tuberous Xanthomas 221
C. Xanthelasma Palpebrarum 221

IV. Malignant and Potentially Malignant Tumors
Actinic Keratoses, Keratoacanthoma 225
A. Actinic Keratoses 225
B. Keratoacanthoma 225
Basal Cell Carcinoma (BCC) 227
Leukoplakia 231
Malignant Melanoma 233
A. Premalignant Changes and Early Types of Malignancy 233
B. Clinical Types of Melanoma 235
Mycosis Fungoides and Other Malignant Lymphomas 237
Squamous Cell Carcinoma 239

V. Selected Commercial Preparations and Prescriptions with Practical Guidelines for Treatment
General Principles 244
Medications and Measures for External Treatment 246
A. Wet Dressings 246
B. Partial Baths (Hand Bath, Foot Bath, Sitz Bath) and Full Baths 246
C. Powders 247
D. Solutions, Tinctures 247
E. Shake Mixtures 249
F. Gels 249
G. Pastes 250
H. Emulsions: Lotions (Milk Type), Creams, Ointments 251
I. Corticosteroid Crystal Suspensions 256
Medications for Systemic Therapy 257
A. Antibiotics 257
B. Antimycotics 258
C. Virostatic Drugs 259
D. Antihistamines 259
E. Corticosteroids 259
F. Retinoids 260
G. Fumaric Acid 261
Compression Bandages 262

Index 263

I. Common General Skin Diseases

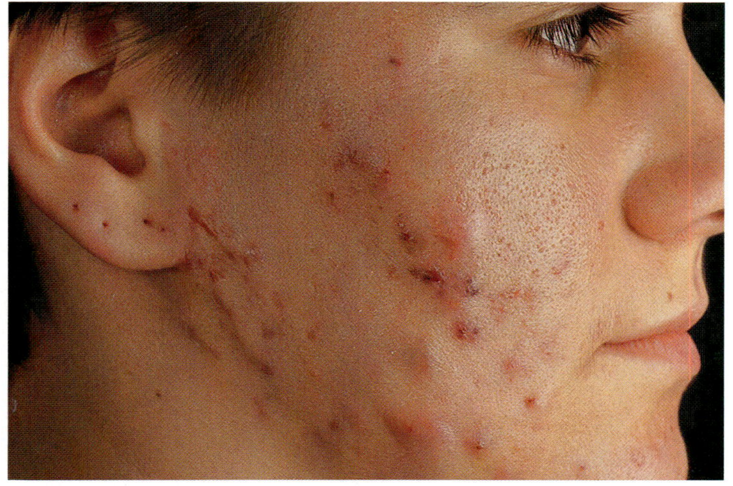

Figure 1 Acne vulgaris. Solitary comedones, inflammatory nodules and isolated pustules on the right cheek. The enlarged follicle openings are clearly visible.

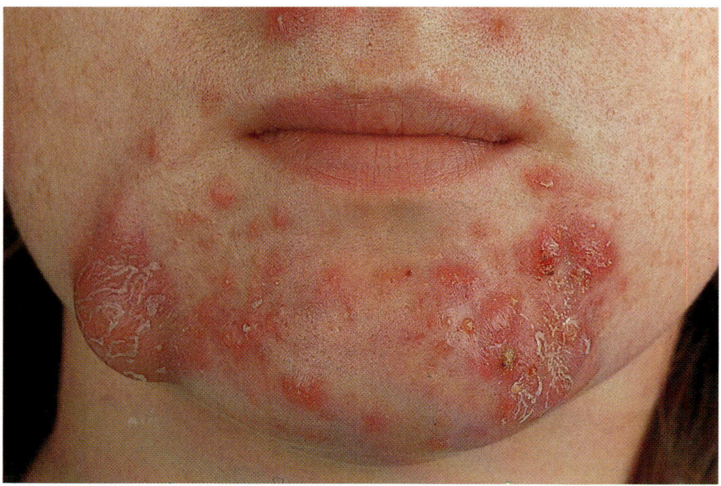

Figure 2 Nodular and cystic acne vulgaris, mainly in the chin area ("chin acne").

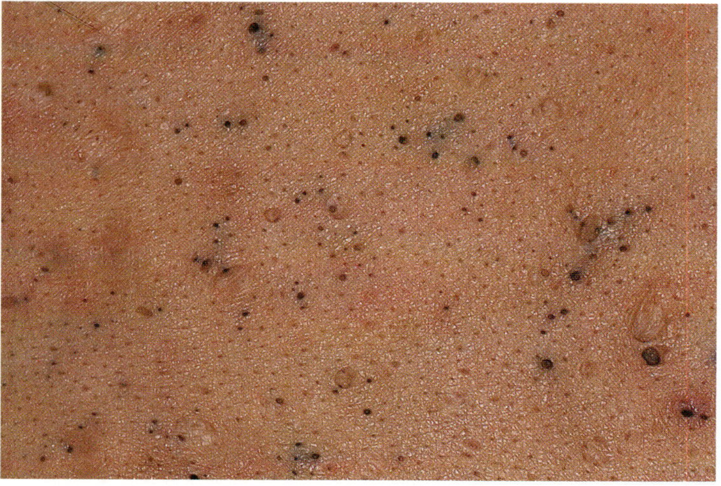

Figure 3 Acne conglobata with numerous clusters of comedones and small scars as sequelae.

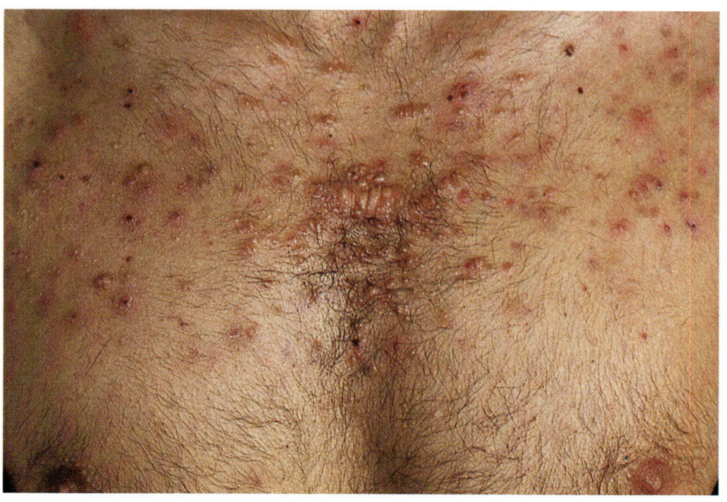

Figure 4 Acne vulgaris. Multiple pustules and keloid formation as they are frequently found in the middle of the chest.

Acne

Acne is one of the most common skin disorders seen by the practicing physician. It occurs during puberty in approximately 75% of all adolescents, but varies in severity. The disorder rarely lasts longer than 10 years and usually disappears in early adulthood. Severe nodular or nodular-cystic involvement occurs mainly in young men. Women 20 to 35 years of age often exhibit nodules in the perioral area or on the chin (chin acne). More severe inflammatory lesions can lead to disfiguring scar formation which makes competent treatment of acne an important task for the attending physician and not just "cosmetic therapy". The etiology is multifactorial and includes heredity, excessive production of sebum (seborrhea) with the formation of free fatty acids, bacterial contamination of the follicles of the sebaceous glands by Propionibacterium acnes, stimulation of sebum production by androgens and altered keratinization of the follicular infundibulum. Psychological factors may also play a role and must be treated appropriately ("Acne excoriée": acne is compulsively scratched open due to agitation).

A. Acne Vulgaris

Clinical Features

Acne presents with a colorful variety of efflorescences.

1. The primary lesion is a comedo without inflammatory changes (blackhead). Its black discoloration is caused by deposited melanin. Secondary inflammation of the follicular apparatus leads to formation of erythematous papules, papulopustular lesions and pustules. In more severe cases, nodules and abscesses with fistulae can develop, often aggravated by the patient's own manipulations. This frequently results in severe scar formation, especially when treatment is inadequate.
2. Acne is primarily located on the face. In more severe cases, the chest and upper back may also be involved.
3. There is generalized seborrhea with oily facial skin and a disposition for greasy hair.

Therapy

Treatment is symptomatic and must be continued as long as comedones and inflammation are present, usually for a period of several years.

External

1. The skin must be cleansed with a mild soap **(R. 5)** to remove the grease.
2. Benzoyl peroxide is effective against papular and pustular lesions. The base of the medication must be chosen according to the condition of the skin (alcohol gel for very oily skin **[R. 25a],** water-based gel for less oily skin **[R. 25a]** and emulsions for sensitive skin, especially for the face **[R. 44a]).** For very sensitive skin, treatment can be given in the form of short-contact therapy (effective time period 5–10 minutes).
3. Tretinoin (vitamin A acid) solutions are more effective than gels **(R. 25b)** or creams **(R. 44b),** but also irritate the skin more easily. They are effective against comedones, less effective against papules and pustules.
4. Topical therapy with antibiotics in a mildly fatty base, primarily erythromycin and tetracyclines, is effective **(R. 14d).** However, this treatment is not without problems because of the danger of developing resistance to the agents (see **R. 34).**
5. It is important to remove the comedones, but this should be performed by a competent, trained cosmetologist. Excessive pressing and squeezing of nodules by the patient must be avoided.
6. Incision of cysts and purulent nodules should only be performed by a physician.
7. Intralesional injection of a corticosteroid crystal suspension into larger nodular lesions can occasionally be helpful. It is not recommended for the face (see **R. 46).**
8. After the inflammatory changes have subsided, scars can sometimes be successfully treated by cosmetic surgery such as cryotherapy, dermabrasion, excision of scars or collagen injection. The decision to perform these procedures should be made by a dermatologist experienced in these treatments. It is more desirable, however, to prevent scar formation by early and appropriate treatment of acne lesions.

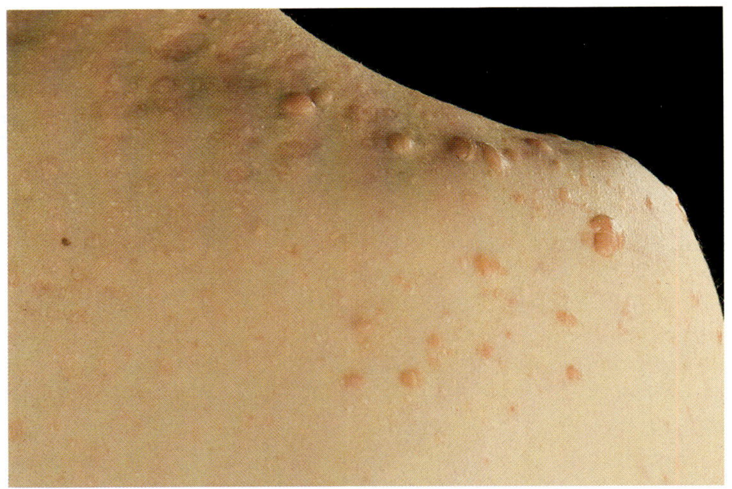

Figure 5 Acne vulgaris. Scars and keloids on the right shoulder.

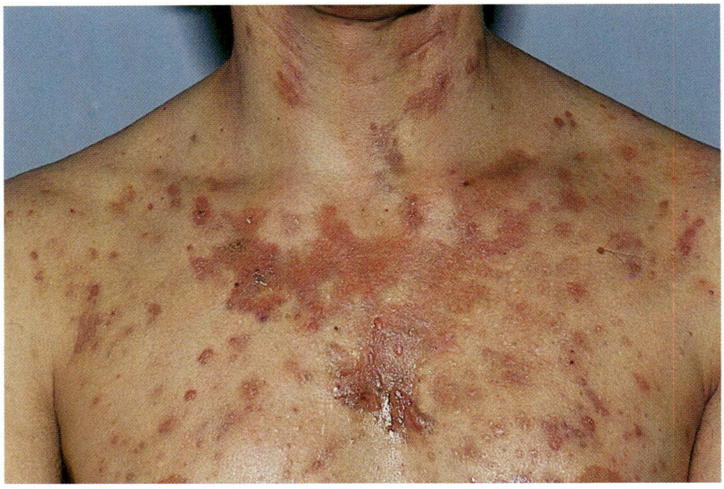

Figure 6 Acne conglobata. Deep folliculitis and extensive fresh scarring with beginning keloid formation on the mid-chest.

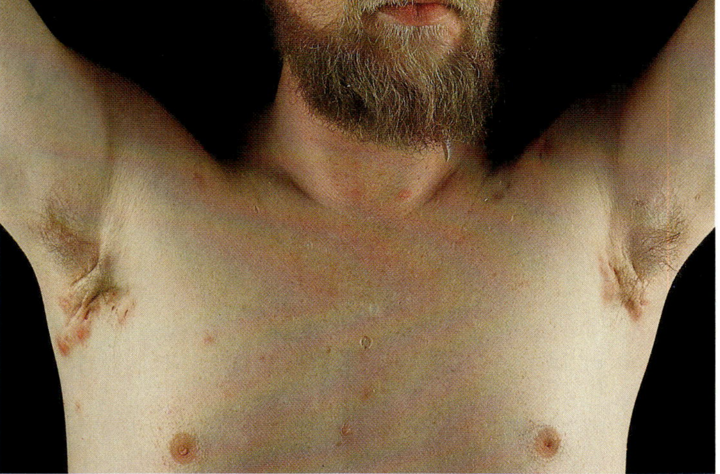

Figure 7 Chronic abscess formation with extensive scarring in both axillae in a patient with acne conglobata.

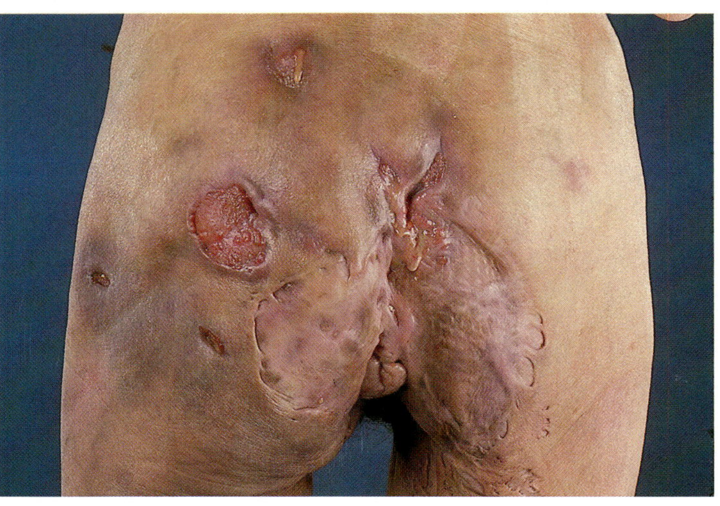

Figure 8 Acne conglobata. Severest form after many years of recurrent development of nodules, abscesses and fistulae, as well as extensive scarring in the perianal and gluteal regions. Condition after several operations with skin grafts.

Internal

1. The role of diet in the treatment of acne is often emphasized in the media, but there is no evidence to support its effectiveness. Many acne patients are already influenced psychologically by their disease and should not be burdened by a useless diet.
2. Female patients may benefit from a supplemental therapy with anti-androgens. Due to the teratogenic effects of anti-androgens, a contraceptive agent should be combined (for example Diane, as recommended by the original German text, which contains cyproterone acetate 2 mg and ethinyl estradiol 0.5 mg). Despite its risks (tumors of the liver, etc.), this therapy can be tried in cases which cannot be treated with other measures.
3. Systemic antibiotics, such as tetracyclines **(R. 49)** or erythromycin **(R. 51)** are indicated especially when marked inflammatory changes are present. One begins treatment with a usual dose per day until significant improvement has been achieved. Treatment is then continued with a reduced maintenance dose for another 1–2 months. The influence of this treatment on the intestinal flora is minimal.
4. Isotretinoin **(R. 65)** at a dose of 0.25 to 1 mg/kg body weight for 16 weeks should be used only for severe cases.

B. Acne Conglobata

It is practical to discuss this severe form of acne separately from acne vulgaris. In contrast to acne vulgaris, acne conglobata occurs more frequently in men. Its course is usually much more prolonged.

Clinical Features

1. The comedo is the primary lesion as in acne vulgaris. Additionally, there is clustering of comedones and giant comedones. Inflammatory changes with formation of abscesses and fistulae are more extensive than in acne vulgaris.
2. In addition to the sites usually affected by acne vulgaris, acne conglobata can also involve the entire trunk, the arms and the back of the neck. In severe cases, the axillae, the groin and the perianal region can also be involved (acne triade, acne tetrade).
3. Patients with acne conglobata frequently have a distinct tendency to form keloid scars and display severe seborrhea.
4. The acute course of the disease with high fever and acute immune complex arthritis (acne fulminans) may occasionally require systemic immunosuppressive treatment.

Therapy

External

Topical treatment is the same as that for acne vulgaris (see above).

Internal

Isotretinoin, a derivative of vitamin A **(R. 65),** is the treatment of choice for acne conglobata. The daily dose is 0.5 to 1 mg/kg body weight and is given in treatment cycles of 16 weeks.
Plastic surgery is occasionally necessary for treatment of chronic fistulae or extensive scars which cause restriction of motion, especially in the axilla. Systemic medical treatment of the disease, however, takes precedence.

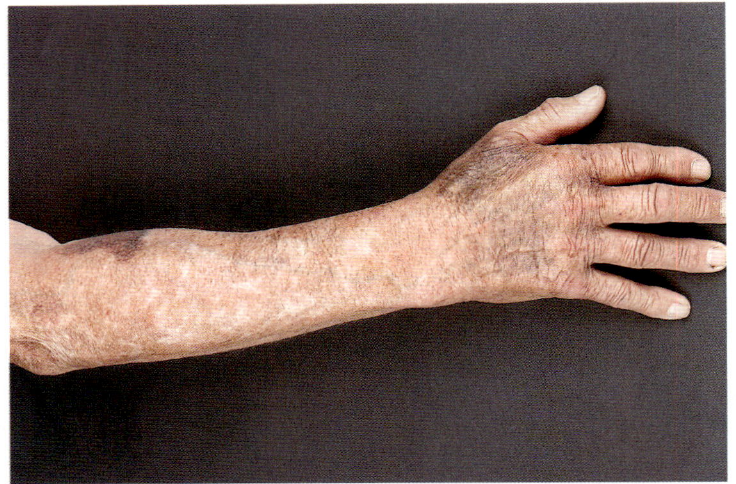

Figure 9 Star-shaped pseudoscars ("pseudocicatrices stellaires") of aged skin on the forearm. Result of light-induced damage to the connective tissue. Note senile purpura.

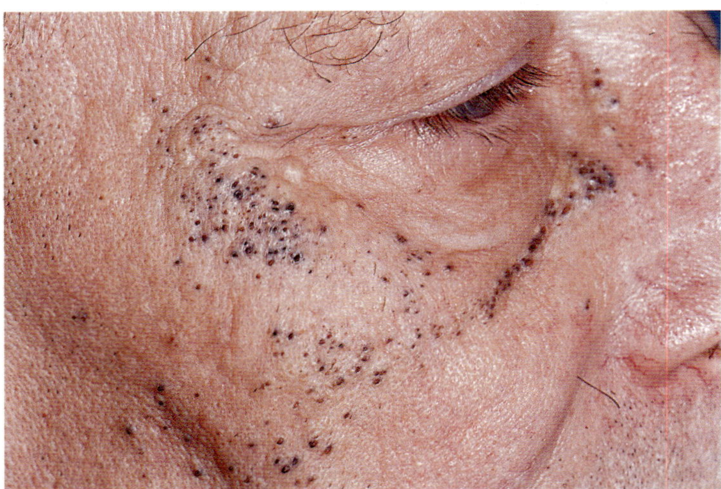

Figure 10 Senile comedones lateral and below the right eye.

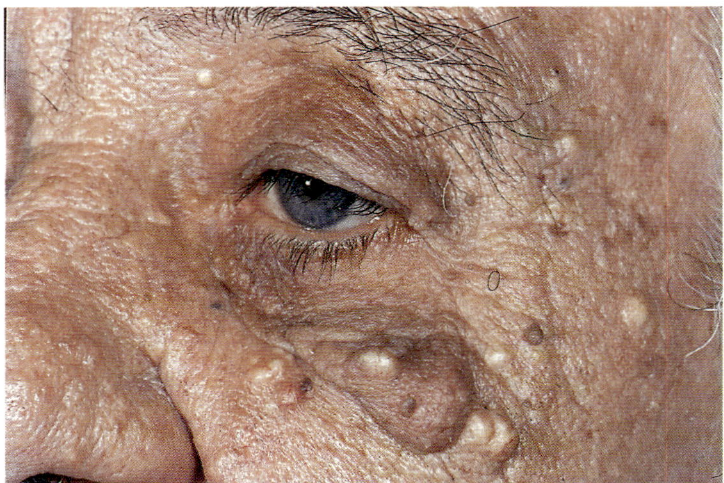

Figure 11 Light-induced pseudocysts of the connective tissue in the periorbital area (so-called Favre-Racouchot's disease).

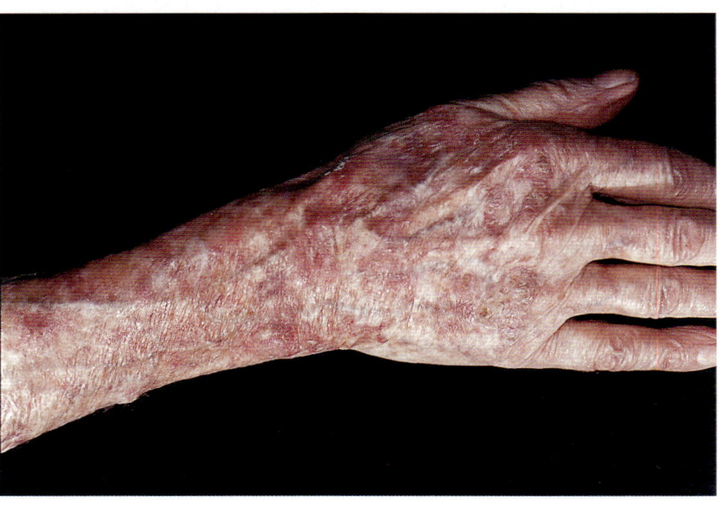

Figure 12 Senile purpura and actinic keratoses.

Age-Related Skin Changes

A. Senile Atrophy of the Skin

Human skin undergoes natural changes with age. The morphological alterations caused by advancing age alone are best recognized in areas of the skin which are not exposed to light. In these areas the skin is thin, dry and is easily wrinkled. The skin of older people also tends to be dry and desiccated, which makes senile pruritus one of the most frequent complaints of the elderly (> 80 years). Dermatitis due to dry skin (see page 149) occurs frequently during winter because of the low humidity of the air. Loss of elasticity of the senile skin is evident. Various benign tumor-like skin proliferations often develop with advancing years, such as pigmented and non-pigmented skin tags, senile angiomas, seborrheic keratoses, senile lentigines and hyperplasia of the seborrheic glands.

B. Changes in the Senile Skin due to Prolonged Exposure to Sunlight

There are many changes that occur in the skin from exposure to sunlight over a period of decades. They, too, generally occur in the elderly, but must be distinguished from age-related changes in areas of the skin which are not exposed to light. These changes include actinic keratoses, hypo- and hyperpigmentation, senile lentigines, wrinkles, star-shaped pseudoscars, elastosis (formation of amorphous material in the skin), loss of elasticity, enlarged blood vessels, senile purpura, senile comedones, hyperplasia of the seborrheic glands, as well as chronic actinic cheilitis in the red area of the lips.

a) Pseudoscars, Senile Comedones and Senile Cysts

Star-shaped pseudoscars are the result of tears in the light-aged connective tissue of the skin, so they are actually genuine scars. These changes are seen most frequently on the forearms, where they form bizarre, depigmented areas with serrated borders. Treatment is not possible and not necessary.

Senile cysts and senile comedones are other clinical signs of light-induced aging of the connective tissue. They are known as Favre-Racouchot's disease (nodular elastosis with cysts and comedones). They are the result of light-induced collagen changes and cause a collection of yellowish, histologically amorphous material in the upper corium. Pseudocysts, i.e., cyst-like collections of this amorphous material, as well as senile comedones can most frequently be observed lateral of the eyes. In senile comedones, the external opening of the follicle is enlarged; the surface shows a black discoloration. Senile comedones can be treated topically with vitamin A acid.

b) Senile Purpura

A better name for senile purpura (purpura senilis) would be actinic purpura, since it is the result of connective tissue changes in skin that has been exposed to light. There is an increased tendency to hemorrhage, especially on the back of the hand and on the forearms, rarely in the face. Irregular wine red to purple-colored, coin-sized hematomas can occur in the atrophic skin after even the most minor injuries, or sometimes in severe cases spontaneously. The lesions are asymptomatic. Usually it is merely a cosmetic problem that is caused by a loss of elasticity in the small blood vessels combined with aging of the surrounding connective tissue.

The hematomas disappear after a few weeks. Skin discoloration is not as pronounced as it is after a traumatic hematoma.

No effective external or systemic therapy is known. Prophylactic protection against pressure, for example, when shaking hands, is indicated.

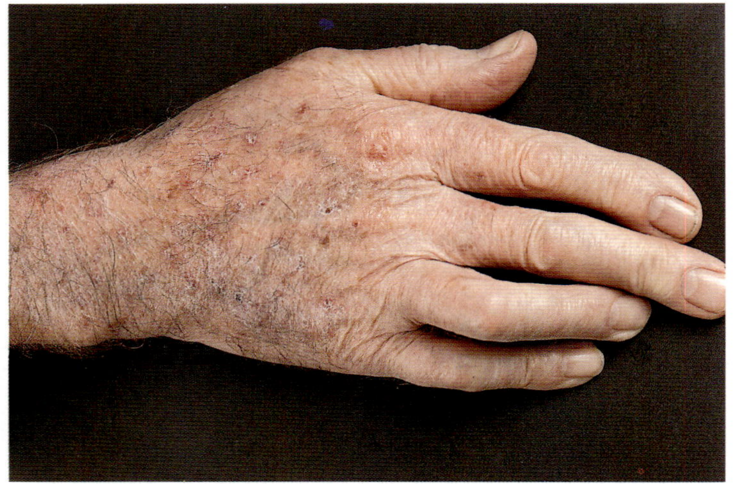

Figure 13 Actinic keratoses. Multiple keratoses on the back of the hand after exposure to sunlight for many years.

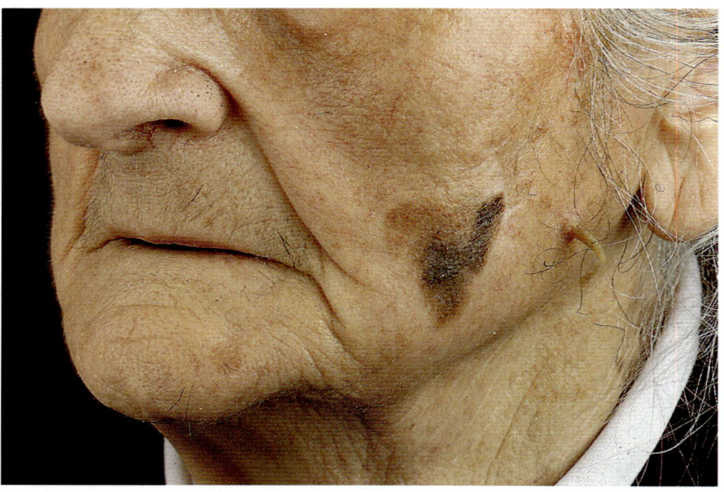

Figure 14 Senile skin with lentigo maligna (left cheek), cornu cutaneum and multiple senile lentigines.

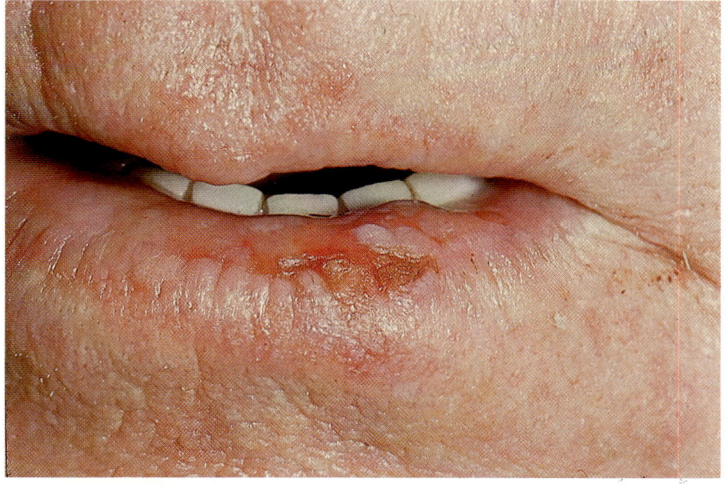

Figure 15 Chronic actinic cheilitis. Erosive, crusty lesions and leukoplakia-like foci on the lower lip after exposure to sunlight for many years.

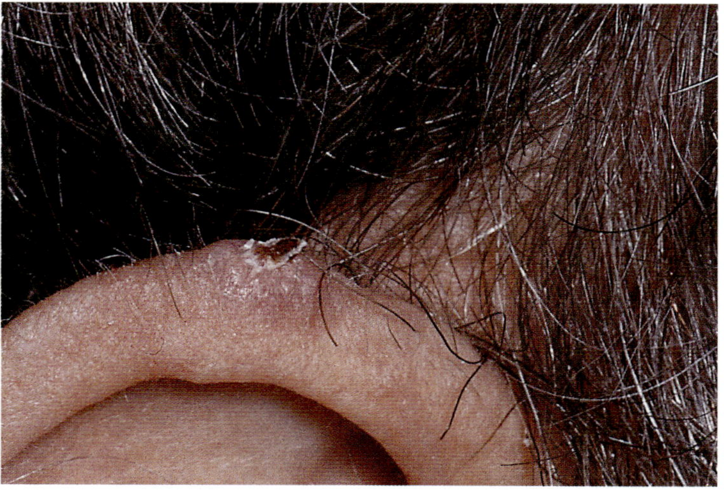

Figure 16 Chondrodermatitis helicis. Keratotic nodule on the upper margin of the helix, pressure sensitive.

c) Chronic Actinic Cheilitis (Chronic Light-Induced Inflammation of the Lips)

Chronic actinic cheilitis develops primarily in older men after years of exposure to intense sunlight, especially in those who work outdoors, such as farmers, masons, seamen, etc. Chronic actinic cheilitis must be regarded as a facultative precancerous lesion.

Clinical Features

1. The complete clinical picture of the disease develops after years of dryness and discrete scaling of the lower lip. The lower lip becomes thickened with a greyish-white discoloration of the red of the lip so that the border between it and the surrounding skin becomes indistinct. Scaling, fissures and vertical rhagades are present to various degrees and worsen in cold and windy weather. Leukoplakia may occur in small areas, while in other areas distinct keratoses may develop. In addition, round, or more frequently, oval-shaped erosions are seen.

2. Usually only the lower lip is involved; the upper lip is rarely involved, and then in addition to the lower lip. This is because the lower lip is exposed more extensively to sunlight.

Therapy

1. The early stage of this condition can extend over many years. Frequent lubrication of the lips as well as reduced exposure to sunlight and light-protective measures **(R. 45)** are sufficient therapy.

2. The presence of erosions, keratoses and leukoplakia-like changes make more intensive treatment necessary.

a) Carcinoma of the lip must be excluded by biopsy.

b) Partial or complete excision of the red of the lip with its subsequent replacement (according to von Langenbeck) may be indicated. This is a relatively easy and effective method and is also of prophylactic importance in severe cases. This procedure can remove the chronically light-damaged tissue completely. The long-term effect is usually lasting; the cosmetic result is very good in most cases.

c) Topical treatment with 5-fluorouracil in a 1 to 5% solution or a 5% ointment over a period of 2 weeks is a conservative measure which frequently has only a temporary effect. In the beginning, this treatment causes a marked inflammatory reaction, accompanied many times by erosions; it may require the use of a corticosteroid cream. The actinic cheilitis disappears after 2–3 weeks. Regular check-ups must be repeated since relapses occur.

3. These patients must be followed carefully. The risk of developing squamous cell carcinoma is much higher.

d) Chondrodermatitis Helicis

This condition is also known as "painful ear nodule". It occurs as a single lesion on the border of the helix, rarely on the anthelix. The condition occurs mainly in older men, more frequently on the right auricle than on the left. Histologically it appears as a circumscribed cartilage necrosis with an overlying chronic necrotizing inflammatory reaction.

Many causes of the condition are suspected. The most likely cause appears to be pressure-damage of skin with actinic changes (the right side is the preferred side on which the elderly sleep).

Clinical Features

1. The lesions are pressure-sensitive round nodules which cannot be distinguished from the surrounding cartilage by palpation. They usually develop a central crust or ulceration after being present for a longer period of time.

2. They are found most frequently on the upper part of the helix of the right ear, less often on the anthelix.

Therapy

Wedge excision with removal of all of the involved cartilage is the treatment of choice. Protection from sunlight and pressure (soft pillow) are necessary prophylactic measures.

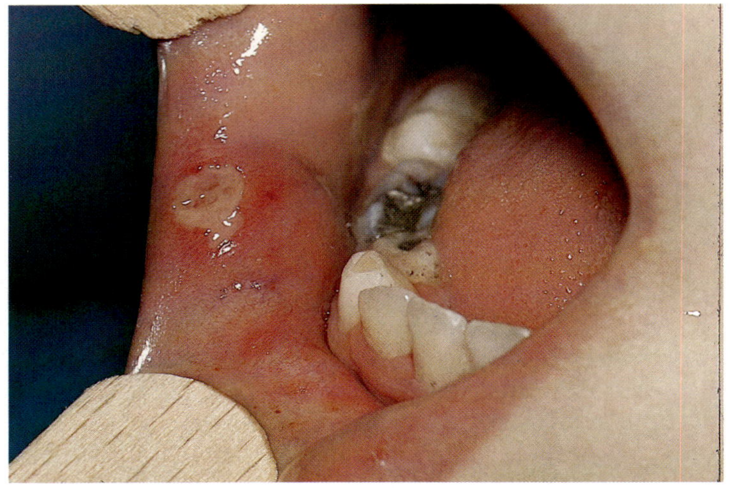

Figure 17 Recurrent aphthae. Fresh aphtha with yellow fibrin coating and erythematous border.

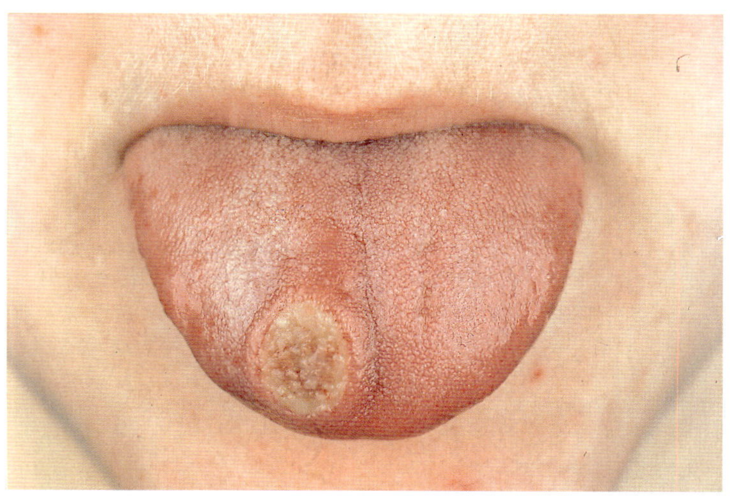

Figure 18 Recurrent aphthae. Aphtha of the tongue with adherent fibrinous coating and raised margin.

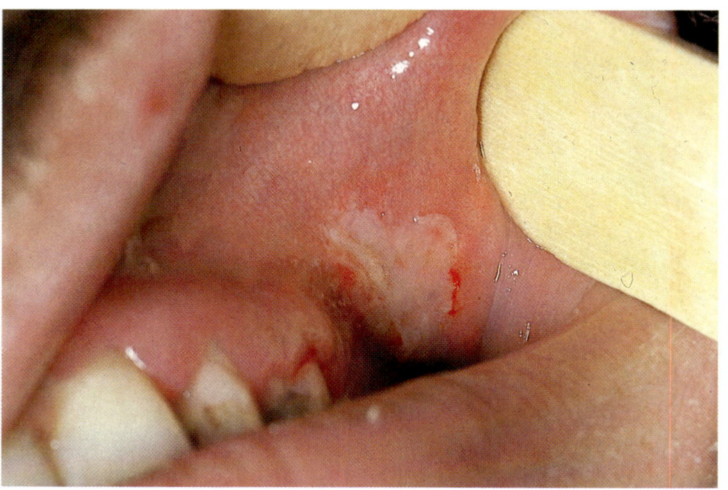

Figure 19 Recurrent aphthae. Large fresh aphtha with curvilinear border in the upper mucobuccal fold.

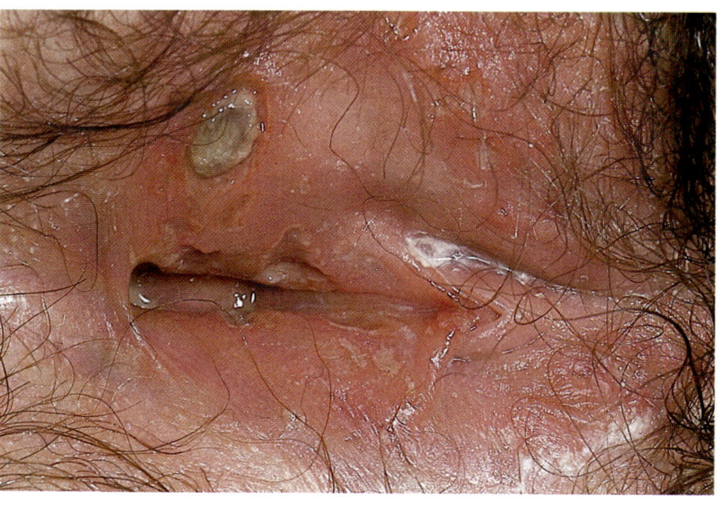

Figure 20 Recurrent aphthae. Deep genital aphthae on the labia minora and majora.

Aphthae

Recurrent Aphthae

Recurrent aphthae (habitual or familial aphthae) are painful erosions or ulcers of the mucous membrane of the mouth. They last only a few days and their etiology is unknown. Certain foods (nuts, chocolate, tomatoes, etc.) can occasionally cause an acute attack. An attack can also be initiated or aggravated by menstruation. It is important to distinguish recurrent aphthae from other diseases with aphthoid stomatitis, such as intraoral recurrent herpes simplex (rare), herpetic gingivostomatitis (initial manifestation of a herpes simplex infection), adverse drug reactions, infections with enteroviruses, bacterial gingivitis (see page 143) and pemphigus. With the exception of pemphigus (see page 23), these diseases are characterized by a one-time, simultaneous appearance of multiple aphthoid lesions. They do not show the typical protracted course with multiple recurrences of only a few aphthae at a time.

Clinical Features

1. Recurrent aphthae are characterized by the sudden appearance of painful erosions, generally 3–4 mm in size, which are covered by a white or yellowish fibrinous coating surrounded by an erythematous zone. They run a protracted course. Initially the lesions often appear transiently as nodules.
2. The disease involves mainly the mucous membranes of the cheeks and lips, the tongue and the gingiva.
3. Individual aphthae heal within a few days to 2 weeks. They occur in batches of a few aphthae at a time and recur over a period of several months or even years.
4. Special forms include solitary aphthae, giant aphthae, simultaneously or alternatively appearing genital aphthae, and very deep ulcerous aphthae (slowly healing over a period of several weeks or months. Consultation with a dermatologist or stomatologist may be necessary to exclude Behçet's or other diseases).
5. In some patients, Crohn's disease, ulcerative colitis or a deficiency of iron, vitamin B_{12} or folic acid is an underlying disorder.

Therapy

Treatment is still unsatisfactory. The therapeutic goal is reduction of pain and quicker healing of the lesions. At the present, treatment has not been able to prevent recurrences or prolong the symptom-free intervals. Nuts or sweets containing nuts should be avoided if they provoke attacks of aphthae.

1. In most cases the symptoms are minor and do not require treatment. The patients should not be burdened with a treatment that is more bothersome than the disease. Occasionally, sucking malt sugar or liquorice can alleviate the symptoms.
2. Sour and spicy foods, citrus fruits and alcoholic beverages can increase the discomfort and should be avoided. Mouthwash and toothpastes that cause pain should not be used.
3. Topical corticosteroid preparations can be beneficial in patients with extensive involvement and increased pain (application of adhesive pastes such as Kenalog in Orabase). We have found the following preparation of an adhesive gel useful: Betamethasone valerate 0.04, polymethacryl acid sodium 1.0, glycerol (85%) 4.0, water, to make 20.0.
4. Topical anesthetic preparations may be indicated for severe pain (e. g., anesthetic lozenges). The accompanying temporary numbness of the surrounding area must be accepted.

Topical antibiotic solutions or systemic antibiotics, cauterization with silver nitrate and antiseptic solutions such as chlorhexidine, hexetidine or gentian violet solution are not effective against recurrent aphthae.

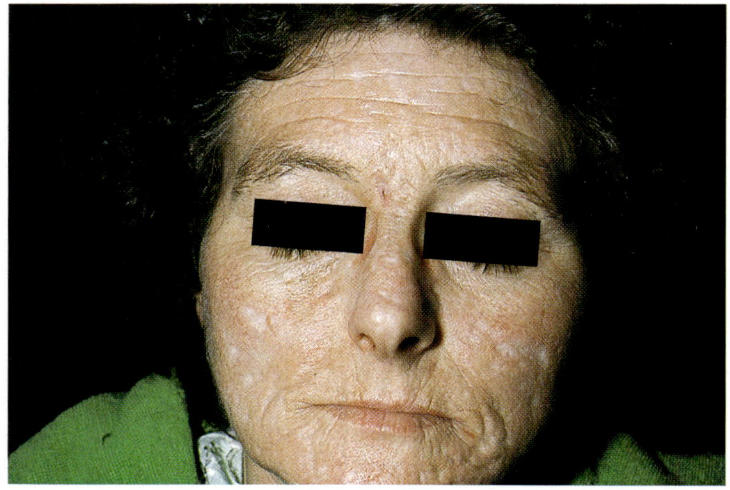

Figure 21 Self-induced skin lesions. White indented scars resulting from habitual excoriations in the face.

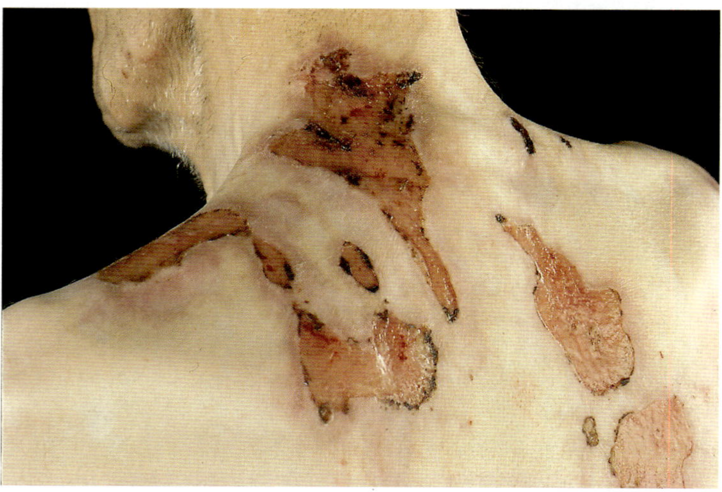

Figure 22 Self-induced skin lesions. Shallow fresh and older erosions and ulcerations caused by repeated scraping with a knife.

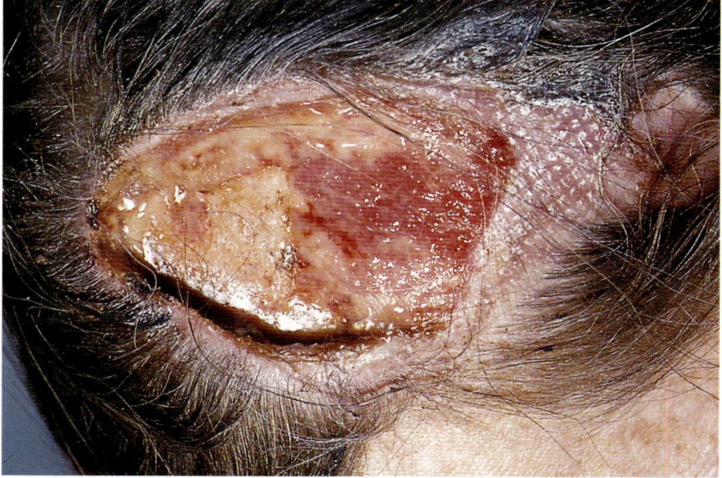

Figure 23 Self-induced skin lesion. Scalp defect after months of repeated trauma with a knife.

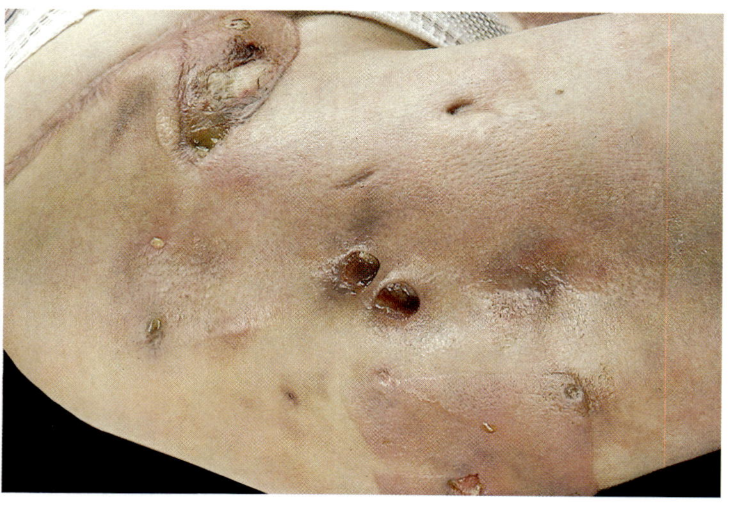

Figure 24 Self-induced skin lesions. Abscesses, fistulae and their sequelae treated by multiple plastic surgical procedures in the right gluteal and thigh regions.
Cause: Self-injection of soap solution into the subcutaneous tissue. The 18-year-old girl was hospitalized continuously in several hospitals for a period of 5 years.

Self-Induced Skin Lesions

Self-inflicted skin lesions are signs of an aggressive treatment of the patient's own body. They are typical of various syndromes pertaining to different medical specialties. Sooner or later the physician always becomes involved in the patient's actions, and the physician-patient relationship becomes part of the disease. The patients try to deceive the physician by producing symptoms and by a tendency to interrupt treatment or to change physicians frequently, especially if discovery is imminent. Physicians who have not treated such patients before experience a feeling of helplessness and narcissistic insult.

It is important for successful treatment to diagnose or suspect the underlying severe personality disorder as early as possible, based on the morphology of the lesions. The dermatologist is faced with so-called dermatitis artefacta, as well as Münchausen syndrome (vivid description of symptoms and/or incorrect information on past history in order to obtain invasive diagnostic procedures, hospitalization and even surgery). On rare occasions, self-traumatization is seen, such as compulsive cutting of the skin.

The disorder is seen almost exclusively in adolescents or young adults. In one large study of 1185 patients, 71% were female and 70% worked in so-called helping professions. The larger percentage of women was explained by the fact that women have a tendency to self-inflict damage while men would show violent behavior toward others if in similar conflict situations. Additionally, sexual abuse in early childhood, which occurs more frequently in girls, often plays an important role in self-induced skin lesions.

Special forms of self-induced skin lesions are so-called "neurotic excoriations" (that is, compulsive scratching due to unbearable itching with or without skin changes such as acne), self-mutilation in mentally retarded or schizophrenic patients, as well as trichotillomania (see page 71), onychophagia (habitual nail biting) and epidermotillomania (injuries to the skin using fingernails, teeth or other mechanical devices).

Dermatitis Artefacta

These patients inflict skin lesions by mechanical, chemical or thermic methods; most frequent are mechanically inflicted lesions.

Skin mutilations caused by scratching with the fingernails are the most common. They manifest themselves as linear excoriations or small ulcerations. Many times already existing wounds from various sources are kept open by mechanical irritation with the fingernails. Rubbing, scraping or scratching with various objects can produce erythemas, erosions and ulcerations. Relatively simple manipulations, such as intensive rubbing with a pencil, can produce injuries which extend into the corium. The shape and appearance of the wound (punctate, oval-shaped, linear, etc.) depend on the instrument used.

A typical method used for the creation of artifacts is the delaying of wound healing (even operative wounds) by scratching, applying caustic solutions, or introducing or injecting tissue-toxic materials (soap solutions, urine, etc.). This often leads to misinterpretation of symptoms as "disturbed wound healing" and thus often results in an extensive, unnecessary and expensive search for suspected immune defects. Manipulation of wounds frequently produces new foci of disease, as well as repeated hospitalizations.

Chemical methods include the use of caustic substances. One sees chemical burns with acids or lye, especially with household chemicals (see page 157). Thermic lesions are seen less frequently than chemical or mechanical self-injuries. They include burns from lighters, stove burners, irons and cigarettes. Frostbite is created by application of ice packs, freezer elements, etc.

Clinical Features

1. The symptoms are manifold and depend on the mechanism of injury. Symptoms include contact dermatitis, circumscribed edemas, erosions, ulcers and deep abscesses. These lesions (e.g., erosions or ulcers) are often placed in a linear fashion or have sharp corners, in contrast to "natural diseases".

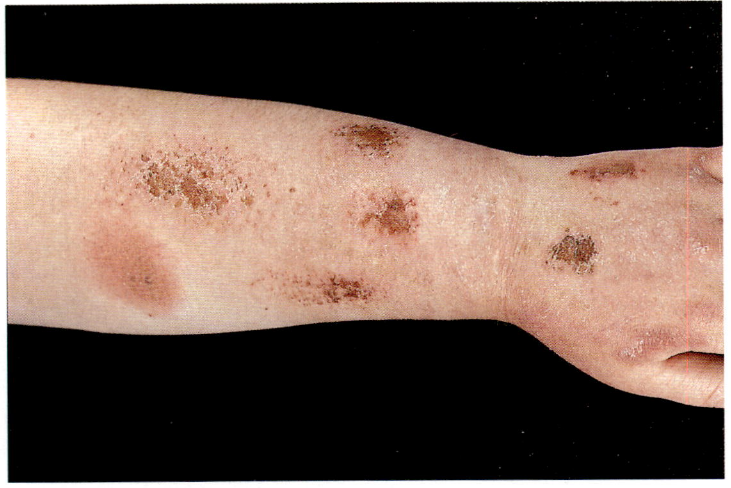

Figure 25 Self-inflicted injury by repeated application of a caustic fluid.

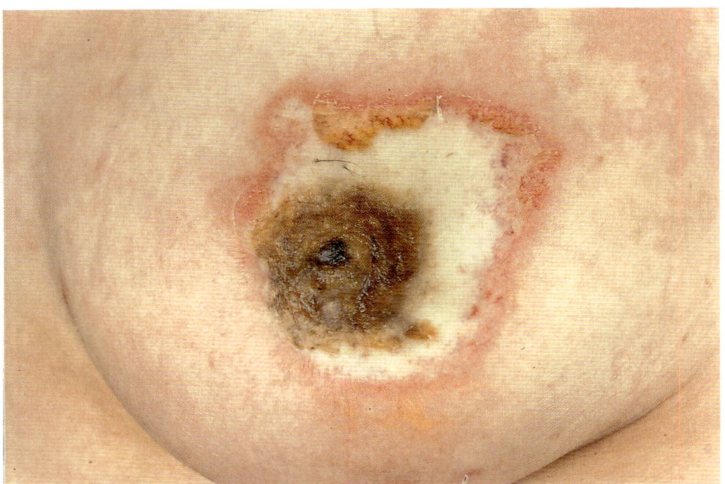

Figure 26 Self-inflicted injury. Sharply demarcated burn from an iron in the perimamillary area.

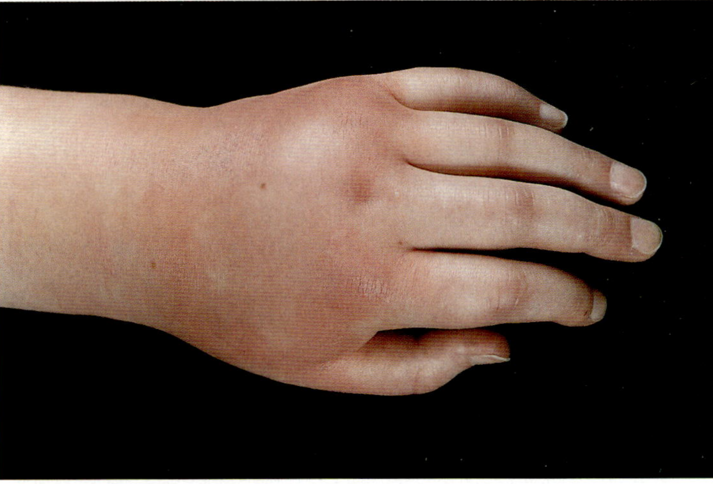

Figure 27 Self-induced skin lesion. So-called traumatic edema of the hand. Induction of a chronic edema by repeated binding of the arm.

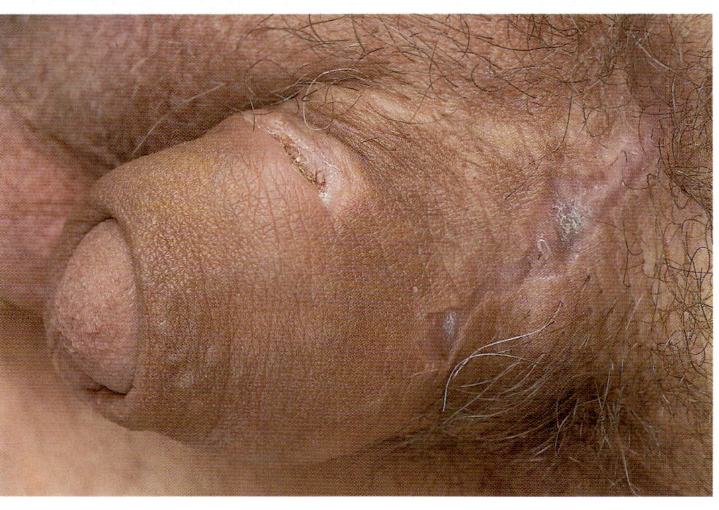

Figure 28 Self-induced skin lesions. Chronic inflammation with fistulae on the shaft of the penis after injection of paraffin oil (paraffin granuloma).

2. Self-injuries are primarily located in areas the patient can reach with his or her own hands. They are rarely found on the middle of the back, for example. They predominate on one side, in right-handed persons on the left, in left-handed persons on the right.
3. In patients with a prior self-injury history, we often find several or numerous scars.
4. The so-called "chronic traumatic edema of the hand" can be produced by repeated and prolonged tapping of a specific area of the skin, e.g., the hand. Prolonged manipulation is only necessary in the beginning to produce this swelling. Later, only occasional tapping of the dorsum of the hand for a few minutes is sufficient. A similar syndrome with production of an artificial lymphedema can be induced by tying off an extremity without interrupting the arterial blood supply. This type of edema is usually found on the forearm or hands and can often be recognized by the persistence of the groove from the tourniquet.
5. These patients are often intimately knowledgeable about how their bodies react to trauma and are able to discover ways of manipulating which the attending physician would not think of. Many of the patients acquire significant knowledge by studying the appropriate literature. Self-induced diseases are of variable physical severity. Superficial forms of dermatitis artefacta are occasionally disfiguring, but they are usually not dangerous. Interference with wound healing can lead to life-threatening sepsis and may necessitate amputation of the involved extremity. Patients with multiple auto-destructive tendencies (self-injuries, addictive diseases, frequent operations and accidents) usually have a poor prognosis.

Therapy

The diagnosis can be substantiated by the patient's own admission, by observation of self-mutilation attempts or by the discovery of the devices used for self-traumatization. At the same time, this information usually is available only after the physician has gained the patient's confidence, or if the patients seek help and are assured that no problems will arise if they disclose this information. In most cases, however, the physician cannot obtain such access without appropriate psychotherapeutic training.

1. Success of local therapy is usually prompt in the beginning, provided the tendency to self-traumatize can be overcome. The patients must either stop self-traumatization on their own or it must be prevented by external measures, e.g., appropriate bandages (starch bandage).
2. These physical methods, however, are not the most important; the patients must receive psychotherapy. Primary care physicians usually do not have the necessary training and are unable to treat these patients.
   Good cooperation between the attending physician and the psychotherapist from the moment the diagnosis has been made is paramount, as these patients tend to split the somatic and psychotherapeutic professionals from one another (the doctor present is good, the absent doctor is bad). Manipulations of the patient's body (removal of necroses, surgical coverage of skin defects, etc.) should be avoided as soon as diagnosis has been made, since these procedures can produce new artifacts and can make treatment more difficult.
3. As long as the diagnosis is unclear, an interview with relatives regarding the patient's situation can be helpful. These interviews can clarify possible conflict situations which the patient would not divulge on his own.
4. "Inconspicuous" observation of the patient by nurses or fellow patients in the same room, or a clandestine search of the patient's belongings in his hospital room can destroy the patient's confidence in his physician.

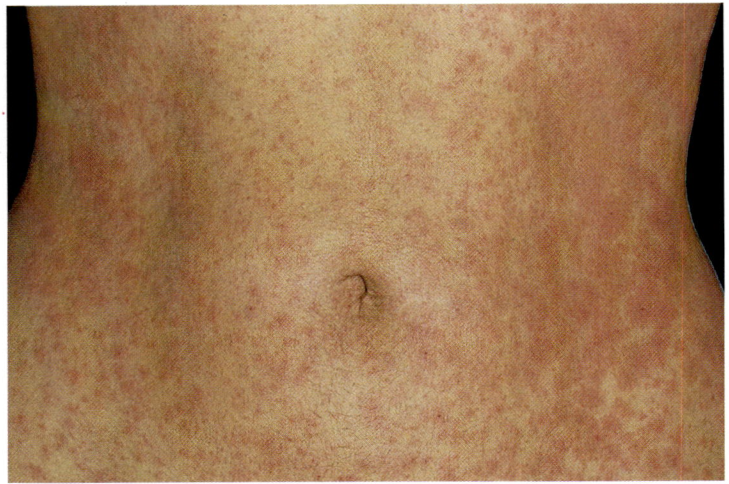

Figure 29 Maculopapular drug eruption on the trunk, caused by sulfamethoxydiazine.

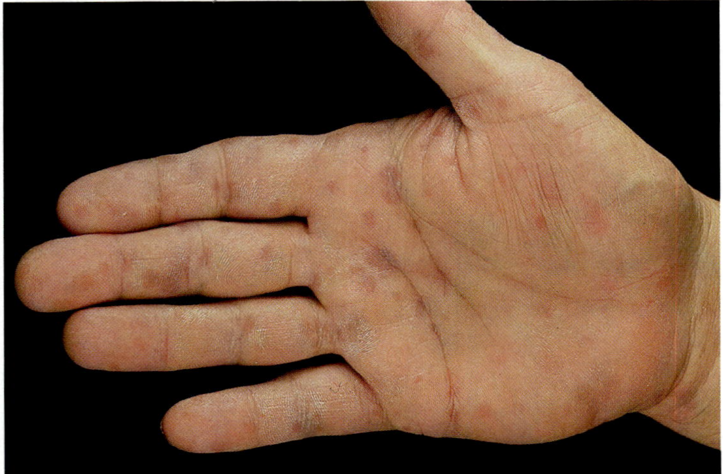

Figure 30 Macular drug eruption caused by diclofenac. Typical appearance in the palm of the hand.

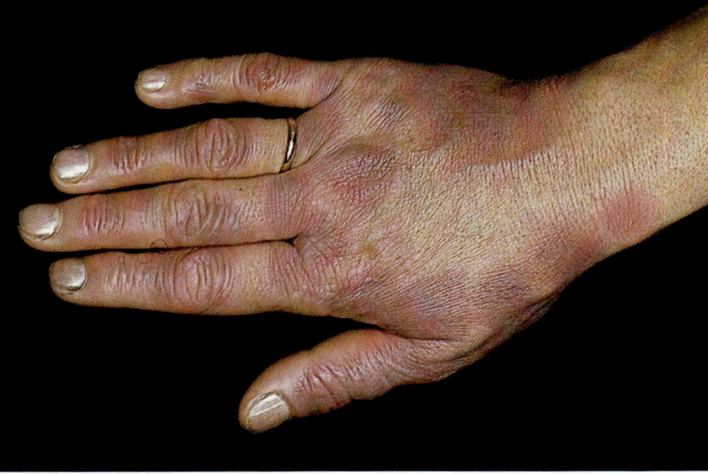

Figure 31 Macular drug eruption caused by metamizole. Penny-size lesions on the dorsum of the hand and fingers.

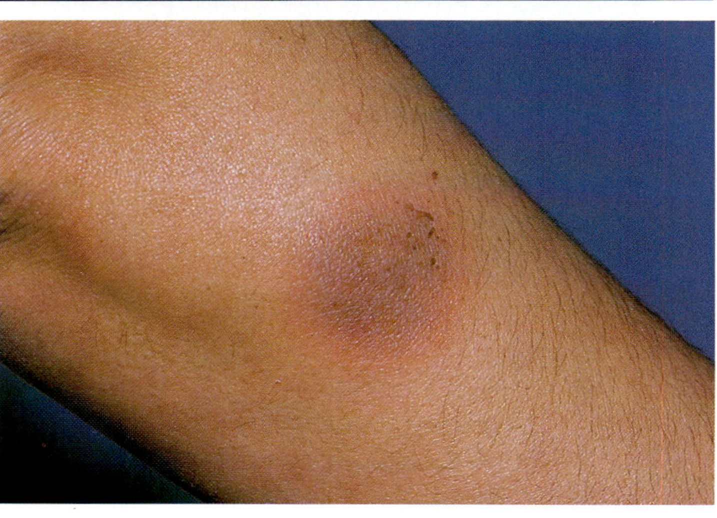

Figure 32 Fixed drug eruption. Brownish livid discoloration with erythematous margin without central vesicular eruption, caused by metamizole.

Side Effects of Drugs

Undesired effects of drugs are most often observed in the skin. These symptoms are usually harmless and transient. Occasionally, however, they can develop into life-threatening systemic diseases, such as toxic epidermal necrolysis, anaphylactic reactions with anaphylactic shock, or purpura. The symptomatology of side effects of drugs is extremely varied. The most frequent eruptions are macular drug exanthemas, drug-induced urticaria, dry skin, drug-induced photosensitivity and itching. There are numerous, less frequent reactions such as fixed drug eruptions, skin discolorations, hair loss, nail disorders and skin atrophy.
It is important to recognize these symptoms as adverse reactions to drugs and to determine which drugs are at fault. This is often difficult, especially when multiple drugs have been given. An accurate history is extremely important; it must include the point at which the medication was first given and the point when the symptoms began for each drug, since generally this provides the most useful information on the culprit. It must also be determined whether subsequent administration of the same or similar drugs will cause adverse reactions. This information must be entered on the patient's medical identification card, and the patient must be apprised of this. The diagnostic value of skin tests or of in vitro tests is limited. Skin tests are indicated only for an allergic pathogenesis. At the present, in vitro tests with a few exceptions generally do not provide reliable information regarding certain drugs as the offending agents. Indication for and performance of an oral or other systemic provocation must be left to an experienced allergist, especially since this re-exposure can endanger the patient.

A. Macular Exanthemas

Clinical Features

1. Macular or maculopapular exanthemas usually develop within the first three days following administration of the drug. The common ampicillin exanthemas are exceptions. They normally develop 7 to 9 days after drug administration. Other exceptions are exanthemas caused by allopurinol, carbamazepine and phenytoin, which often develop 2–4 weeks after administration of the drug.
2. Clinically, drug eruptions can resemble infectious exanthemas, especially measles (morbilliform), German measles (rubelliform), or scarlet fever (scarlatiniform). The skin eruption alone is therefore not sufficient to warrant the diagnosis of a drug eruption. History and other symptoms must also be taken into consideration.
3. Fever (drug fever), enlarged lymph nodes, and eosinophilia are occasionally concomitant symptoms of macular exanthemas.
4. Progression to toxic epidermal necrolysis (within hours) or to an erythroderma or exfoliative dermatitis (within days or weeks) is possible. Macular drug eruptions must be differentiated from the macular exanthemas of infectious diseases.

Therapy

The causative drug or drugs must be discontinued.

1. In most cases the symptoms are transient and not very pronounced, so that systemic or local therapy is not necessary.
2. Itching can be treated with systemic antihistamines **(R. 61, 62)**, provided these drugs did not cause the eruption.
3. Other symptoms (fever, enlarged lymph nodes, arthralgia) may require systemic corticosteroid therapy **(R. 63)**.
4. The allergy or intolerance must be entered on the patient's identification card to avoid future administration of this or similar drugs (cross-reacting allergy).

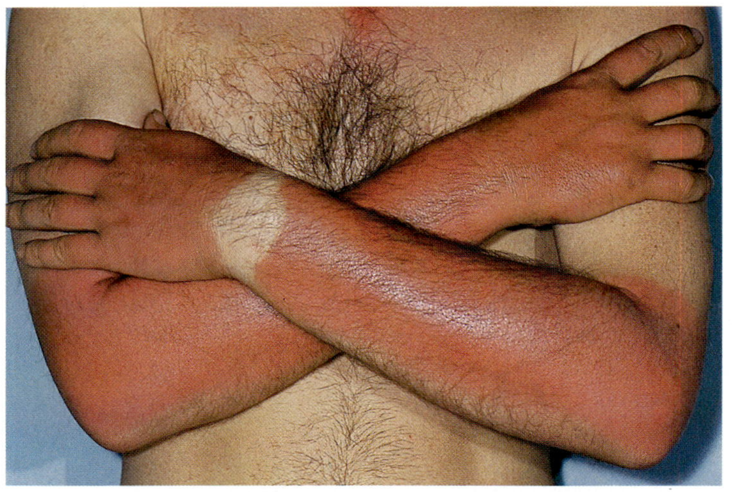

Figure 33 Phototoxic drug reaction caused by demethylchlortetracycline; acute inflammatory erythema limited strictly to the areas exposed to sunlight.

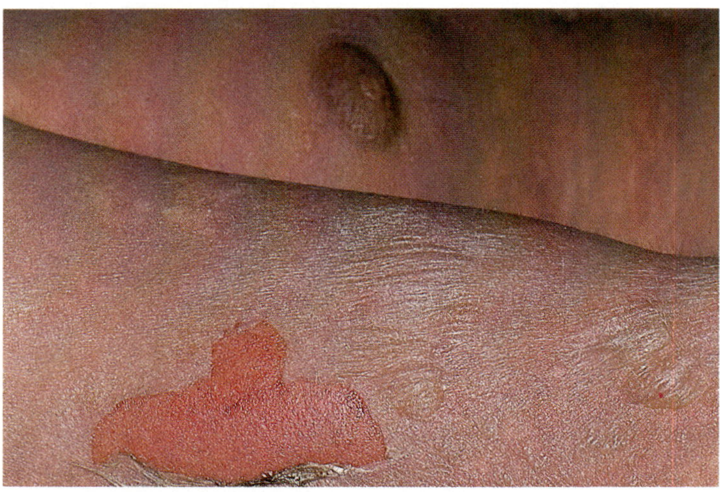

Figure 34 Toxic epidermal necrolysis. Extensive sloughing of the upper epidermal layers with erosions and bullae as in second-degree burns.

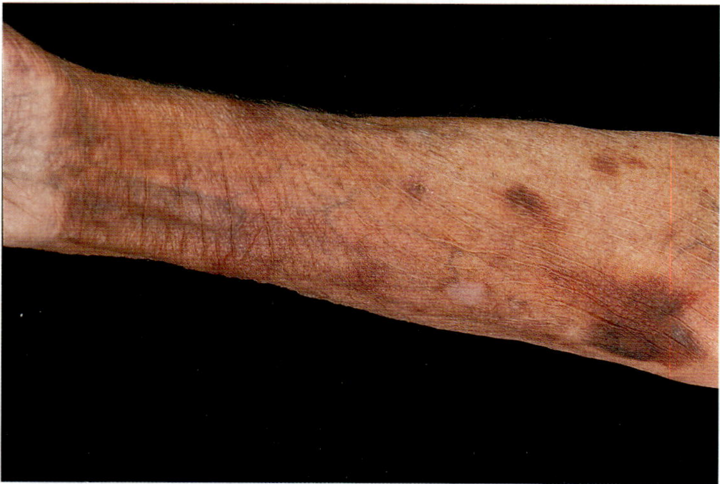

Figure 35 Typical cortisone purpura and cortisone atrophy of the skin in a patient who received systemic corticosteroid treatment for bronchial asthma for many years.

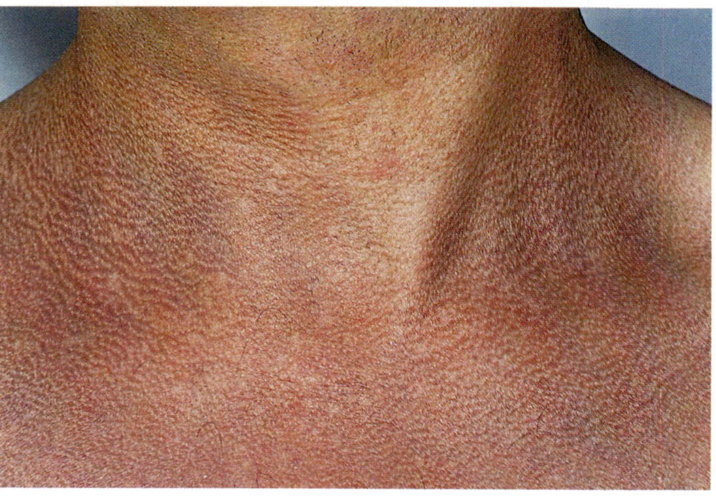

Figure 36 Cortisone skin with telangiectasias and brownish erythema between the follicles on the lower neck.

B. Fixed Drug Eruptions

Clinical Features

1. One or more fairly large, grey-blue to reddish-brown, round or oval spots occur in the same location every time the drug is given. The formation of bullae is possible.
2. A typical residual brownish discoloration can persist at the site of the lesion for months or even years.

Therapy

The causative drug must be identified and eliminated from the patient's therapy. Bullae may be evacuated and dabbed with a disinfective solution **(R. 17)**. No other treatment is necessary.

C. Toxic Epidermal Necrolysis

Toxic epidermal necrolysis (drug-induced Lyell's syndrome) is the most severe cutaneous drug eruption. It is a rare occurrence with an annual incidence of approximately 1:1,000,000. The most frequent causative agents are co-trimoxazole, allopurinol, phenytoin, carbamazepine as well as antibiotics and nonsteroidal anti-inflammatory drugs. A spotty and a planar form can be distinguished. The mortality rate is approximately 30% despite intensive care.

Clinical Features

1. Influenza-like prodromes and a spotty skin eruption are followed by extensive sloughing of the epidermis, causing large erosions like those seen from scalding.
2. General symptoms consist of pain and severe malaise, as well as symptoms resulting from the extensive loss of epidermis: Circulatory failure with symptoms of shock, kidney failure, sepsis and toxic damage to the internal organs are possible.
3. Late symptoms and sequelae are loss of hair and nails, pigmentation and adhesions of the conjunctiva (symblepharon).

Therapy

The disease must be treated like a severe burn. The patient must be hospitalized and severe cases treated in the intensive care unit.

D. Light-Provoked Drug Reactions (see pages 95–97)

Clinical Features

1. Erythema, scaling, occasional blistering, thickening of the skin and itching are symptoms.
2. The eruptions are limited to areas of the skin exposed to light, especially the face and hands.

Therapy

1. The causative drug must be identified and its administration avoided.
2. Topical treatment with a steroid cream (for acute symptoms) or ointment (for subacute and chronic changes) **(R. 38)** is appropriate.
3. Excessive exposure to light must be avoided until all symptoms have subsided.
4. A sunscreen may be indicated.

E. Urticaria and Angioedema (see pages 153–155)

Urticaria is one of the most frequent drug eruptions of the skin. It can be either an allergic or a non-allergic reaction, or it can be part of an anaphylactic or anaphylactoid reaction of the entire organism; it can be associated with the symptomatology of shock. Urticaria is most often seen after administration of analgesics or antibiotics, but can be caused by almost any medication. The causative agent must be avoided since the symptoms of allergic urticaria can increase in severity with repeated administration of the drug. Angioedema is rarely caused by drugs, mainly by aspirin or ACE inhibitors.
Clinical features and treatment will be discussed on page 153.

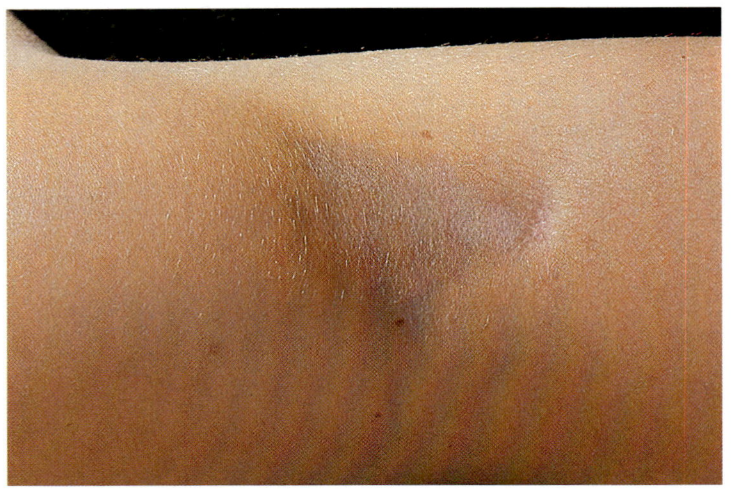

Figure 37 Lipoatrophy by inadvertent subcutaneous instead of intracutaneous injection of a corticosteroid crystal suspension.

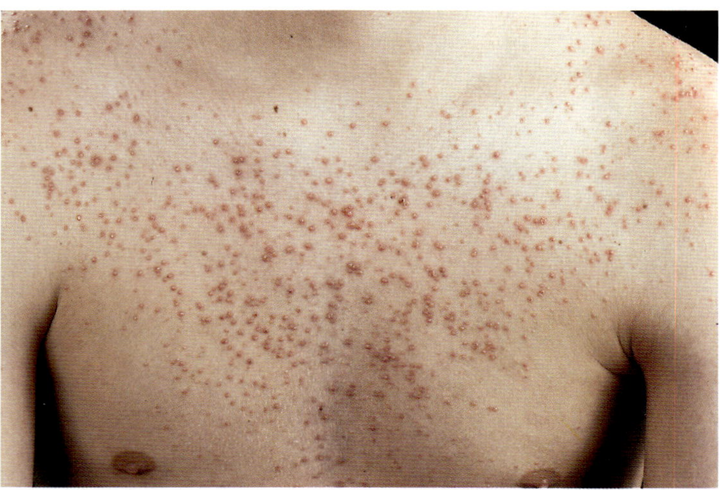

Figure 38 Steroid acne.

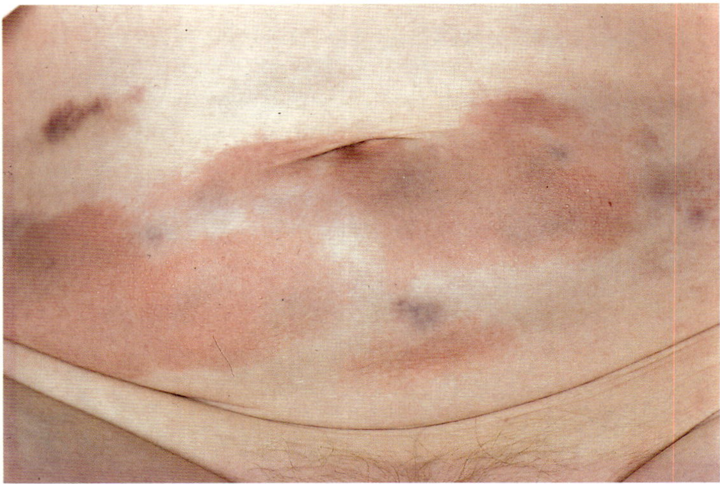

Figure 39 Allergy to heparin. Erythemas and shallow infiltrates at the site of injection in the lower abdomen. The hematomas caused by heparin are clearly visible at the injection sites.

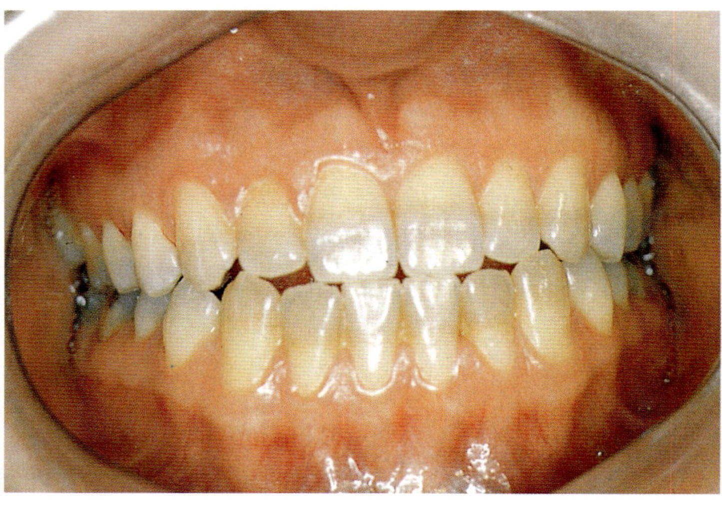

Figure 40 Tetracycline discoloration of the teeth. Band-shaped greyish discoloration of all teeth.

F. Purpura, Cutaneous Hemorrhages

Cutaneous hemorrhages can be caused by drug-induced allergic and non-allergic thrombocytopenia (cytostatic and analgesic drugs), clotting disorders (cephalosporins) or as part of a vasculitis (Henoch-Schönlein disease).

Clinical Features

1. Depending on the severity of the disorder, one may see a variety of symptoms ranging from petechiae to extensive hemorrhage in the skin and mucous membranes.
2. Areas of the skin exposed to mechanical forces are often involved first.

Therapy

Treatment is determined by the clotting and platelet activity and by the pathomechanism of the disorder. In severe cases, replacement of clotting factors or platelets may be necessary. Administration of systemic corticosteroids may also be indicated.
Progressive pigment purpura is a special form with vascular involvement and a chronic course.

G. Cortisone-Induced Skin Changes

Prolonged use of corticosteroid creams or ointments can produce local skin changes, such as erythema, thinning of the skin, increased hair growth, striae and cutaneous hemorrhage. Topical cortisone application over large areas of the skin can lead to increased steroid absorption with generalized symptoms (see **R. 38**).

H. Acneiform Eruptions

Drugs can produce acneiform eruptions or can aggravate an existing acne vulgaris. Steroid acne is the most frequently occurring form of drug-induced acne. It usually presents with bright red papules on the forehead, upper chest, shoulders and upper back. Comedones are absent. Steroid acne is the result of therapy with high doses of corticosteroids, often dexamethasone. The condition subsides when the medication is discontinued. Testosterone can lead to massive acne when used for retardation of growth in tall boys. Occasionally, one sees an increase of an existing acne in athletes or body builders who use anabolic steroids.

I. Skin Changes at the Site of Injections

Numerous adverse drug reactions are possible at the site of injections of systemic drugs. Granulomas, indurations, ulcers and necroses with subsequent atrophy can occur as a result of faulty injection techniques or difficult injection conditions that produce perivascular distribution of the drug. In particular, this occurs with toxic agents, such as cytostatic drugs or irritating solutions, such as strong alkaline solutions. Allergic reactions, erythemas and inflammatory infiltrates can develop only at the site of injection without any systemic allergic reactions. However, systemic reactions can be seen after repeated application of the drug if these warning signs are ignored. Since the drugs are present at higher concentrations at the site of injection, they are more likely to produce reactions here than in the rest of the body where the substance has been diluted. These reactions include damage to the venous wall which can develop into thrombophlebitis. Other local complications include discolorations, granulomas, atrophy and the induction of benign tumors.

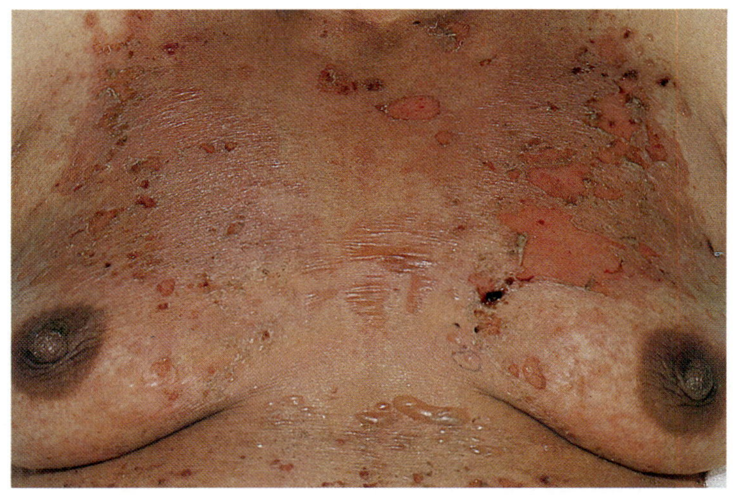

Figure 41 Pemphigus vulgaris. Flaccid bullae and extensive erosions on erythematous base.

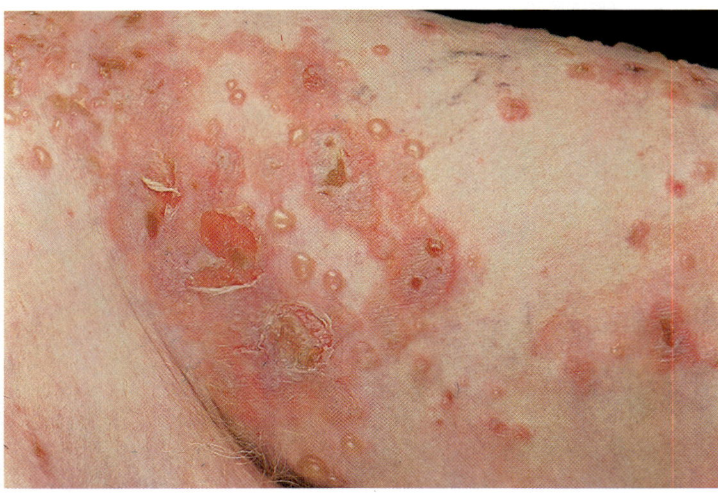

Figure 42 Pemphigus vulgaris on the left thigh. Bullae originating on an initially normal skin, followed by erosions.

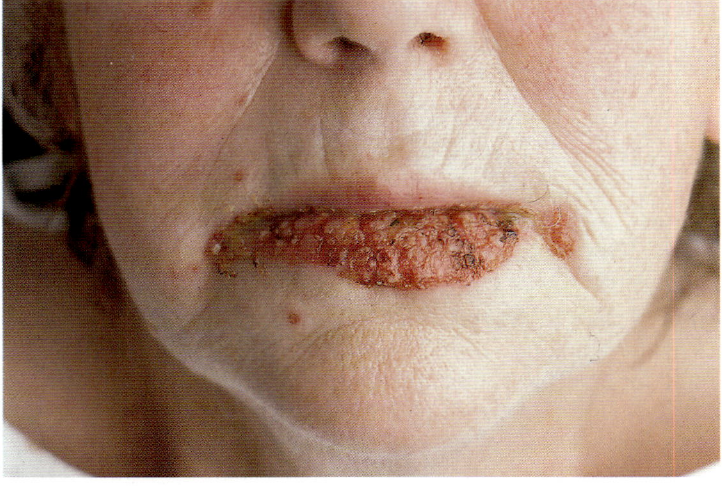

Figure 43 Pemphigus vegetans of the lips.

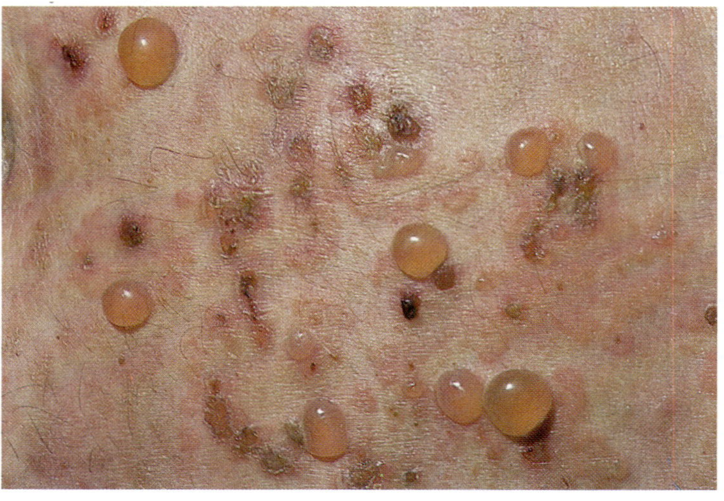

Figure 44 Bullous pemphigoid. Individual and crops of tense and flaccid bullae in various stages of development.

Vesiculobullous Diseases

Bullae and vesicles are symptoms which have different etiologies and thus can occur in diseases unrelated to one another, such as mosquito bites, contact dermatitis, erythema multiforme and certain viral diseases, such as herpes simplex and herpes zoster. The so-called vesiculobullous diseases are chronic diseases with generalized blistering. The patient may have to be hospitalized for a diagnostic work-up that includes histologic and immunofluorescence examinations and possibly electron microscopic studies. The therapeutic program is usually determined during hospitalization.

A. Pemphigus Vulgaris

This autoimmune disease is caused by the production of antibodies to the intercellular junctions of the epidermis without a recognizable cause. This makes the junctions defective and leads to the formation of spontaneous or traumatic fissures and blisters. Histologic examination reveals a detachment of the individual keratinocytes from each other (akantholysis). Direct immunofluorescence reveals the bound IgG antibodies (also C3) with their reticulated pattern (because they are located between the cells). The antibody titer in the blood serum can be determined by indirect immunofluorescence; it runs approximately parallel to the activity of the disease.

Clinical Features

1. Blisters, remnants of blisters and erythema can be seen, occasionally with residual brown pigmentation.
2. The mucosa of the mouth is often involved; in more than 50% of the cases, this precedes the skin lesions. Eating is painful, and the patients often lose weight.
3. There is a chronic course over many months or years with acute attacks of the disease. Without proper treatment the disease can be fatal.

Therapy

1. In severe cases, the patients must initially be treated in the hospital.
2. Immunosuppressive treatment with high doses of corticosteroids in combination with azathioprine, methotrexate or cyclophosphamide until antibody formation is completely suppressed (3-5 weeks). The dose is then reduced until a maintenance dose is reached, which often means a compromise between minor skin changes and still tolerable drug side effects. Treatment can extend over many years. The indication for this form of systemic treatment depends on the extent of the cutaneous symptoms and the involvement of the oral mucosa. The risks of long-term treatment with corticosteroids (see **R. 63**) and the risks of long-term immunosuppression must be taken into account (risks of tumor development, infections).
3. Topical treatment with corticosteroid creams or fatty gauze is possible, but is less important than systemic treatment.

B. Bullous Pemphigoid

This is the most frequent of all blistering diseases in elderly individuals. The blisters occur subepidermally. As in pemphigus vulgaris, autoantibodies appear (most frequently IgG) for reasons unknown. However, they are not directed against the intercellular junctions but against certain antigens in the region of the basal membrane (major bullous pemphigoid antigen 230 kD, minor bullous pemphigoid antigen 180 kD). Direct immunofluorescence shows a linear deposition of C3 in the region of the basal membrane, and usually also IgG, less often other immunoglobulins. The diagnosis is made by histologic and immunofluorescence examination of biopsy material.

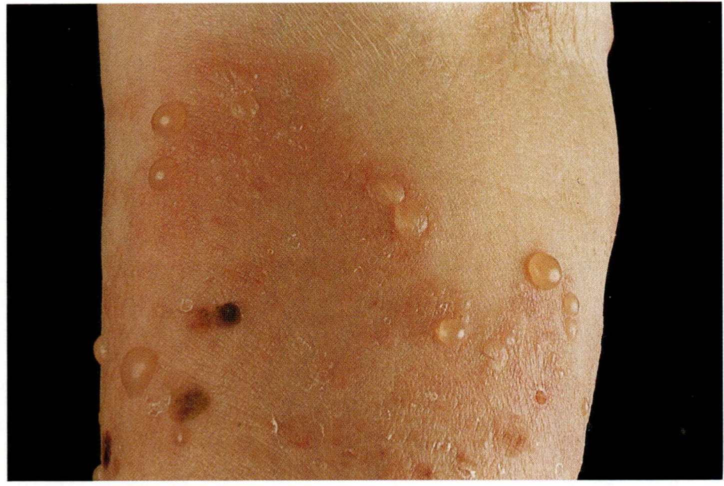

Figure 45 Bullous pemphigoid. Erythematous area with peripheral bullae and remnants of bullae on the flexor side of the left forearm.

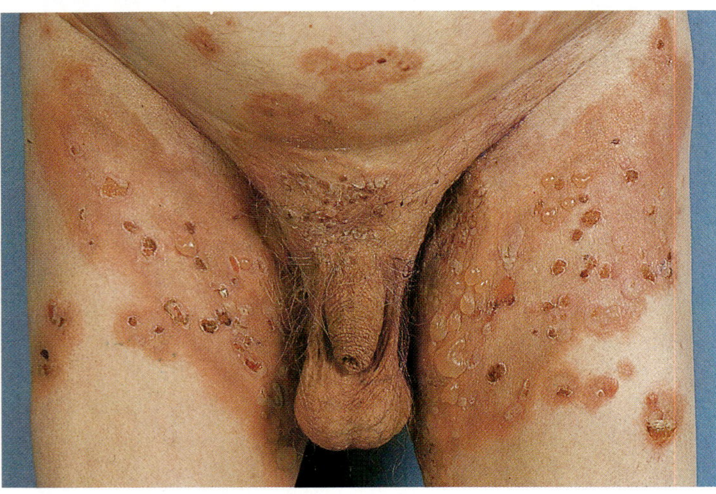

Figure 46 Dermatitis herpetiformis. Symmetric urticarial erythemata with fresh and ruptured bullae. Circinate borders surround the lesions.

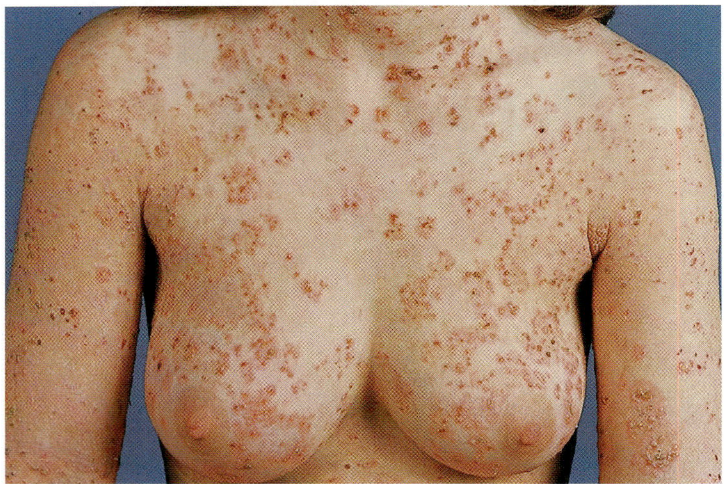

Figure 47 Dermatitis herpetiformis. Generalized symmetric appearance of urticarial lesions. Formation of vesicles and crusts around the periphery.

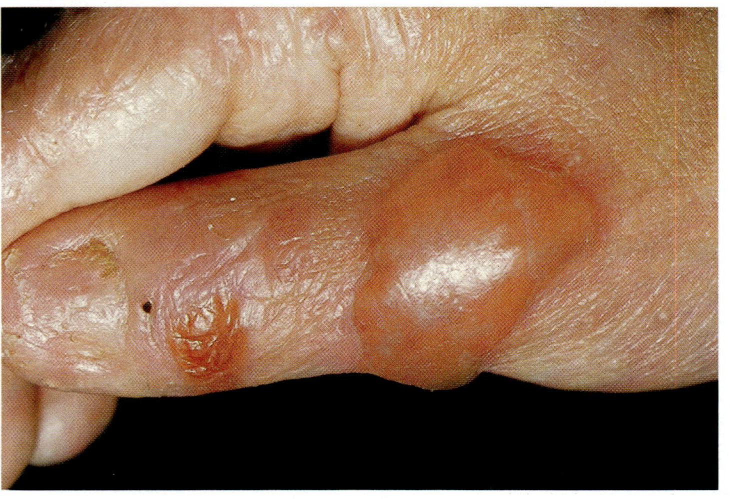

Figure 48 Epidermolysis bullosa hereditaria dystrophica. Vesicle formation in areas under mechanical stress or after trauma. Nail dystrophy typical of the condition.

Clinical Features

1. This disease lasts many months or even years in the elderly.
2. The disorder is characterized by the appearance of bullae on normal or erythematous skin; the erythema can be raised as in urticaria. In addition, there are remnants of bullae, erosions, erythemata and brown discolorations. Often, there are unpleasant skin sensations, from itching to burning of the skin.

Therapy

1. The disease usually responds well to high doses of corticosteroids that can soon be reduced to a maintenance dose. Response is usually better than in pemphigus vulgaris. It is important that the steroid dose is held as low as possible (the patients are usually elderly individuals). Corticosteroids may be supplemented by azathioprine.
2. Local therapy consists of evacuation of bullae and application of corticosteroid cream and disinfectant solutions (**R. 17**).

C. Dermatitis Herpetiformis

This is a rare, chronic, relapsing disease that can occur at any age, most frequently in the 2nd to 4th decade; it then lasts for the rest of the patient's life to varying degrees. The cause is still not clear. Genetic factors play a role (high incidence of HLA-B8, -DR3, -Dqw2). Ingestion of glutens, and frequently iodide (seafood, etc.), leads to an exacerbation of symptoms in almost all patients. The diagnosis is confirmed histologically (deposition of eosinophils in the tips of the papillae) and especially by fluorescence microscopic findings (granular IgA deposits in connective tissue papillae). The disease is distinguished from linear IgA dermatosis, a condition with similar symptoms, but with linear IgA deposits along the basal membrane and without the special HLA pattern or the gluten-sensitive enteropathy.

Clinical Features

1. The clinical picture is polymorphic. Typically, one finds symmetrically grouped or peripherally located vesicular lesions on urticarial erythemata.
2. Subjectively, the patients complain of a burning sensation that is frequently more severe than the itching.
3. Occasionally the oral mucosa is involved.

Therapy

1. The treatment of choice for suppression of symptoms is prolonged systemic administration of dapsone (diaminodiphenylsulfone), usually over the course of many years, at a daily dose of 50–100 mg. Before initiating therapy, glucose-6-PDH must be determined, and during therapy, methemoglobin must be monitored regularly.
2. Topical treatment of blisters consists of corticosteroid creams **(R. 38)** or white shake lotion **(R. 20)**, occasionally supplemented by oil baths **(R. 7)**.
3. Strict adherence to a gluten-free diet and avoidance of iodized salt can support the therapy.

D. Epidermolysis Bullosa Hereditaria

This is a group of rare genetic disorders resulting from inadequate fixation of the epidermis to the dermis. Slight pressure, a mild blow or shearing forces can lead to the formation of blisters. There are several subgroups that can be differentiated by clinical and electron microscopic criteria. Forms without creation of scars (formation of vesicles above the basal membrane) include the epidermolysis bullosa simplex group (this frequently has autosomal dominant inheritance) and two forms with autosomal recessive inheritance. A late form (epidermolysis bullosa tarda [Weber-Cockayne]) presents with mildly or markedly increased blister formation from mechanical stress (hiking, marching, manual labor) in comparison to healthy individuals. The forms with scar formation (blister formation below the basal membrane, defect of the anchoring fibrils) can be recognized by the absence of fingernails and of course by the scars in the skin. Mutilations are possible.

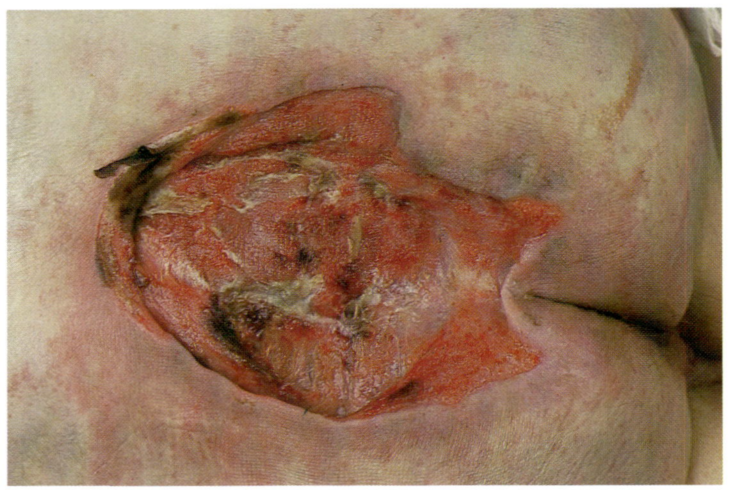

Figure 49 Deep sacral decubitus ulcer.

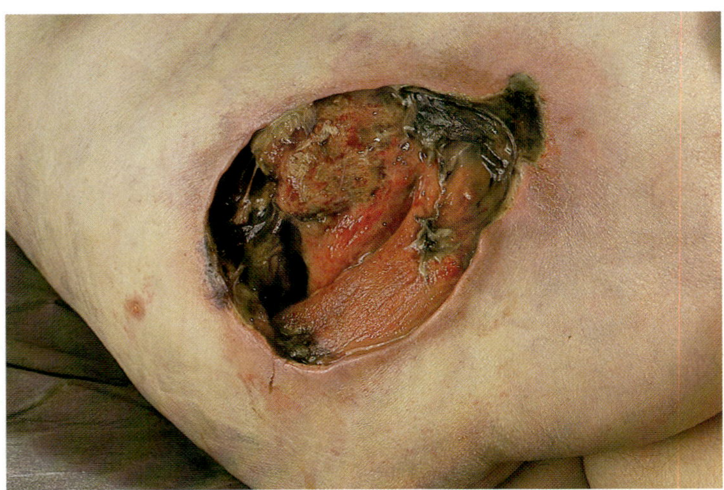

Figure 50 Decubitus ulcer, right hip. Deep ulcer with necrotic tissue and exposed musculature.

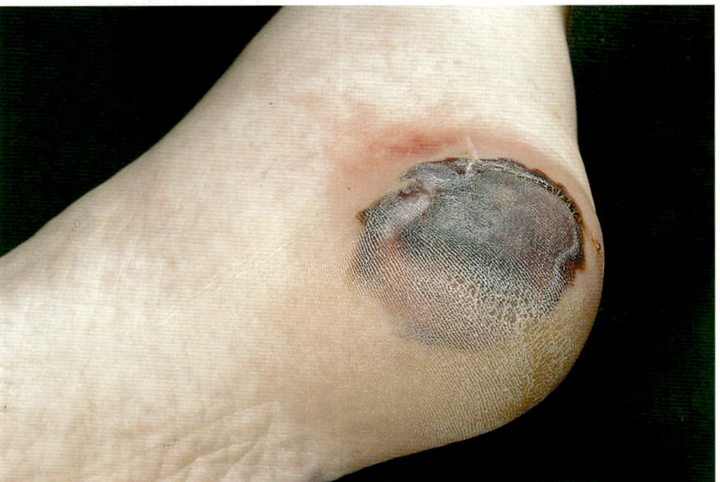

Figure 51 Acute decubitus necrosis. The patient was in a deep coma for a long time following a suicide attempt with barbiturates.

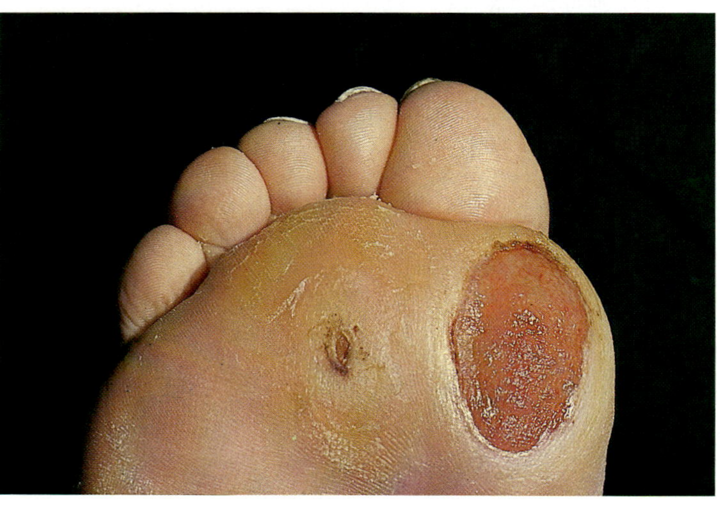

Figure 52 Malum perforans. Ulcers on the ball of the forefoot in a patient with polyneuropathy.

Decubitus Ulcer

Decubitus ulcers occur as a result of pressure on individual areas of the body in patients who are unable to move adequately. This constant pressure produces atrophic changes and finally pressure necroses. The patients are usually bedridden and suffer from generalized weakness and cachexia due to chronic disease, neurologic disorders or severe disorders of the musculoskeletal system. In addition, sensory disturbances can prevent normal, physiologic shifts in position and thus result in decubitus ulcers. This occurs in diseases such as multiple sclerosis, paraplegia and polyneuropathy (malum performans on the ball of the big toe) and in comatose patients with inadequate padding who are unable to change position, e. g., those suffering from poisoning with barbiturates or other hypnotics, or during prolonged operations and deep anesthesia with inadequate padding. For this to occur, tissue hypoxia that lasts several hours can be sufficient. Patients with poorly developed subcutaneous fat are especially at risk for developing decubitus ulcers.

Clinical Features

1. Erythema with occasional inflammatory infiltration can be seen. The skin becomes less resistant to shearing forces, and shearing can easily lead to detachment of the epidermis. This can rapidly cause erosions and shallow ulcers.
2. In hyperkeratotic areas, a decubitus injury to the deeper layers of the skin sometimes initially causes a blister which often becomes hemorrhagic.
3. Prolonged pressure can cause deep, purulent ulcers with undermined margins and fistulae, followed by exposure of muscles, fasciae, tendons and bone.
4. Ischemic changes are initially limited to the pressure areas, especially the sacral region, the heels and the shoulders.

Therapy

General

The most important measure is relief of pressure on the affected regions. For sacral decubitus, these patients must be maintained as long as possible in a lateral or prone position. The use of decubitus mattresses, alternating air circulating mattresses, rotating frame beds, soft bedding (sheep skin, etc.), is important for even distribution of pressure. The use of a blow dryer for periods of 10 minutes to areas of maceration and careful massage with ice cubes for several minutes several times a day are additional measures.

Systemic

It is important to increase the patient's body weight as much as possible with tasty food, rich in calories, as well as good emotional care by the nursing staff.

External

Local therapy is secondary to relief of pressure and depends on the extent of the decubitus ulcer.

1. The only topical treatment necessary for an erythema, in addition to pressure relief, would be a silicon spray or a soft zinc oxide paste **(R. 30)**.
2. Erosions and shallow ulcers should receive normal wound care, including debridement of the necrotic tissue and prevention of desiccation of the wound with semipermeable synthetic bandages (see page 33).
3. When crusts and deep ulcers are present, the wound should be cleaned and if necessary dressed with wet dressings **(R. 1)**, debriding agents should be applied **(R. 43)**, and later medication to enhance the formation of granulation tissue can be tried (see page 33). As much of the crusts and necrotic tissue should be removed mechanically as possible, followed by irrigation with H_2O_2 and disinfectant solutions. This may require the use of a bulbous cannula when the margin is undermined or a fistula is present.
4. Appropriate plastic surgery can shorten treatment time significantly for those patients whose underlying disease can be expected to permit mobilization, for that matter, it can facilitate rehabilitation. The success of such procedures depends on many factors which should be clarified carefully preoperatively.

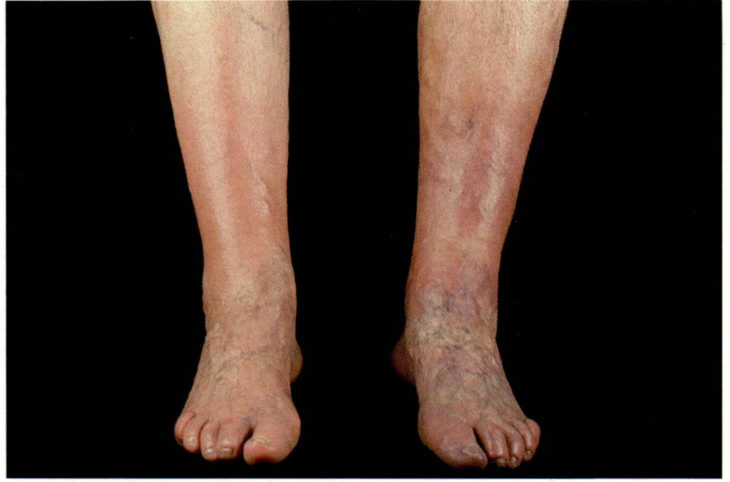

Figure 53 Arterial occlusive disease. Condition following arterial embolus of the lower left leg several days prior. Bluish discoloration of the toes.

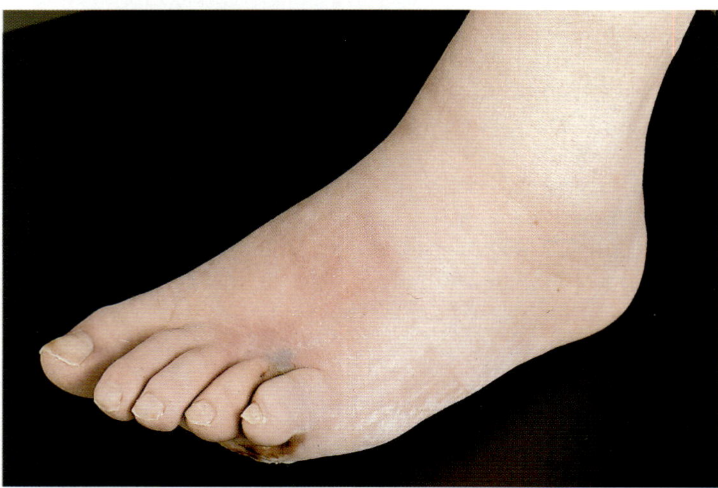

Figure 54 Arterial occlusive disease. Erythema of the forefoot and beginning gangrene.

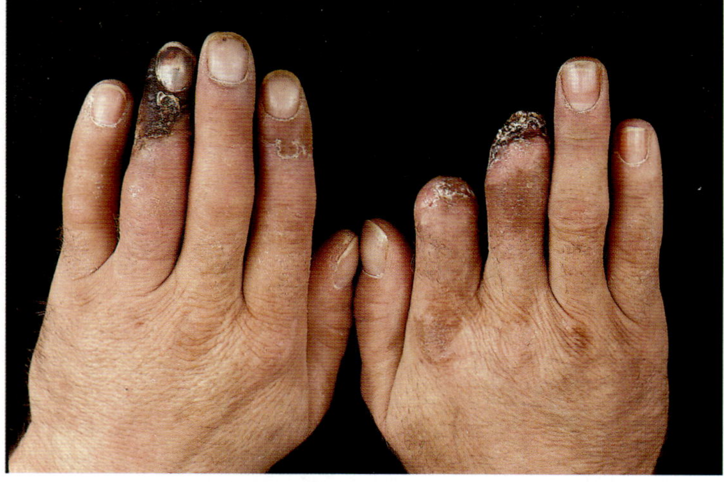

Figure 55 Endangitis obliterans with necroses of the distal phalanx of several fingers.

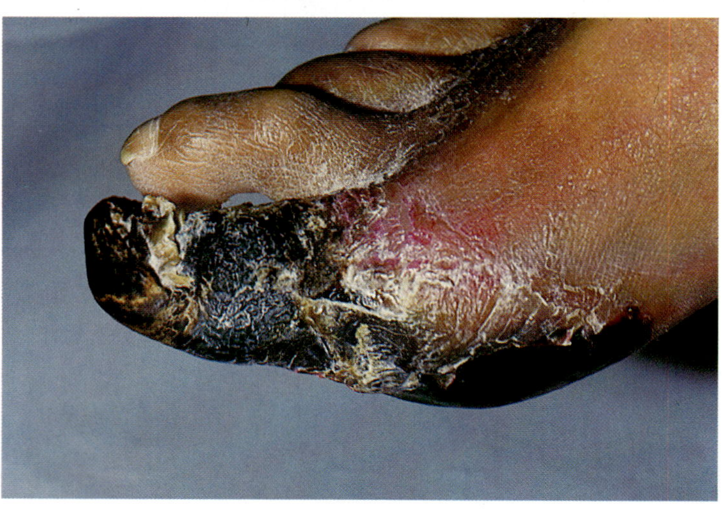

Figure 56 Diabetic gangrene. Dry gangrene of the right big toe with mummification.

Vascular Disorders

A. Obstructive Arterial Diseases

The causes of obstructive arterial diseases are manifold. The arterial blood supply can be cut off by tight bandages. It can be obstructed by arteriosclerosis obliterans, which can also be a complication of diabetes mellitus; by deposits on the vessel walls with resulting narrowing of the lumen; or complete occlusion caused by arterial thrombi or drugs such as epinephrine, norepinephrine or ergotamine preparations. Acute arterial occlusions require immediate hospitalization and treatment. The practicing physician encounters arteriosclerosis obliterans much more often as a chronic vascular disorder. This widespread, epidemic arterial disorder is usually a generalized vascular disease with reduction of blood supply to the heart (coronary artery disease), kidneys, brain, abdominal organs and legs.

Clinical Features

Peripheral arteriosclerosis obliterans can be subdivided into four clinical stages.

Stage 1: *No symptoms.* The occlusion can be diagnosed only by angiography or occasionally by Doppler examination.
Stage 2: *Pain from exercise.* Increased oxygen demand by the musculature produces pain with intermittent claudication. The painfree walking distance is an important indicator of the degree of vascular obstruction.
Stage 3: *Resting pain.* Blood supply is already impaired to the degree that pain is present even at rest. The patient often lets his leg hang out of the bed to ease the pain.
Stage 4: In addition to the previous symptoms, *necroses* develop in the areas with impaired blood supply.

The skin is involved only in arteriosclerosis obliterans of stage 4 or in acute complete arterial obstruction. Thin, dry skin of the legs as well as a pale color, reduced skin temperature and hair loss already suggest upon inspection that the blood supply to that area is impaired.

Therapy

The most important principle is to eliminate all risk factors as early as possible (overweight, lack of exercise, smoking, arterial hypertension, diabetes mellitus, disorders of fat metabolism and gout). Vascular training with exercise is useful in stages 1 and 2. Combined arterial and venous disorders, which are frequently present in older patients, are more difficult to treat. Compression therapy impairs arterial blood supply even more. In stages 2, 3 and 4, it must also be determined whether a circumscribed stenosis can be removed surgically or by catheter dilatation. In advanced stages, amputation of the involved extremity is often the last resort. Surgery is indicated when moist gangrene with impending sepsis is present or when pain is so severe that it can no longer be relieved with medication.

Internal

Vasodilator drugs (caution: "steal phenomenon", i.e., reduction of blood supply in the involved region through redistribution of blood), drugs that prevent platelet aggregation, or anticoagulants are less important in comparison to the above-mentioned therapeutic measures.

External

Topical therapy is limited to preventing infection of the necroses. Dressings can produce moist chambers with anaerobic infection and should be avoided. Treatment with dry powders and disinfectant solutions is preferable until necroses are demarcated. Mechanical removal of necroses must be carried out with great care to avoid additional tissue damage.

B. Venous Disorders, Ulcus Cruris (Leg Ulcers)

Statistical studies have shown that approximately 20% of all citizens of the Federal Republic of Germany have varicosis of the saphenous system. Approximately 1 million patients are suffering from venous leg ulcers, and there are some 16,000 fatal pulmonary emboli annually, most of which are due to thrombosis of the leg veins. These figures show the significant impact of

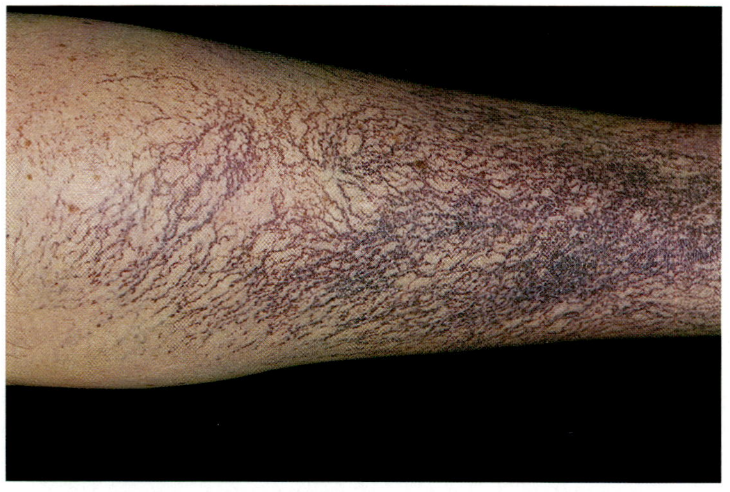

Figure 57 Fans of intracutaneous varices on the lower leg.

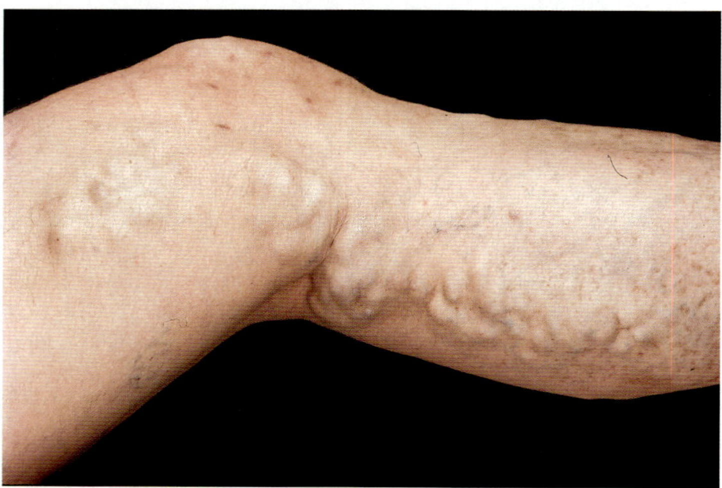

Figure 58 Varicosis caused by insufficiency of the greater saphenous vein.

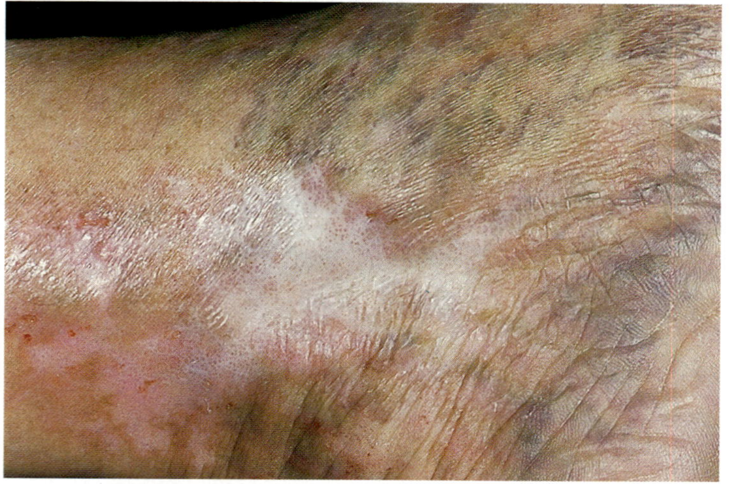

Figure 59 Atrophie blanche in chronic venous insufficiency. Circumscribed white sclerotic foci with punctate blood vessels, left medial malleolar region.

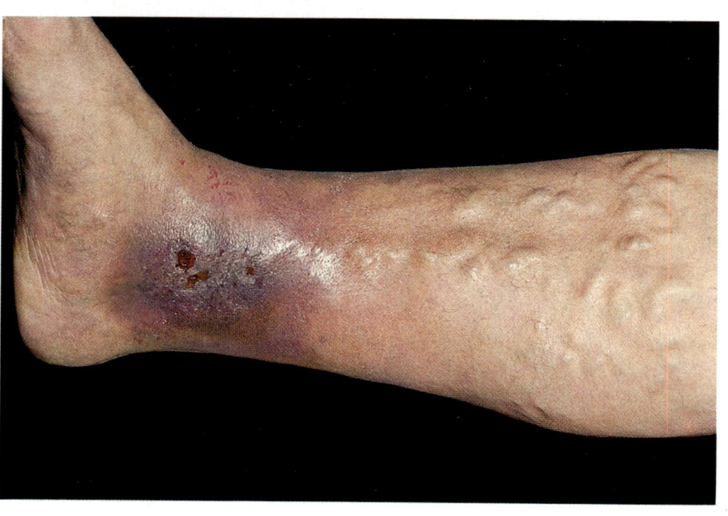

Figure 60 Venous leg ulcers in a patient with chronic venous insufficiency. Several ulcers in the area of the medial malleolus. Dermatosclerosis, deposition of hemosiderin. Massive varicosis.

venous disorders. In addition to a familial disposition, there are individual factors such as overweight, a predominantly sitting or standing occupation, inappropriate shoes (elimination of the calf muscle pump by high heels) and hormonal factors such as ovulation inhibitors and pregnancy that can be responsible for manifestation of the disorder. Women are afflicted more frequently than men; incidence and severity of the symptoms are higher in the older age groups. The causes of chronic leg vein insufficiency include primary varicosis, recurrent thrombophlebitis, primary insufficiency of the perforating veins and prior thrombophlebitis. Dermatologic symptoms develop independently of the causes of chronic leg vein insufficiency.

Clinical Features

1. One of the earliest symptoms is the patient's complaint of "heavy legs". The earliest dermatologic sign of chronic incompetence of the leg veins is edema at the ankles, which initially occurs only in the evening after prolonged standing or in hot weather.
2. Varices occur at the same time or somewhat later. Depending on the size of the involved veins, these can be fan-shaped, intracutaneous varices (purely cosmetic), reticular varices, or varices of the saphenous system (small saphenous vein or great saphenous vein).
3. Persisting edemas lead to protein deposits in the interstitium with increased formation of connective tissue. The skin is firm and difficult to compress (dermatosclerosis). This frequently leads to the development of stasis dermatitis (see page 49).
4. Prolonged stasis can lead to extravasation of erythrocytes (stasis purpura). Hemoglobin is metabolized into hemosiderin, which remains in the tissues for a long time and causes brown discoloration of the skin.
5. Incompetence of the perforating veins often produces atrophie blanche distal to their point of entry. These are whitish areas of atrophic scarring that develop spontaneously without trauma, usually in the ankle region.
6. Increasing nutritional disturbance of the skin frequently leads to leg ulcers, either spontaneously or as a result of minimal trauma, erysipelas or thrombophlebitis.
7. Areas of predilection for venous leg ulcers are the ankle region and the distal part of the lower leg.
8. The morphology of leg ulcers is manifold. It includes shallow ulcers that are often painful and develop on the basis of atrophie blanche, as well as ulcers involving the lower leg in a sleeve-like fashion and developing as a result of extensive thrombotic obstruction of varicose skin veins.
9. The development of a squamous cell carcinoma is a rare complication that may occur after long-standing leg ulcers (after decades). Rapidly proliferating granulation tissue with necrotic decomposition is a suspicious finding and should be examined histologically.

Therapy

Exact phlebologic diagnosis is necessary before optimal long-term therapy can be established (light reflexion rheography, ultrasound, phlebography).

General

Of primary importance is correction of the impaired venous blood flow. There are three ways to achieve this: support stockings (see page 262), injection with sclerosing solutions and vein stripping. These methods complement each other to a certain degree, or they overlap for certain indications. In addition, specific dermatologic therapy may be necessary for accompanying cutaneous symptoms, especially leg ulcers. The previously mentioned therapeutic measures may have to be supplemented by systemic drug treatment. Since chronic stasis conditions have a tendency to develop eczematous reactions, the routine use of "vein ointments" (OTC ointments) should be avoided. Contact allergies to the medications, preservatives, or bases of these ointments often develop and may make topical treatment of an ulcer very difficult at a later date. Exercise, such as swimming, bicycling or running, is useful in enhancing the musculovenous pump. Proper footwear with low heels is also important.

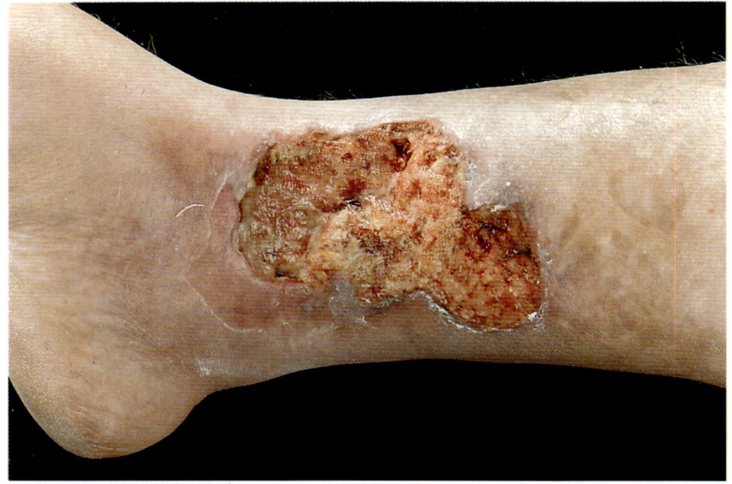

Figure 61 Venous leg ulcer in a patient with postthrombotic syndrome.

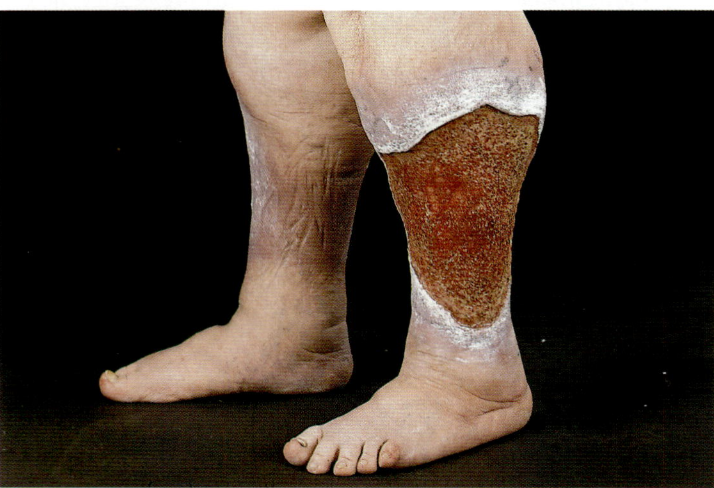

Figure 62 Venous leg ulcer. Severe postthrombotic syndrome with extensive cuff-like ulcer.

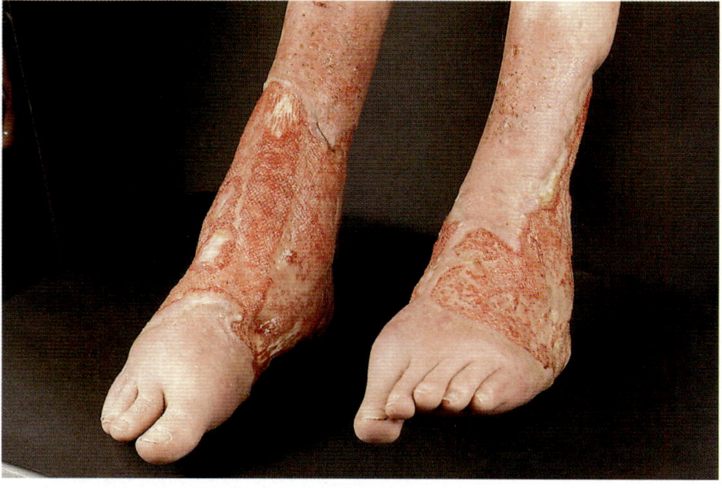

Figure 63 Cuff-like ulcers on both lower legs and forefeet in a patient with chronic venous insufficiency. The extensive stasis sclerosis is clearly visible.

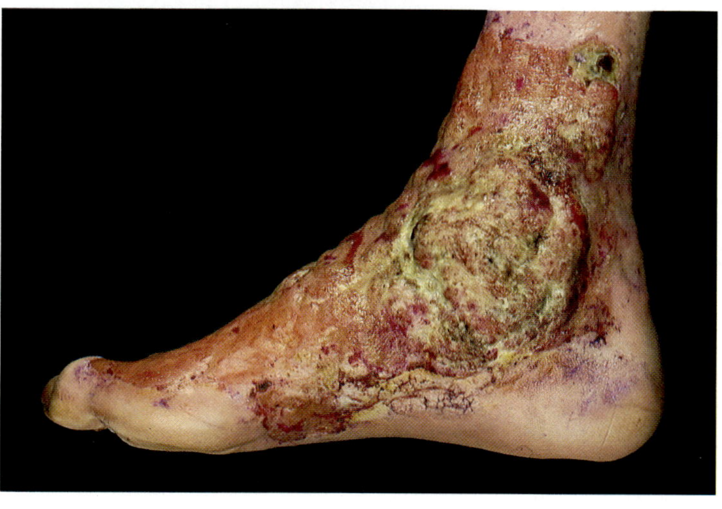

Figure 64 Squamous cell carcinoma on a venous leg ulcer that had persisted for 12 years (in a patient with generalized morphea).

External

Topical treatment of leg ulcers is carried out in several stages: cleansing, promoting production of granulation tissue, and epithelial coverage.

1. Disinfecting leg baths, e.g., with addition of potassium permanganate and the application of moist compresses with antiseptic solutions **(R. 2)** for hour intervals may be helpful.
2. Necrotic tissue should be removed with debriding medications. These medications can be applied in combination with moist compresses or the necrotic tissue can be removed with a surgical spoon (which may be painful).
3. Thick fibrinous or necrotic crusts are always heavily contaminated with bacteria. These crusts must be removed to eliminate the growth medium for bacteria. Significant bacterial infection requiring local or systemic treatment rarely occurs in venous leg ulcers.
4. Porous foam rubber materials, as well as hydrocolloid bandages are useful, especially when they are applied with mild pressure. Examples are Op-Site, Bioclusive, Vigilon and Duoderm. In contrast to mixed ointments, which often contain neomycin or balsam of Peru, these materials almost never cause contact allergies. These dressings can be also left in place for several days to avoid tearing off the newly formed epithelial tissue.
5. Once clean granulations are present, antimicrobial powder **(R. 12)** can be applied to promote epithelialization.
6. Application of a compression bandage (see page 262) and mobilization of the patient are absolutely necessary as part of the therapeutic program. Compression bandages achieve their optimal effect only when the patient is ambulatory.
7. Large ulcers should be debrided and covered according to Reverdin's or meshgraft technique to shorten the healing time.

Internal

Systemic medications cannot replace the above-mentioned therapeutic measures for chronic leg vein insufficiency. They can only supplement them in individual cases. Diuretics can be useful to treat edema but are not recommended for prophylaxis of edema. Medications to increase the venous tone may be helpful. These include hydroergotamine, which, however, may damage arterial blood flow (ergotism) and rheologic drugs (pentoxifylline), as well as drugs that "seal" blood vessels, such as horse chestnut extract.

C. Other Common Vascular Disorders

These are primarily diseases of the small vessels, and they have an abnormal reaction to cold in common. The clinical severity of these disorders varies from functional problems (acrocyanosis) to severe illnesses, such as Raynaud's disease.

a) Acrocyanosis

Clinical Features

1. Poorly defined, bluish-red discolorations of the acra, frequently associated with hyperhidrosis. The so-called "iris diaphragmatic phenomenon" is of diagnostic importance.
2. The symptoms are localized to the hands and feet and occasionally on the arms, legs, nose and cheeks. In obese patients, the gluteal area and mammae may be involved. Sometimes there are transitions to chilblains (see page 65).
3. The cold moist hands and feet are often conspicuous; occasionally there are complaints of paresthesias. These patients have a disposition for other skin diseases, such as warts (see page 215), fungal infections (see pp. 113–121) and pyodermas (see pp. 131–133). Acrocyanosis occurs mainly during puberty and adolescence and almost always in women. The disorder disappears spontaneously after a few years and is no longer present in middle-aged persons.

Therapy

Vascular training with contrast baths, sauna and athletic activities is important. Nicotine must be avoided.

Internal

Systemic drugs to improve blood supply and increase the tone of the vessel walls are often prescribed. Their effect on acrocyanosis, however, is questionable.

External

Protection from cold is very important.

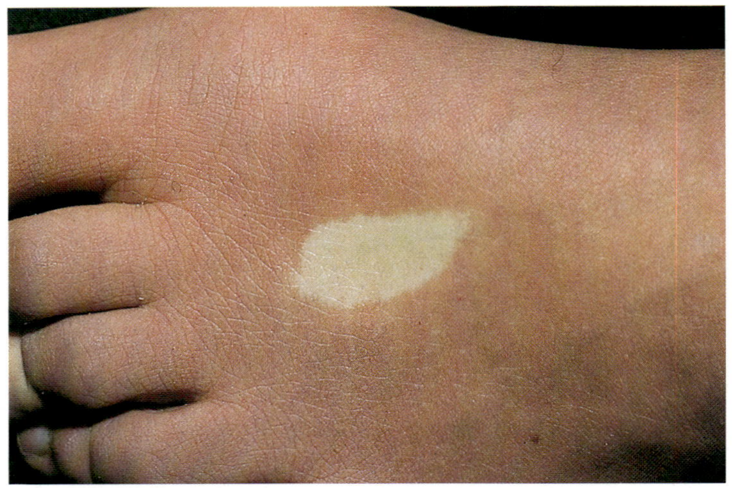

Figure 65 Acrocyanosis. Iris diaphragmatic phenomenon, i.e., blanching on finger pressure with subsequent refilling from the periphery.

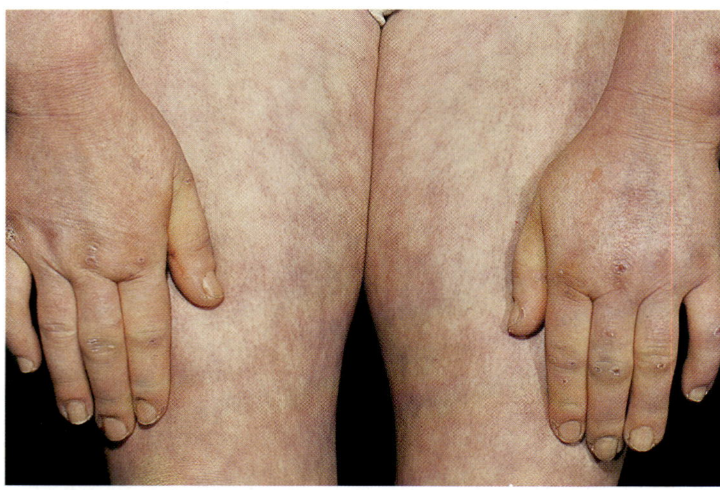

Figure 66 Livedo reticularis. Reticulate dusky vascular markings.

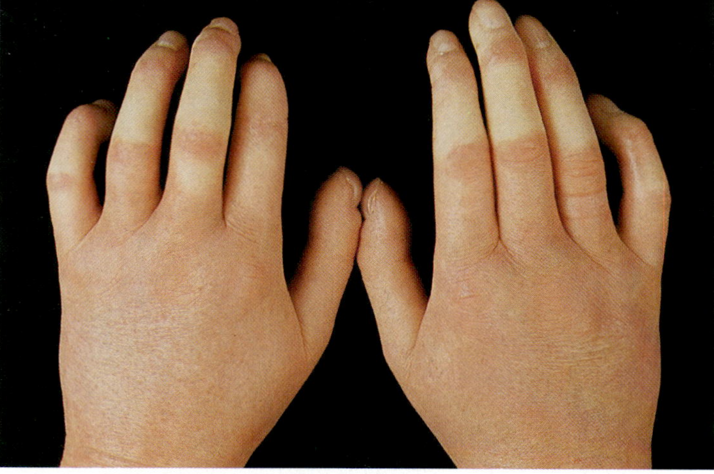

Figure 67 Raynaud's phenomenon. Blanching of the fingers induced by cold.

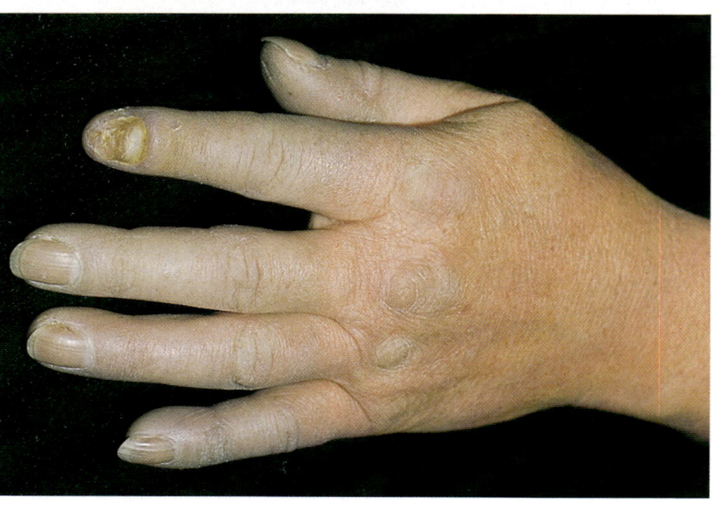

Figure 68 Raynaud's phenomenon in a patient with progressive scleroderma. Phase of venous atonia with edematous swelling and mild cyanosis. Candidal infection of nail and nailbed of the index finger secondary to impaired blood supply.

b) Livedo Reticularis

Clinical Features There is reticulated bluish discoloration of the skin on the arms, legs and trunk that increases with exposure to cold (cutis marmorata). These symptoms appear in infants and adolescents, especially in females. It does not represent a genuine disease process.

c) Raynaud's Disease/Raynaud's Phenomenon

The disorder is characterized by intermittent spasms of the small arteries of the fingers and toes, mainly as a result of exposure to cold. It occurs especially in the winter months. A number of causes or factors have been identified, including diseases such as progressive scleroderma, lupus erythematosus, cold agglutination disease and cryoglobulinemia, vibration injuries, certain chemicals or drugs (PVC, ergotamine, bleomycin). Conditions for which a cause cannot be identified are classified as Raynaud's disease. The disease occurs much more frequently in women than in men. Prognosis is determined primarily by the underlying causative mechanism.

Clinical Features Sudden blanching of one or more fingers occurs on exposure to cold. After a few minutes, a dark cyanotic discoloration occurs and gradually changes to a long-lasting red color (reactive hyperemia). These attacks can occur several times a day, depending on the severity of the disease.

Therapy It is important to treat an underlying cause, if known. Measures must be taken to protect against cold (mittens, muff, pocket heater) and smoking is prohibited. Warm hand baths can help, preferable shortly before going outside.

Internal Systemic calcium channel blockers (e.g., nifedipine 10–20 mg daily) can be used preferably in the morning and in the evening, depending on the symptoms. Other "blood vessel active" drugs are less effective.

External Nitrates (e.g., nitroglycerin 2% ointment) have been found to be effective.

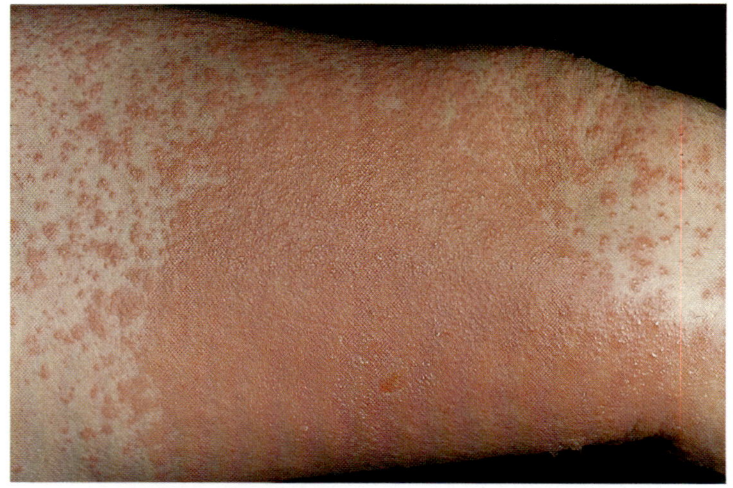

Figure 69 Acute allergic contact dermatitis caused by an ointment for chilblains. Erythema, papules, vesicles and central erosion with ill-defined borders on the right thigh.

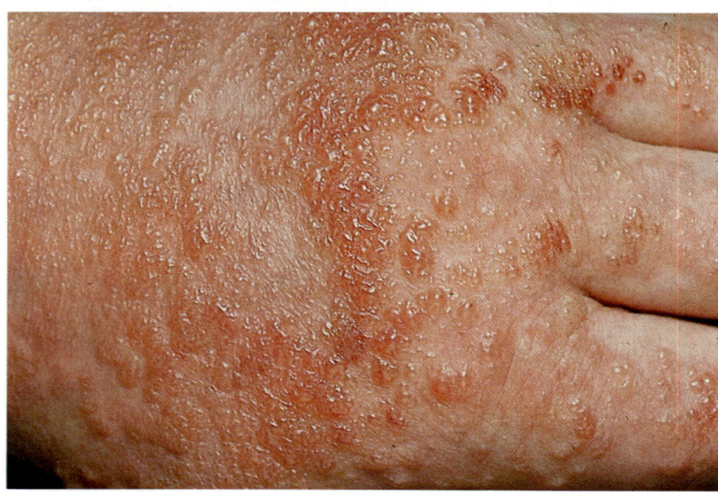

Figure 70 Acute contact dermatitis caused by benzoyl peroxide. Vesicular stage.

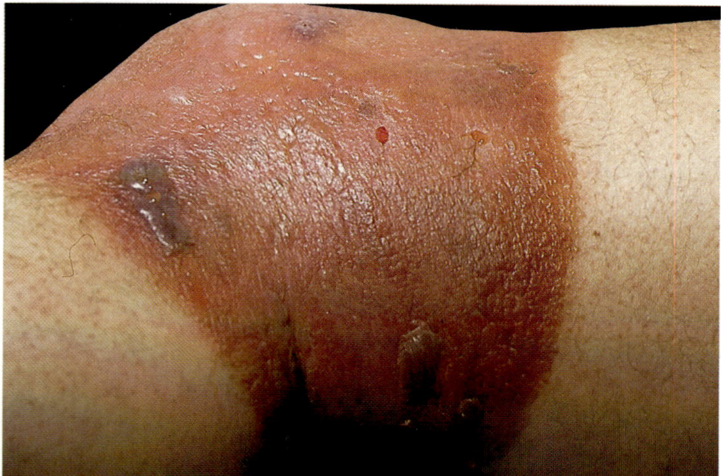

Figure 71 Acute allergic contact dermatitis caused by heparin ointment. Erythema and vesicles, some of which are hemorrhagic. The lesion is sharply delineated.

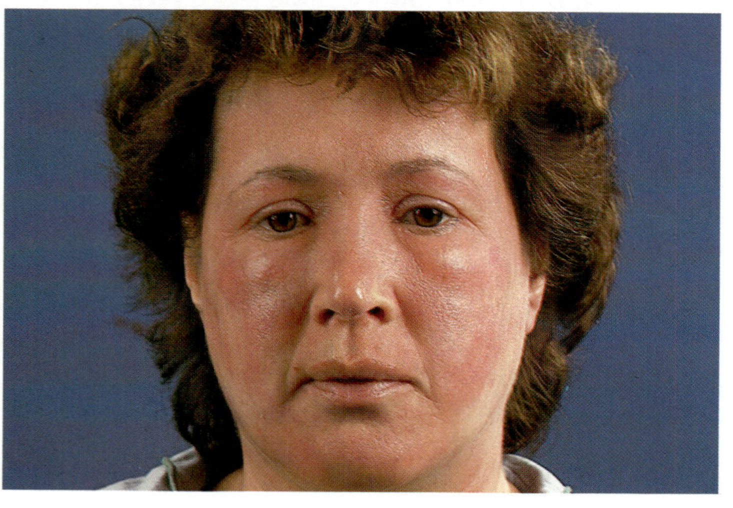

Figure 72 Acute contact dermatitis caused by shampoo. Erythema and marked edema.

Eczematous Diseases

Individual eczematous diseases can ordinarily be differentiated from one another by their clinical symptoms and the course of the disease. A contact eczema is due to the external action of an injurious substance. Non-allergic contact eczemas occur much more frequently than allergic ones, especially chronic non-allergic contact eczema which results from repeated exposure to toxic substances over a long period of time. Acute toxic contact eczema is due to substances that primarily irritate the skin, such as alkali or wound secretions. Other eczemas, such as eczema due to dry skin (see page 149), diaper rash and stasis eczema on the lower legs of patients with venous insufficiency, may be considerably influenced by exogenous factors. In contrast, other forms of eczema are mainly or completely caused by endogenous factors: atopic dermatitis, vesicular palmoplantar eczema (pompholyx), chronic hyperkeratotic eczema of the palms and the soles of the feet, seborrheic dermatitis, bacterial ear eczema, nummular eczema and lichen simplex chronicus.

Occupational eczemas are important because of their effect on the patient's personal situation (disability with subsequent pension claims). The condition, acquired at the workplace, is a long lasting, allergic or non-allergic contact eczema, usually on the hands. It is the task of the physician (with the help of cooperating specialists in occupational medicine and dermatology) to identify the causative allergens and irritating agents and see to it that they are eliminated. Otherwise such conditions can lead to absences from work, change of the workplace or even loss of occupation. Skin protection is thus part of occupational protection. If a vocational skin disease is suspected, it is advisable to consult a dermatologist as soon as possible to perform further tests (patch tests, alkali tolerance tests). If the suspicion is confirmed, the condition should be reported to the trade association, also by the employer. This may necessitate long-term observation to make sure that an existing skin disease does not develop into an occupational disease. An existing atopic dermatitis of the hands is often aggravated by the patient's work. This aggravation must be avoided by the above-mentioned measures.

A. Acute Allergic Contact Dermatitis

The patient must have been previously sensitized by exposure to contact allergens and thus have a certain disposition. Common contact allergens are nickel (fashionable jewelry), topical medications (antibiotics, balsam of Peru), many industrial materials (nickel, chromium salts, rubber additives), textiles, as well as plants (primrose, chrysanthemums). The capacity of the individual substance to sensitize varies. Children under the age of 10 years rarely develop allergic contact dermatitis. They do, however, develop non-allergic eczema. The same is true for elderly patients.

Clinical Features

1. Erythema, nodules, vesicles, erosions, weeping surfaces and crusts characterize an acute contact dermatitis. All these symptoms can occur simultaneously, or just one or several may be present at the same time. The patient almost always complains of pronounced itching. With prominent facial involvement, many times the patient also develops edema of the eyelids and the periorbital region.
2. The symptoms evolve slowly, at least several hours later, but usually 1–3 days following contact with the causative agent. The lesions heal within 2–3 weeks.
3. Frequently, the affected area corresponds to the area in contact with the allergen, but occasionally it exceeds the contact area.
4. Disseminated reactions are possible with rapidly developing scattered papules that exceed the contact area and involve other regions of the body.

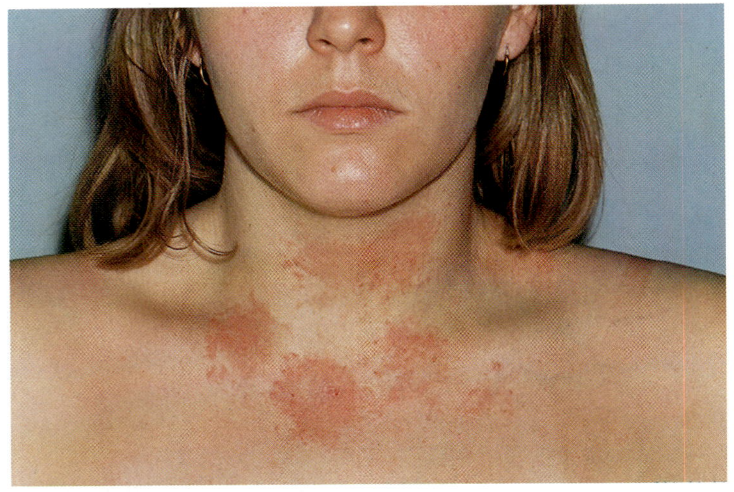

Figure 73 Allergic contact dermatitis caused by jewelry in a patient sensitized to nickel.

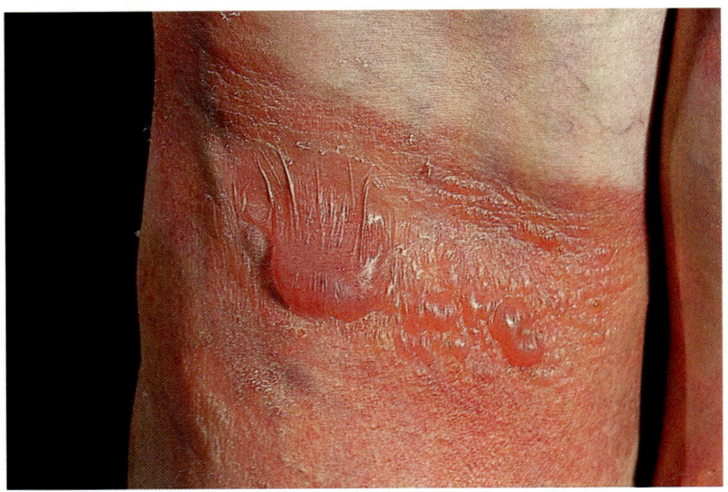

Figure 74 Acute allergic contact dermatitis caused by stocking dye. Erythema and blisters in the left popliteal area.

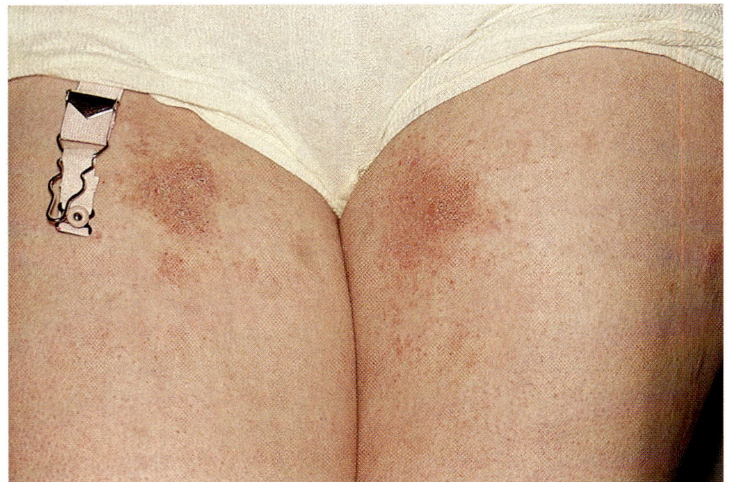

Figure 75 Allergic nickel dermatitis caused by the patient's garters. Papular eczema with indistinct border.

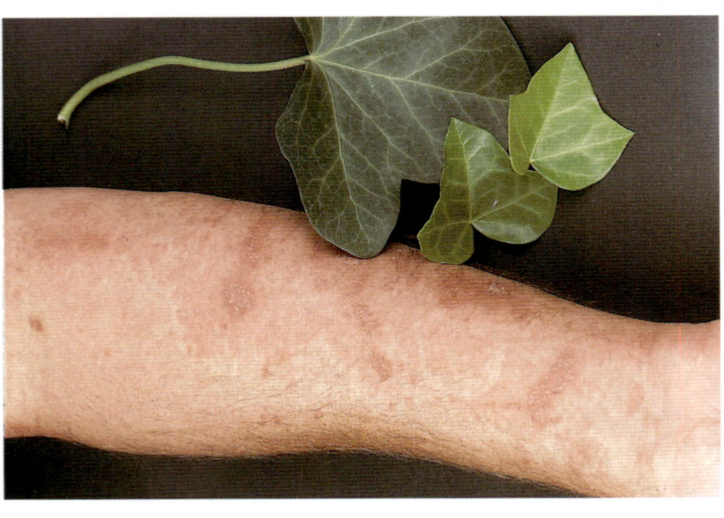

Figure 76 Allergic contact dermatitis caused by ivy.

Therapy

It is important to identify and eliminate the causative agent, usually with the help of a dermatologist (patch test, etc.).

1. Wet dressings **(R. 1)** are the treatment of choice for acute weeping contact dermatitis. In addition, creams containing corticosteroid **(R. 38 b, c)** are applied thinly.
2. For non-weeping lesions, a shake mixture **(R. 20)** or corticosteroid creams **(R. 38)** are used, the latter only for short periods (no longer than a few weeks).
3. Antihistamines are useful for relief of pruritus **(R. 61, 62)**. A brief treatment period with systemic corticosteroids does not shorten the healing period but may be sometimes justified in severe cases **(R. 63)**.

B. Chronic Allergic Contact Eczema

This is an eczema caused and maintained by prolonged exposure to contact allergens, such as nickel (jewelry), rubber (underwear, gloves) or leather (shoes). The causative agents can be found in the home, but also at the place of occupation. Many times the etiology is the combination of a chronic occupational irritation of the skin and a contact allergy acquired and maintained by occupational exposure to an industrial substance (see above).

Clinical Features

1. Pruritus, thickening of the skin, coarsening of surface markings, occasionally hyperkeratosis and rhagades are the symptoms of a chronic allergic contact eczema. There is frequent recurrence of acute eczematization with papules and crust formation.
2. Healing occurs slowly and with scaling. Occasionally, residual pigmentation remains.

Therapy

Recognition and elimination of the contact allergen are important for long-term success in treatment.

1. Corticosteroid-containing creams and ointments **(R. 38)** shorten the course of the disease significantly.
2. Tar or urea-containing ointments in combination with corticosteroids **(R. 39 b)** are useful for thickened and lichenified lesions.
3. Protective ointments **(R. 33 b, c)** are indicated as prophylaxis against occupational contact allergies.

C. Chronic, Non-Allergic Contact Eczema (Toxic Degenerative Eczema, Cumulative Toxic Contact Dermatitis)

This is an important and frequent form of eczema. Constant contact over the course of months or years with weak caustic solutions, excessively concentrated detergents, organic solvents or occasionally, just plain water can cause damage to the skin. The skin reacts to this cumulative toxic irritation with chronic eczema. It is mainly observed in housewives, members of medical or paramedical professions, cleaning and kitchen personnel (skin damage from water and detergents), masons (damage from alkali) and other construction workers. It is particularly frequent in patients with atopic dermatitis. Later, a contact allergy can develop secondarily.

Clinical Features

1. Dryness and thinning of the skin with fissures, scaling, rhagades and itching are seen. Later, the skin thickens, and the skin markings become coarse. There is recurrent acute eczematization with vesicles, erosions and crusts (see page 37).
2. The symptoms are limited to the area exposed to the chronic trauma, almost exclusively the hands. Normally, disseminated reactions do not occur.
3. Irritability of the skin is increased. Even minor trauma or stress situations can exacerbate the eczema.

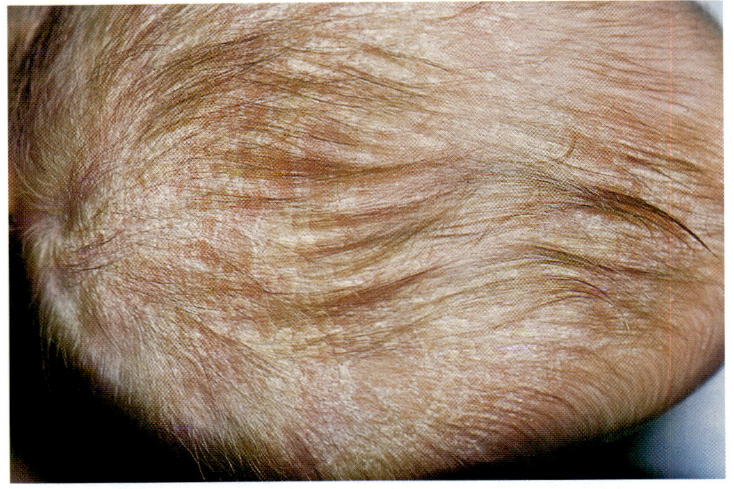

Figure 77 Atopic dermatitis, crusta lactea (cradle cap). White and yellowish, slightly "fatty scaling".

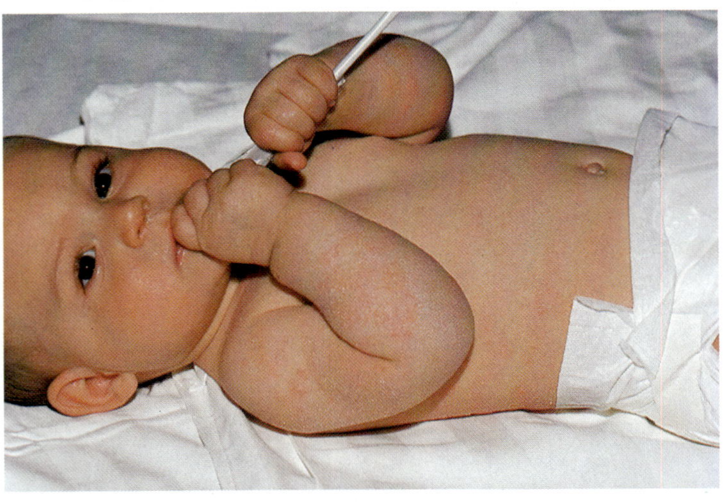

Figure 78 Atopic dermatitis. Numerous, mostly round, eczematous lesions of varying size, located on abdomen and arms.

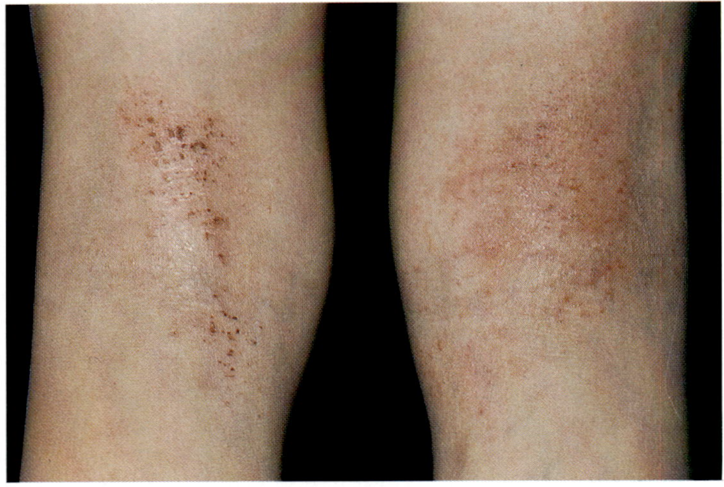

Figure 79 Atopic dermatitis. Characteristic location in the popliteal regions.

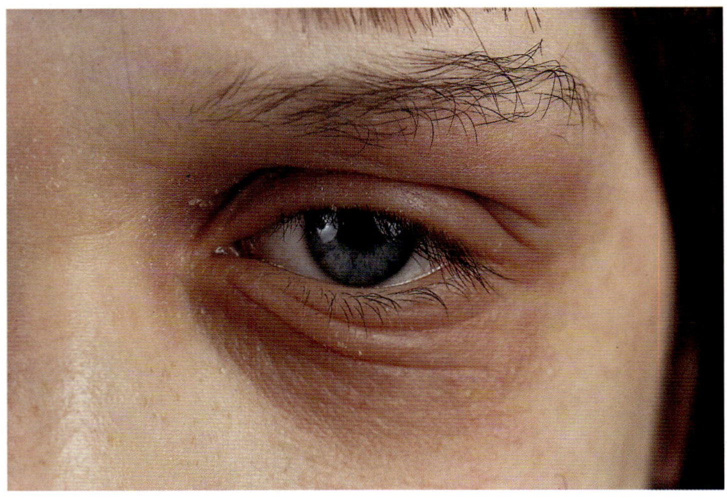

Figure 80 Atopic dermatitis. Chronic dermatitis of the eyelids with typical double folds on the lower lid.

Therapy

1. The most important measures are recognition and elimination of the causes. Housewives should wear vinyl gloves with cotton gloves underneath whenever working with water or strong irritants (floor and household cleaners).
2. Topical therapy consists of applying ointments containing corticosteroids **(R. 38)**, urea **(R. 39b)**, or tar substances **(R. 39c)**. Occlusive dressings should not be used.
3. Skin-protective ointments can be used prophylactively (e.g., ointments with acid pH).
4. Experience shows that therapy is more successful if the patient gets enough sleep.
5. Systemic treatment is usually superfluous.

D. Atopic Dermatitis (Atopic Eczema; Disseminated Neurodermitis)

This skin disease is part of the atopic syndrome that also includes such disorders as bronchial asthma, allergic rhinitis, and occasionally food allergies. Atopic dermatitis is a genetically fixed disease, which means that the skin disorder or the disposition for it can be present to varying degrees during the patient's entire lifetime. The patient remains afflicted with atopic dermatitis whether skin changes are present or not. There are typical symptoms for certain age groups, such as crusta lactea in infants, flexural eczema and other eczematous lesions in childhood and finally prurigo in adults. Itching as well as the other symptoms can be present to varying degrees, occasionally in an abortive stage. Pruritus, however, is generally the most agonizing symptom of the disease. Scratching aggravates the eczema and plays an important role in the development and continuation of chronic eczematous skin changes. Frequently, the asthma worsens as the skin disorder improves and vice versa. The skin changes often disappear in childhood, during puberty or adolescence, and never recur, but in many patients the eczema persists in adulthood. Atopic dermatitis, however, is rare in elderly patients. The point at which symptoms will finally disappear can not be predicted for individual patients.
Laboratory tests often show eosinophilia and elevated total IgE, as well as an increase of allergen-specific IgE antibodies that can be demonstrated by RAST. Nevertheless, diagnosis is determined by the symptomatology and the history, not by laboratory tests. Since cell-mediated immunity is disturbed in patients with atopic dermatitis, bacterial, mycotic and viral skin infections are more frequent for them than in the general population, especially pyodermas such as impetigo. The immune disorder of these patients is particularly significant for infections with the herpes simplex virus, which can lead to a life-threatening condition, the eczema herpeticum (see page 75).

Clinical Features

1. Infantile eczema (cradle cap) is characterized by fine yellowish scales and dry skin on the scalp and face. The condition begins in the first few months of life, usually at the beginning of the third month.
2. In children, the eczema typically involves the flexor regions, such as the antecubital area, the popliteal space and the flexor surfaces of the feet.
   In these areas, the eczematous lesions develop with the clinical signs of chronic eczema (thickening of the skin, coarse skin markings, brownish post-inflammatory pigmentation), frequently together with the symptoms of an acute dermatitis (erythema, papules, weeping areas). Linear erosions and crusting from scratching are seen very often.
3. Other eczematous lesions can be found as patches or spots, occasionally as nummular lesions, on the sides of the face, the neck, the trunk and the extremities.
4. An important feature of atopic dermatitis, especially with regard to the patient's occupation, is an eczema of the hands, usually manifest as erythema, thickening of the skin and scaling. Occasionally, vesicular palmar eczema (pompholyx) of the skin is also present (see page 45).
   In these areas, the skin is usually more sensitive to chemical, as well as mechanical irritations, the eczema worsens, or another eczematous attack occurs. Patients with atopic dermatitis should be counselled to avoid certain occupations, in particular those as bakers, furriers, hair dressers, restaurant personnel, cleaning occupations, health care, as well as the automobile and building industry.

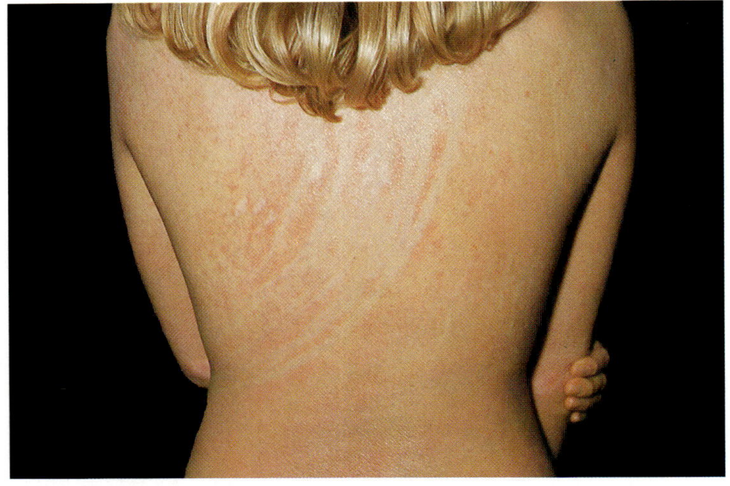

Figure 81 Atopic dermatitis. White dermatographism after scratching. Circumscribed vasoconstriction following linear pressure on the skin.

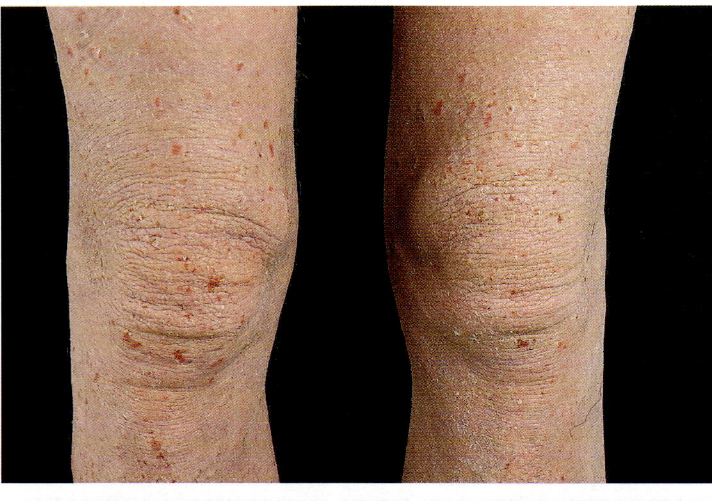

Figure 82 Atopic dermatitis. Long-standing eczema with distinct thickening of the skin (lichenification).

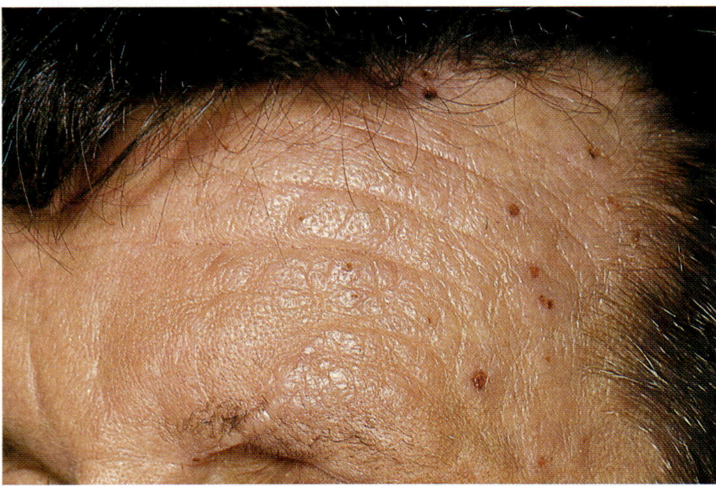

Figure 83 Atopic dermatitis. Thickening of the skin with distinct lichenification (coarser skin markings) and erosions. The lateral parts of the eyebrows are thinned out (Hertoghe's sign).

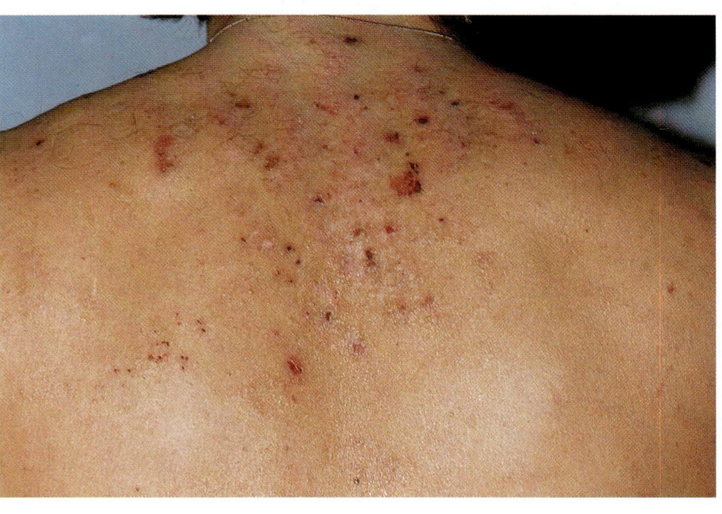

Figure 84 Atopic dermatitis. Prurigo-like in typical hood-shaped arrangement. The nodules have been scratched open. Areas of depigmentation and hyperpigmentation.

5. In adolescents and especially in adults, the disease can develop into prurigo which can completely replace the eczematous lesions (see page 125).
6. Other diagnostic signs of atopic dermatitis are: Herthoge's sign (the lateral aspects of the eyebrows are thinned or absent), wrinkles beneath the lower lid with chronic eczematous changes, and a fur cap-shape of the hair with a low hairline. There is usually "white dermatographism": After strong linear pressure, the initial redness does not persist for a longer period of time, as in healthy individuals, but is replaced by a reflex whiteness after a few seconds.
7. Patients with atopic dermatitis almost always suffer from dry skin that is worse during the winter months.
8. Pruritus is practically always present and can be very annoying. This leads to constant scratching, even during sleep. The patient sleeps poorly and is tired during the day, which further aggravates the itching. Patients with atopic dermatitis cannot tolerate wool, as it causes severe itching.
9. Emotional factors can play an important role. Emotional trauma in childhood can be secondary to the eczema, but may also be due to rejection – many times unconscious – or lack of affection.

Therapy

Since most patients with atopic dermatitis suffer considerably from their skin changes and especially the pruritus, they cooperate well with therapy, as do the parents of the affected children.

General

1. Vacation at the sea or in the mountains usually results in significant but temporary improvement.
2. Breast feeding appears to lessen manifestation of the disease in patients with a disposition to infantile eczema, and we recommend that all infants with a familial tendency to atopic dermatitis (in fact, all infants in general) be breastfed whenever possible for at least 6 months. The commonly recommended diets (buttermilk, sauerkraut and many others) have no effect on the eczema. In some patients, citrus fruits can cause an exacerbation of the disease and should be avoided. The causative role of food allergens has not been proven, contrary to many claims in the literature. The consumption of cow's milk, eggs, tyramine or other food substances rarely leads to an exacerbation of the skin symptoms, but if so, they should be avoided by the affected patients.

Internal

Systemic drug therapy is not without problems, as it must be continued over a long period of time, which requires increased attention to side effects and addiction.

1. Severe pruritus may require the use of antihistamines **(R. 61, 62)**. Antihistamines with a sedative component may be preferable, because they enable the patients, even children, to get a good night's sleep. However, overlapping effects may reduce the patient's functional effectiveness during the day. Long-term use may produce tachyphylaxis; this may reduce the effectiveness of the drug and make higher and higher doses necessary.
2. Systemic corticosteroids should be avoided, if possible. They usually produce prompt improvement, but symptoms recur when the drug is discontinued, and long-term use is not recommended.

External

1. It is important from a therapeutic as well as from a prophylactic point of view to treat the dry skin with regular applications of a water-based ointment without any active ingredients **(R. 33)**. Creams usually do not moisturize sufficiently. Fatty externa should not be applied too thickly, otherwise they can aggravate the skin condition. Urea-containing ointments **(R. 42b)** are useful for treating discrete acute or chronic eczematous lesions that do not require steroids.
2. For acute eczematous lesions, wet dressings are helpful, or corticosteroid lotions (emulsion type) or cremes can be used for several days.
3. For chronic eczemas, interval therapy (see page 245) with corticosteroid-containing ointments **(R. 38)** and additional tar preparations **(R. 39d, e)** is appropriate. In children, only weak corticosteroids should be used topically **(R. 38a)**.

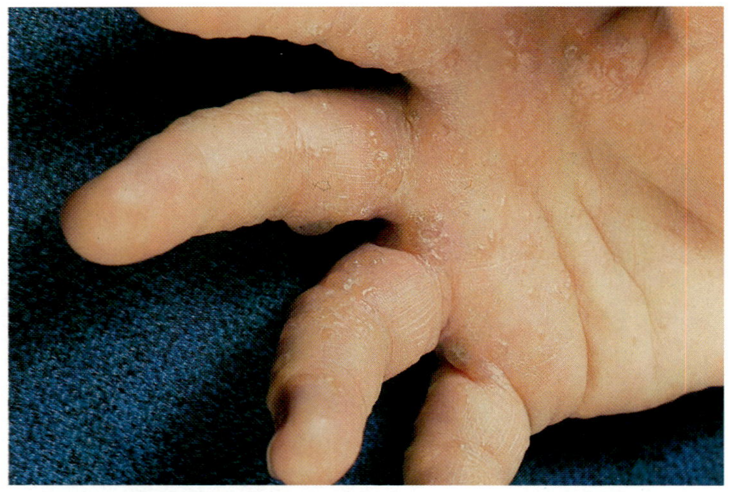

Figure 85 Vesicular palmoplantar eczema (pompholyx). Vesicle formation mainly on the sides of the fingers and on the palm of the hand.

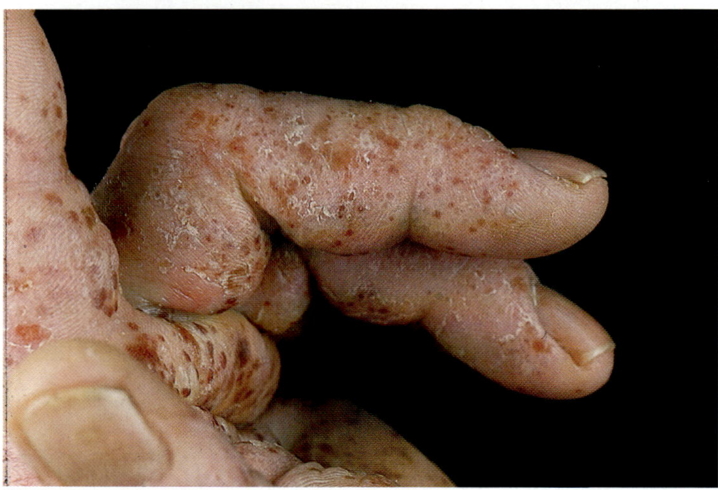

Figure 86 Vesicular palmoplantar eczema (pompholyx). Acute crop of vesicles with hemorrhage into the vesicles.

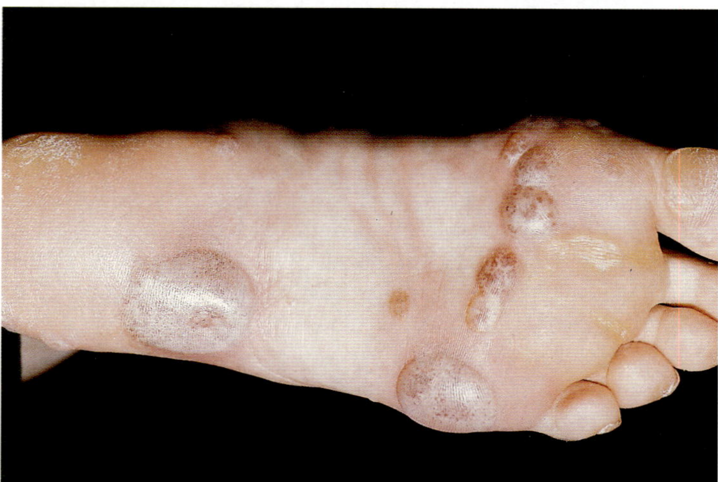

Figure 87 Vesicular palmoplantar eczema (pompholyx). Large blisters on the sole of the foot. This stage is very painful.

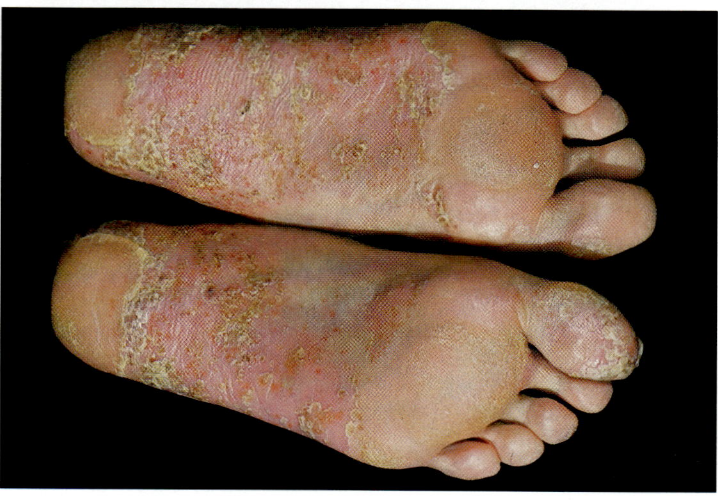

Figure 88 Vesicular palmoplantar eczema (pompholyx). Formation of vesicles, erythema and scaling, especially in the middle of the sole of the foot.

4. A full bath with the addition of bath oil or bath oil with a tar preparation is suitable every day or every other day. To avoid desiccation of the skin, a fatty cream or ointment should be massaged into the moist skin immediately after the bath (**R. 33**).
5. For adolescents and adults, a sauna bath two or three times weekly is often beneficial.
6. Sunbathing or artificial UV-radiation produce significant improvement in many, if not all patients.
7. Relaxation techniques, such as autogenous training, are helpful for many patients. Situations and moods that may — subconsciously — lead to increased scratching should be avoided. Recognition of such situations and appropriate behavioral training can be very useful in the treatment of atopic dermatitis.

E. Vesicular Palmoplantar Eczema (Pompholyx)

This disease is characterized by recurrent vesicular eruptions on the sides of the fingers and toes as well as the palmar and plantar surfaces. The cause of the disease remains obscure in most cases. Hot weather and high humidity can provoke new attacks of vesicular palmoplantar eczema. In some patients, the symptoms are part of atopic eczema; in others, it is due to a contact allergy or a chronic allergic contact eczema (see page 39). Vesicular palmoplantar eczema can occur acutely with an exacerbation of a stasis eczema of the lower legs or as an accompanying symptom of a dermatophytic infection. Mechanical stress and work in a damp environment can increase the symptoms. Especially in adults, vesicular palmoplantar eczema can often develop into "chronic hyperkeratotic eczema of the palms and soles of the feet" (see page 47) and may then be difficult to differentiate from psoriasis.

Clinical Features

1. The disorder is characterized by the sudden appearance of severely itchy papules that rapidly change into small blisters. The vesicles can heal with desquamation. Occasionally, bullae form that can be very firm and painful, especially under the thick horn layer of the palms and the soles of the feet. The lesions often develop into weeping, painful erosions.
2. The lesions are characteristically located on the sides of the fingers and toes, especially at the transition line between the keratotic skin of the palmar and plantar side and the thinner dorsal skin. The palm of the hand and the sole of the foot can be equally affected. Involvement is usually symmetric. Not infrequently, only the hands are affected.
3. Lymphangitis with painful swelling of the regional lymph nodes often complicates the disorder.
4. Hyperhidrosis is often an associated symptom.
5. Sometimes only one attack occurs, but there can also be frequent relapses. The disease can persist for several months or many years.

Therapy

At the present, there is no satisfactory treatment, especially for the chronic form of the disease.

1. Wet dressings (**R. 1**), also with disinfectant solutions (**R. 2**) and corticosteroid pastes (**R. 32b**) or creams (**R. 38b**) are indicated, especially if erosions predominate. Strongly lubricating ointments must be avoided, since the symptoms can thus be exacerbated, also if the lesions are covered by rubber gloves or rubber boots. In subacute or chronic conditions, a tar-containing solution can be brushed on (**R. 16**).
2. Hand baths, preferrably with tannic acid, are beneficial.
3. Systemic administration of antihistamines (**R. 61, 62**) may reduce the itching. An acute attack can be suppressed by systemic administration of corticosteroids, but the disease usually recurs when the medication is discontinued. Therefore, steroids should be reserved for very severe conditions.
4. Photochemotherapy (PUVA) can be successful in the treatment of persistent disease with a chronic course. The patient should be referred to a dermatologist who has experience with this treatment modality.
5. Rubber or vinyl gloves should be used for work with water (dishwashing, cleaning), or with strong irritants (floor or household cleaners). These should be worn over thin cotton gloves and not directly on the skin.

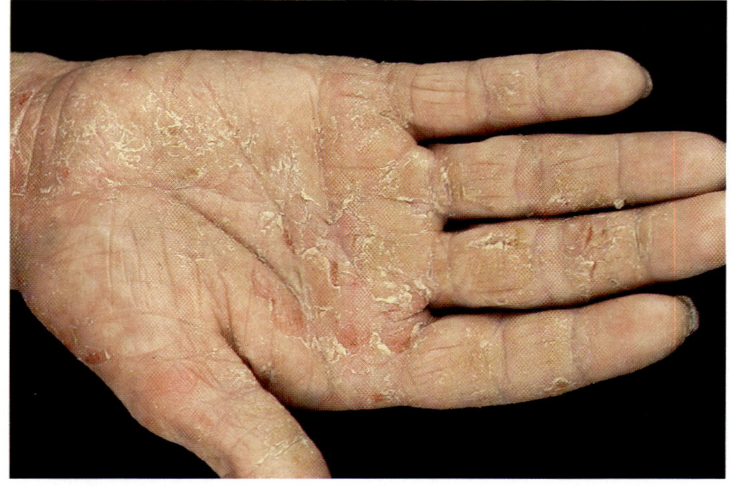

Figure 89 Chronic, hyperkeratotic eczema of the palm of the hand. Typical appearance with erosions, scaling, keratosis and rhagades.

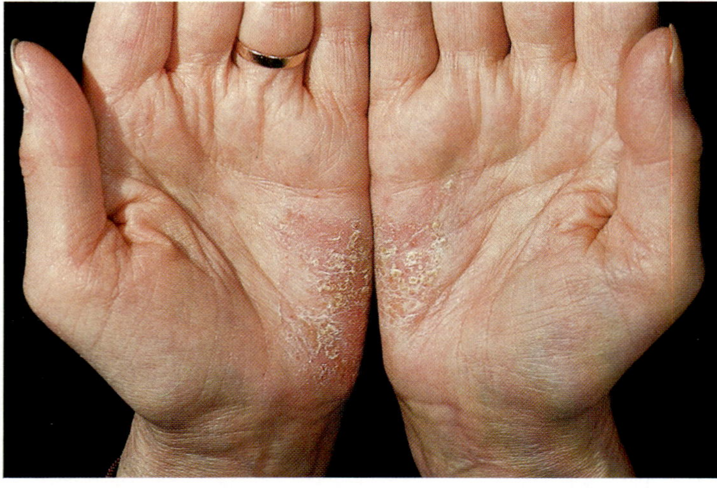

Figure 90 Chronic eczema of the palm. Early, mild form.

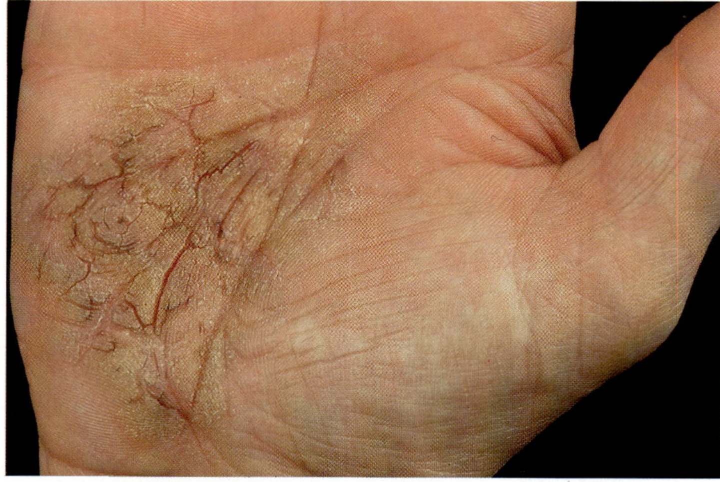

Figure 91 Chronic, hyperkeratotic eczema of the palm of the hand. Hyperkeratotic lesion with deep rhaghades.

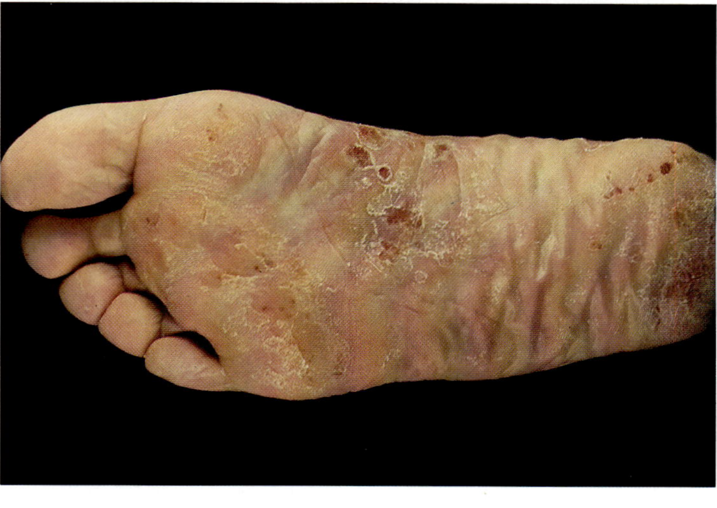

Figure 92 Chronic, hyperkeratotic eczema of the hands and feet. Erosions, scaling and increased keratinization of the sole of the right foot.

F. Chronic, Hyperkeratotic Eczema of the Palms and the Soles

This common disorder affects mainly middle-aged men and is characterized by inflammatory keratosis of the palms of the hands and the soles of the feet. The condition can persist for many months or years and can be a significant handicap for persons who perform manual labor. Not infrequently, the disease begins with a recurrent vesicular palmoplantar eczema which then develops into chronic, hyperkeratotic eczema of the palms and the soles. The course of the disease can extend over many years, and relapses are common. In most cases, no cause can be found, but in some cases, the symptoms can be due to a mycosis, a contact allergy or an atopic dermatitis. Mechanical stress, such as from digging with a spade, and exposure to organic solvents increase the symptoms, but they do not cause the disease. Secondary contact sensitization occurs frequently in long-standing cases, especially for nickel and other metallic ions; this is usually not important for causation or maintenance of this form of eczema. Mechanically stressful work often results in long-standing disability, for example, for lumberjacks.

Clinical Features

1. Extensive keratosis of the central or the entire skin of the palms and the soles of the feet is typical for the disease. Inflammatory changes such as erythema, groups of vesicles, erosions and crusts predominate in some cases but can be absent in others. Deep and and painful rhagades are often present and are caused by stretching of the thick and inelastic skin.
2. The disease involves mainly the palms of the hands and the soles of the feet. Dissemination to distant areas of the skin is rare but can occur in patients with acute eczematization.
3. Itching and pain are present to varying degrees but can be completely absent in the "dry forms" of the disease. Sensation and motor function of the hands and fingers can be disturbed to varying degrees, depending on the extent of hyperkeratosis.
4. The disease runs a protracted course over many months or years. Acute flare-ups with vesicles, etc., recur frequently without a recognizable cause.

Therapy

Treatment is a difficult and thankless task. It is typical for this disease that patients change their physicians frequently. The goals of treatment are prevention of flare-ups of the disease and symptomatic improvement of the eczema. Symptomatic treatment is guided by the existing skin changes.

1. Mechanical pressure must be avoided (the patient may have to take sick days).
2. The most important local treatment, if only hyperkeratosis is present, is frequent application of fatty and water-based ointments **(R. 33b)**. If this is inadequate, ointments containing corticosteroids in combination with salicylic acid or urea **(R. 39b)** can be tried. Tar substances such as coal tar may be useful, especially for chronic cases.
3. Another possibility is the temporary use of a so-called triple therapy (a steroid solution, a strong corticosteroid ointment covered by an occlusive dressing, e.g., polyvinyl gloves).
4. Systemic treatment is usually not necessary. Severe flare-ups may require systemic corticosteroids **(R. 63)** in decreasing doses for a few days.

G. Diaper Dermatitis, Diaper Rash

Clinical Features

Diaper dermatitis develops in the areas in contact with the diaper due to skin irritation from decomposition products of urine and feces, especially in infants with diarrhea or as a result of poor care and in children whose diapers are not changed often enough. Candida infection is superimposed almost always on long-standing cases of diaper dermatitis.

1. Erythema, nodules and occasionally weeping surfaces are characteristic clinical findings.
2. The symptoms originate in the anal and genital regions. Initially, they are limited to areas in contact with the diaper. With severe involvement and in cases secondarily infected with candida, the lesions can spread to other areas of the skin (satellite lesions).
3. In long-standing cases, nodules or firm prurigo-like nodes predominate.
4. General well-being is usually impaired very little, if at all.

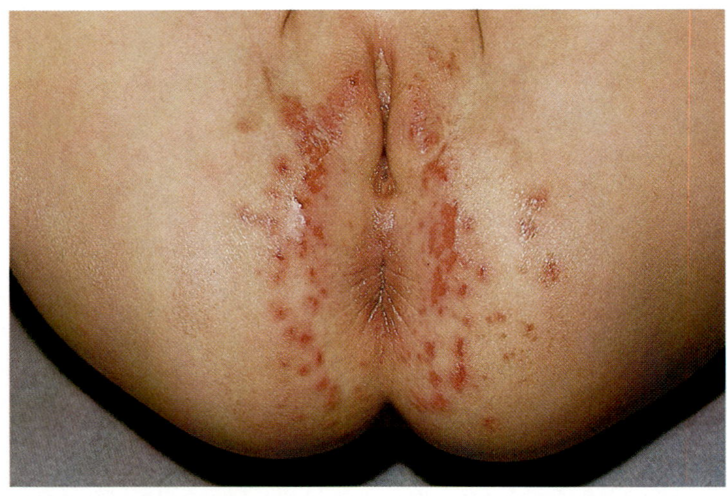

Figure 93 Diaper dermatitis. Erosive nodules in the perianal area.

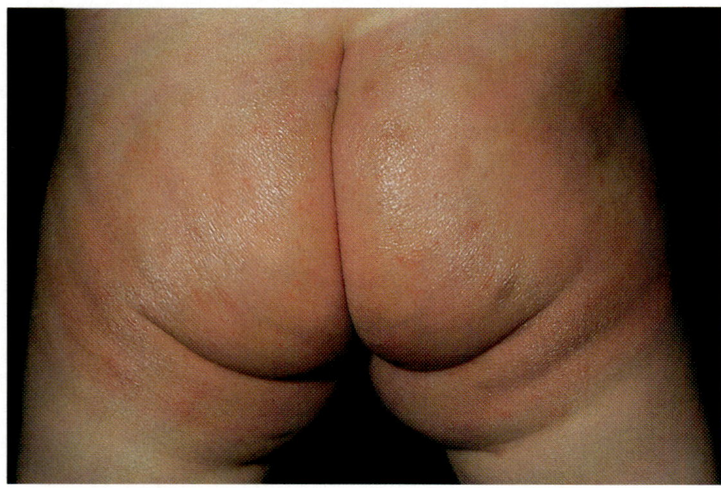

Figure 94 Diaper dermatitis. Erythema and mild scaling, as well as symmetrical papules in the gluteal area.

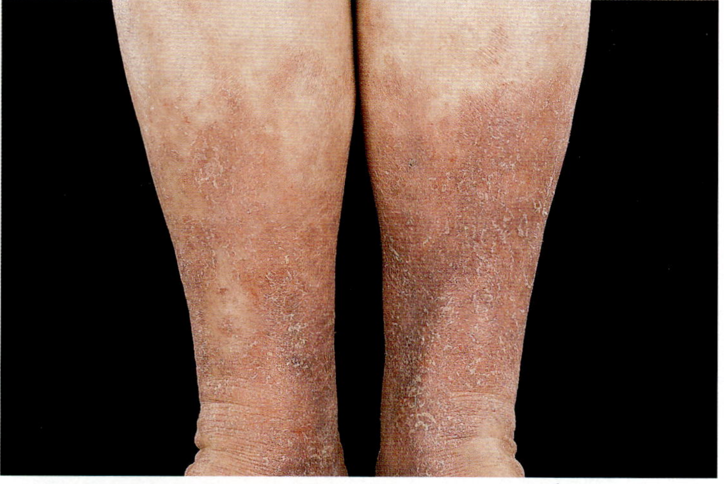

Figure 95 Stasis dermatitis in a patient with chronic venous insufficiency. Erythema, brownish discoloration and scaling on the lower leg.

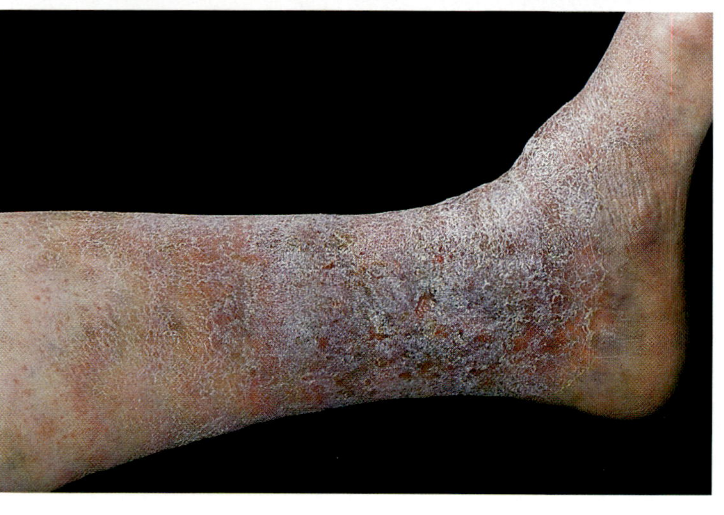

Figure 96 Stasis dermatitis in a patient with chronic venous insufficiency. Considerable scaling, brownish discoloration and erosion on the lower leg and the dorsum of the foot, most pronounced in the malleolar area.

Therapy

1. The involved region must be kept dry, and diapers should be changed frequently. Diapers should be left off for several hours during the day. Absorbent diapers must be used; plastic pants should be avoided.
2. All urine and stool remnants should be removed carefully with oil or baths. After the bath the baby must be dried and powdered well.
3. Nystatin-containing pastes are effective **(R. 31)**.
4. Diarrhea must be treated; sugar and fresh sour fruits must be avoided until the dermatitis is healed; bananas can be given instead. Intestinal candida infection must be treated (reservoir of organisms) (see page 117).

H. Stasis Eczema, Stasis Dermatitis

Acute or chronic eczemas of the lower legs can be found in patients with chronic venous insufficiency. Other symptoms, such as varices, pigmentation, dermatosclerosis, etc., are usually present as well (see page 29–31).

Clinical Features

1. Erythema, nodules, scaling, sometimes with weeping and crust formation, are characteristic of stasis eczema.
2. Large bullae can be found in areas with excessive and rapidly developing edema ("tension blisters", which are also found in patients with cardiac edema).
3. The distal parts of the lower legs, the ankle region, and occasionally the dorsum of the foot are characteristic locations; eventually, the entire lower leg can be involved.
4. Bilateral involvement is seen frequently.

Therapy

1. The most important goal is elimination of the underlying edema by compression with elastic bandages or with rubber stockings (see page 262) and intermittent elevation of the involved extremity. This can be supplemented initially with a mild diuretic and other phlebologic measures (see page 33).
2. Topical therapy consists of moist dressings (3 times daily for 20 minutes) and steroid creams or pastes **(R. 32b; 38b)** to ease itching and reduce other symptoms.
3. Other additives, except corticosteroids, should not be used for topical therapy to avoid the common secondary contact sensitization against substances such as local antibiotics. In particular, local disinfectants and antibiotics are not necessary for the treatment of stasis eczema.

I. Seborrheic Dermatitis

Seborrheic dermatitis occurs frequently and can be found in several typical locations and subvarieties. It is seen mainly in areas with increased activity of the sebaceous glands, especially the scalp, face and chest, less frequently in the axillae and the pubic region. In children, seborrheic dermatitis occurs only until the fourth month of life, probably as a result of maternal hormones. Adults with light skin are afflicted more often. Recurrences are frequent, despite good response to therapy. The cause of seborrheic dermatitis is still unknown. A significant causative role is ascribed to the lipophilic yeast *Pityrosporum ovale*. The incidence of seborrheic dermatitis is approximately 2–5% of the normal population. In patients with AIDS the incidence is much higher, approximately 40–80%.

Clinical Features

1. *Scalp:*
   There is increased desquamation (a few scales are normal). There is itching and occasionally moderate erythema in individual patches or affecting the entire scalp. About 1 cm of the forehead can sometimes be involved too, creating a visible band of eczema below the hairline. There can be extreme itching. Scratching produces erosions and crusts only when there is significant involvement. Physical exertion and emotional stress increase the symptoms.

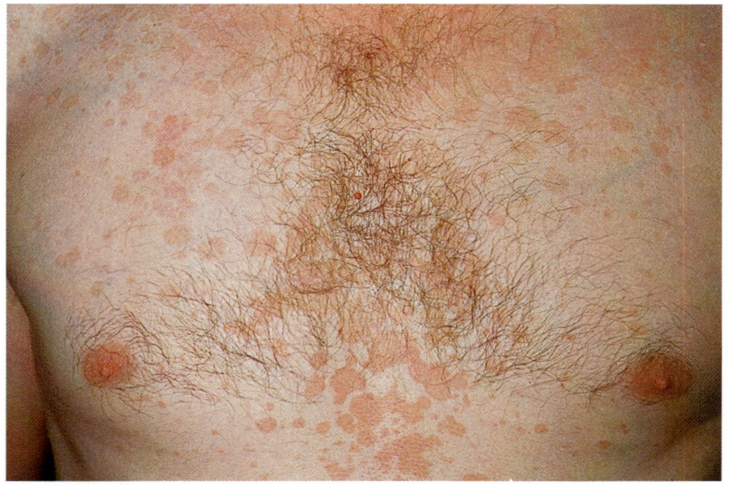

Figure 97 Seborrheic dermatitis. Yellowish-brown, sharply delineated, round lesions with minimal scaling in the middle of the chest.

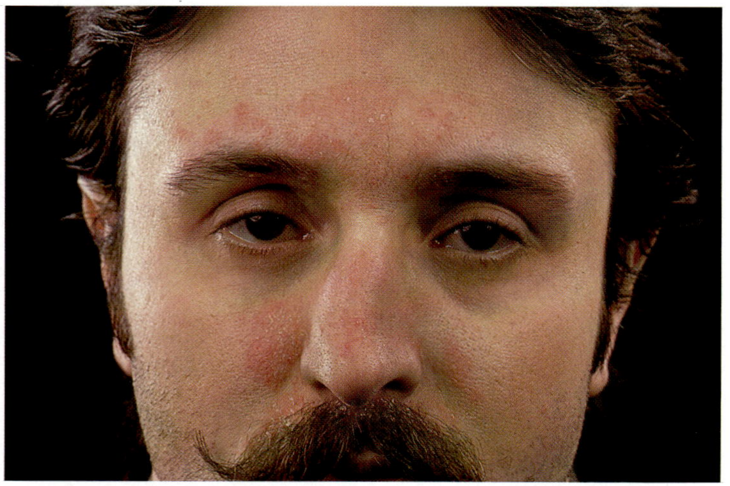

Figure 98 Seborrheic dermatitis. Erythema and scaling in the moustache and nasolabial area, the eyebrows and the mid-forehead.

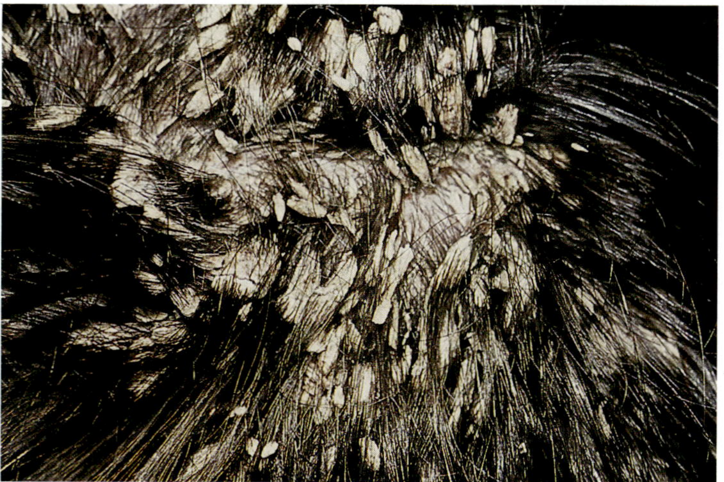

Figure 99 This sheath-like coating of the hairs can occur in patients with squamous diseases of the scalp, particularly in seborrheic dermatitis. So-called "tinea amiantacea".

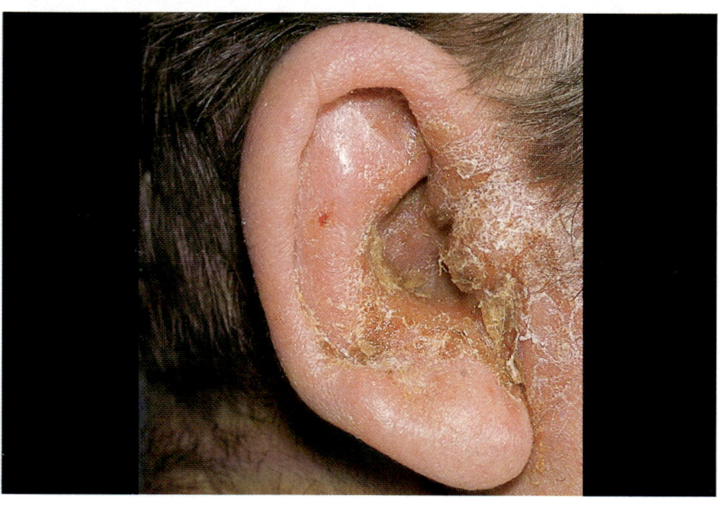

Figure 100 Bacterial ear eczema. Chronic, recurrent eczema of the auditory canal and the auricle with weeping and crust formation. Marked concomitant edema of the auricle.

2. *Face:*
   There are bands of affected skin in and between the eyebrows, in the nasolabial folds and in the vicinity of the eyelashes. The bearded area can also be involved. In other parts of the face, and in and behind the ear, one occasionally finds erythema and desquamation with usually minimal itching.

3. *Middle of the Chest:*
   The chest can be involved with a few light brown or yellowish-red, sharply delineated, slightly scaling patches without a raised margin. Itching is usually absent. The lesions do not cause any subjective discomfort.

Therapy

1. The scalp should be washed with antiseborrheic shampoo (**R. 10**) two to three times a week. The shampoo should contain pyrithione zinc, ketonazole or clotrimazole and should be allowed to take effect for several minutes. Other shampoos are also effective for treatment of scaling. For marked erythematous changes, corticosteroid tinctures should be used (**R. 18**). The hair is parted every 1 to 2 centimeters, and one drop should be applied every 3 to 4 centimeters. If these measures are unsuccessful, application of Keralyt scalp ointment may be indicated. The ointment should be washed out with shampoo the next morning.
2. Lesions of the face and chest can be treated locally with imidazole cream (**R. 35**), also just for periods of minutes. Another possibility is steroid preparations, especially creams (**R. 38a**) for several days until the lesions are healed. Patients with seborrheic dermatitis rarely tolerate ointments with a fatty base, except on the scalp. *Caution*: No long-term topical corticosteroid therapy of the face! This can cause erythema, atrophy and rosacea-like symptoms (see page 139).

J. Bacterial Ear Eczema

This is a recurrent crusty ear eczema that apparently is caused by staphylococcus contamination of this area. Exacerbation by acute generalized disease or ear diseases is typical for this condition. Manipulation of the ear often plays a causative or supplemental role.

Clinical Features

1. Scaling and occasionally erythema of the external auditory canal are often the only symptoms. In more severe cases, weeping, crusts and erosions develop. The external ear shows edematous swelling. Both ears are usually involved to varying degrees.
2. Pruritus is often agonizing.

Therapy

1. Local treatment consists of application of corticosteroid creams in combination with disinfectants (**R. 39a**), and wet dressings (**R. 1**). Corticosteroid-containing ear drops are useful for treatment of the deeper parts of the auditory canal.
2. Otologic consultation may be indicated for removal of crusts and cerumen, as well as exclusion of otitis media.

K. Nummular Eczema

This condition is characterized by coin-shaped or plaque-shaped eczematous lesions that persist for long periods of time and are resistant to treatment. We distinguish a so-called "idiopathic" nummular eczema without detectable cause from nummular eczematous lesions of other eczemas, such as atopic dermatitis and allergic chromate eczema. Nummular eczema in children is practically always a symptom of atopic dermatitis. The cause of "idiopathic" nummular eczema is still unclear. Microbial involvement has been postulated, but has not been confirmed. Frequently, the patients suffer from generalized dryness of the skin. Nummular eczema usually affects middle-aged or older men.

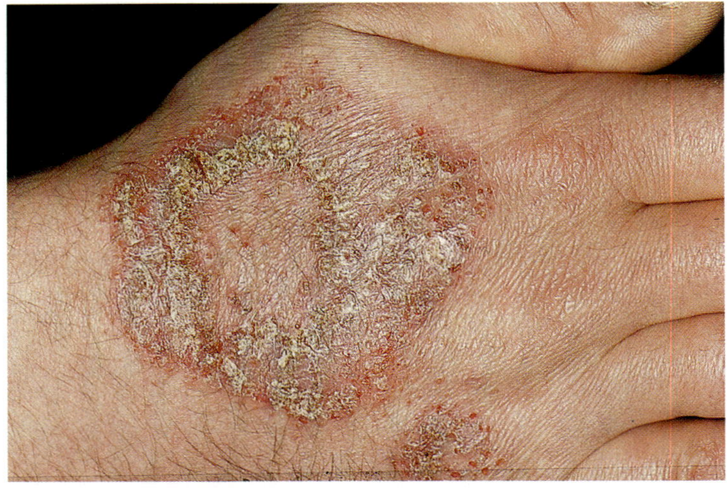

Figure 101 Nummular eczema. Round, sharply delineated, distinctly scaling, crusty, eczematous lesions on the dorsum of the hand.

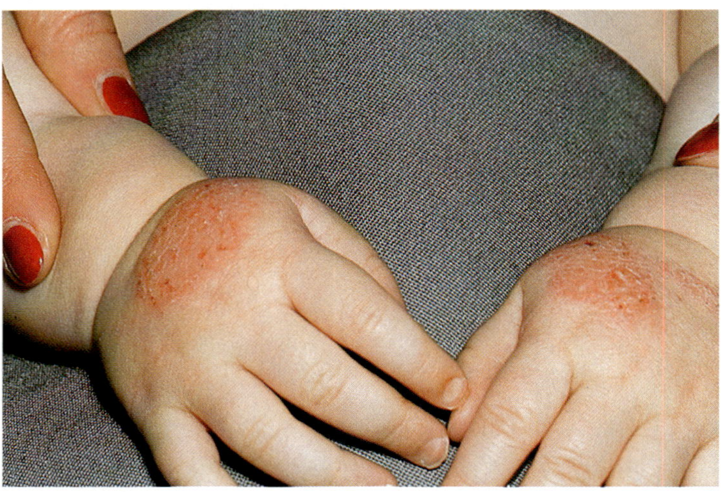

Figure 102 Nummular eczematous lesions in a child with atopic dermatitis. Symmetric appearance of round eczematous lesions on the dorsum of the hand.

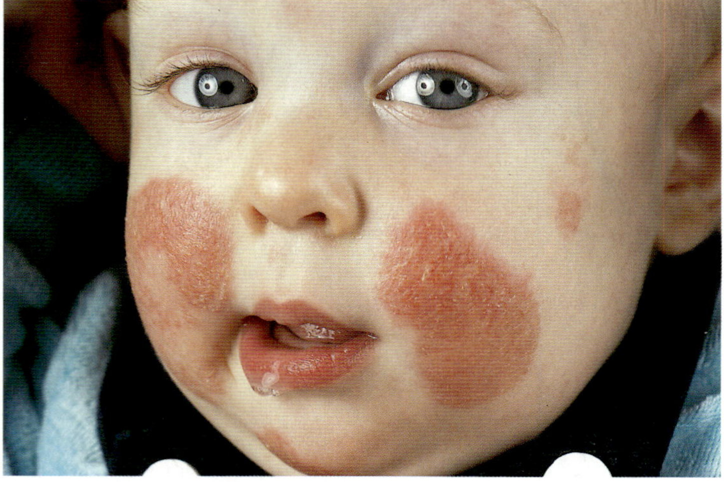

Figure 103 Nummular eczema. Round lesions on the cheeks.

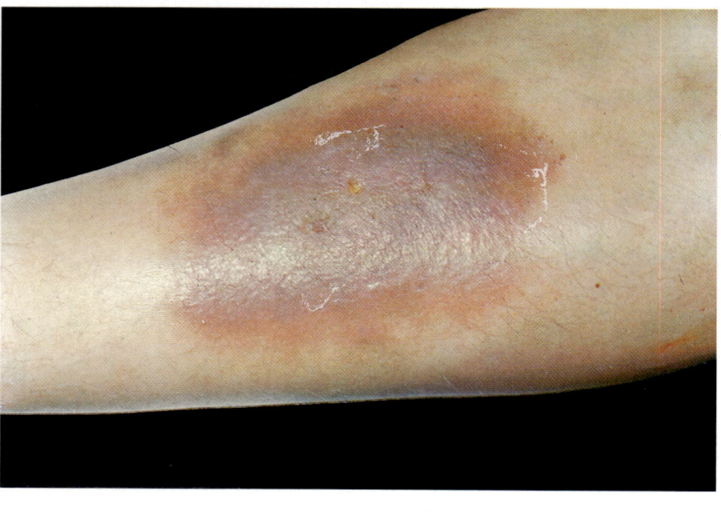

Figure 104 Lichen simplex chronicus. Isolated area of chronic lichenified eczema surrounded by brownish discoloration on the left lower leg.

Clinical Features

1. The lesions consist of coin-shaped foci of varying sizes that are round, sharply delineated and scaling. They are often weeping or covered with crusts and have a raised margin.
2. The extremities and the trunk are mainly involved. There may be only a few lesions, rarely more than 10, 20 or more.
3. The lesions persist for several weeks or months, often despite intensive topical treatment.
4. There is moderate to severe itching.
5. The skin is often dry, a condition often aggravated by frequent washing and bathing and by low humidity in the air (winter, central heating).

Therapy

The prognosis depends on the type of eczema, whether the condition is part of an atopic dermatitis or a chromate eczema or whether it is an "idiopathic" nummular eczema that may be unexpectedly resistant to any therapy for a prolonged period of time.

1. The most important measure is topical treatment with steroid ointments **(R. 38b, c)**. Treatment should be started with a cream when weeping lesions are present. Occlusive dressings may be necessary to improve response to treatment.
2. Coal tar preparations **(R. 41a)** may be used to supplement this regime.
3. The dry skin may also require treatment (see page 149).

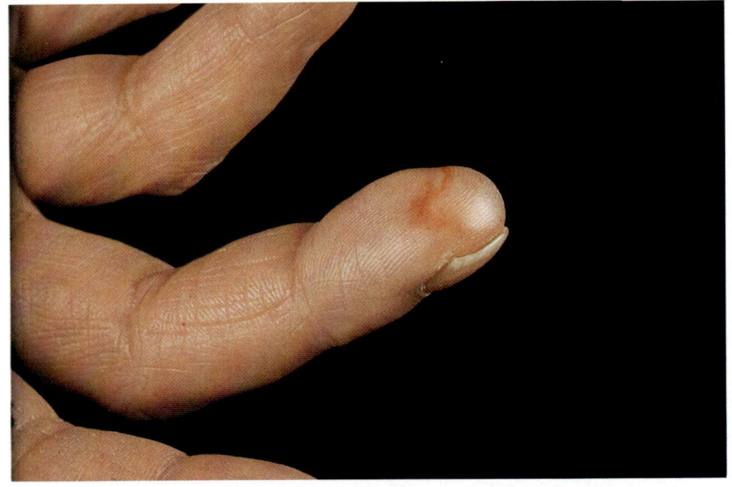

Figure 105 Second-degree frostbite. Bulla on the fingertip with surrounding erythema.

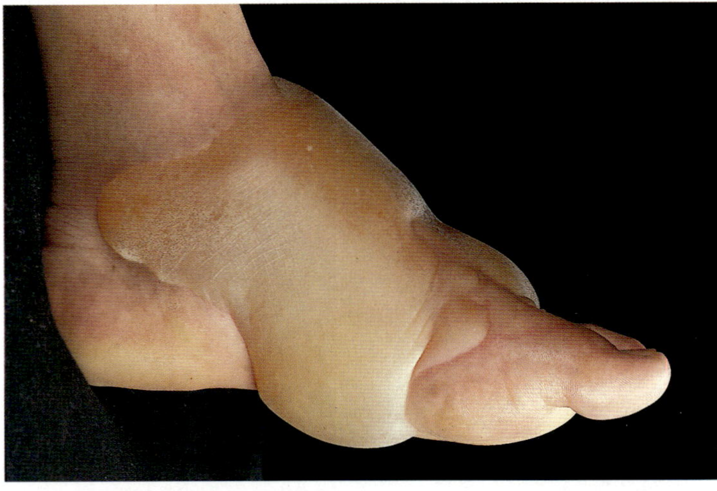

Figure 106 Second-degree frostbite. Monstrous bullae on the foot.

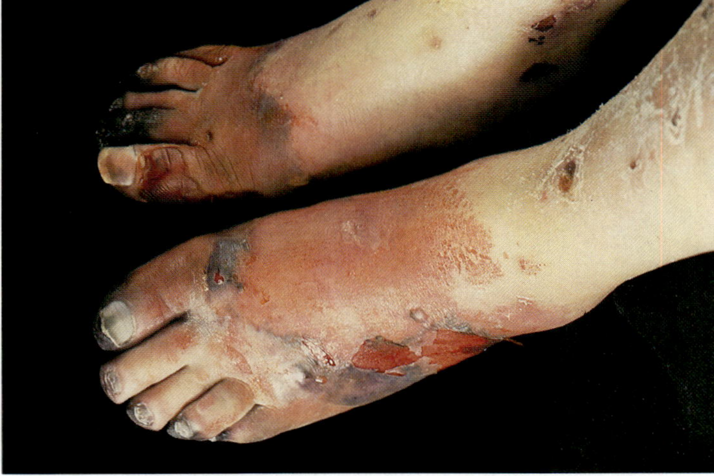

Figure 107 Third-degree frostbite. Erythema, formation of bullae, desquamation of the epidermis, and necrosis of the distal phalanges with mummification.

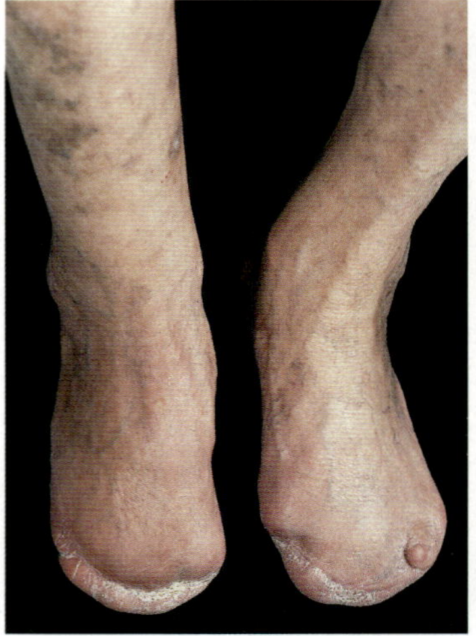

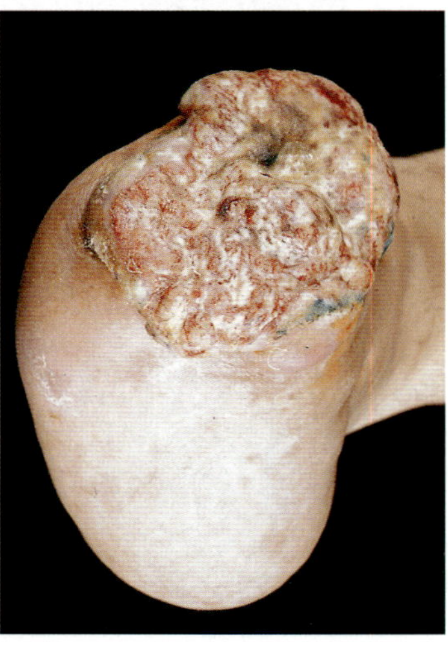

Figure 108 Sequelae of frostbite. Left foot: Loss of all toes. Right foot: Development of a squamous cell carcinoma 40 years later.

Frostbite

Frostbite is sudden, circumscribed tissue damage that occurs at temperatures below the freezing point and predominantly affects the acra. Nowadays, frostbite is seen most often from winter sports, not infrequently in conjunction with increased alcohol consumption. It can also occur during sudden cold spells in persons wearing inappropriate clothing (motorcyclists). Alcohol promotes frostbite by its anesthetic effect and by cooling the body through peripheral vascular dilatation. Various degrees of tissue damage, similar to those distinguished for burns, have been established. Pathogenetic factors include disturbed blood supply, direct injury to the cells from the cold, and possibly injury due to ice crystal formation in the tissues.

Clinical Features

First Degree Frostbite
During cold exposure, the skin of the involved areas is white and much colder than the surrounding skin. Following rewarming, edematous swelling occurs that often itches considerably. This swelling can increase initially due to the liberation of substances that mediate inflammation, but then it slowly disappears over a period of a several days without further sequelae.

Second Degree Frostbite
The skin is waxy and pale. After rewarming, subepidermal blisters appear similar to those seen in burns. These blisters are very painful and can occasionally be hemorrhagic.

Third Degree Frostbite
After third-degree frostbite, the damaged skin remains white following rewarming and sensation is absent. The necrotic area develops a blue-black color, and the hardened tissue is slowly demarcated from the surrounding healthy tissue. Development of wet gangrene with the risk of bacterial sepsis is a serious complication. It is often surprising that only a relatively small defect results after demarcation, despite extensive tissue damage initially. Pain and paresthesias in the affected areas can persist for many years and disable the patient. Development of a carcinoma in the scar of the frostbitten tissue is rare.

Therapy

1. It is important to rewarm the affected areas as soon as possible. Rewarming should be gradual, preferably in a bath of cold tap water that is heated slowly (in approximately $1^1/_2$ hours) to a maximum of 40 °C.
2. The patient should be given warm drinks (but no alcohol) to raise the body temperature, followed by rheologically active medication such as pentoxifylline. Tetanus prophylaxis is also important.
3. Patients who are severely undercooled must be transported carefully. Vasodilatory drugs should be administered with great caution. The sudden return of cold peripheral blood will lower the core temperature of the body even more, with the risk of respiratory and cardiac arrest and irreversible CNS damage.
4. Frostbite should be treated in an open and dry manner. Under no circumstances should wet dressings or ointments be used (danger of wet gangrene). Interdigital spaces are kept dry by insertion of small gauze strips. The involved skin is painted with disinfectant dyes **(R. 14, 17)** and powdered **(R. 12)**.
5. The tissue regenerates extremely well after frostbite, and surgical procedures such as excision of necroses and amputations should be delayed as long as possible. Patience is the most important therapeutic principle.

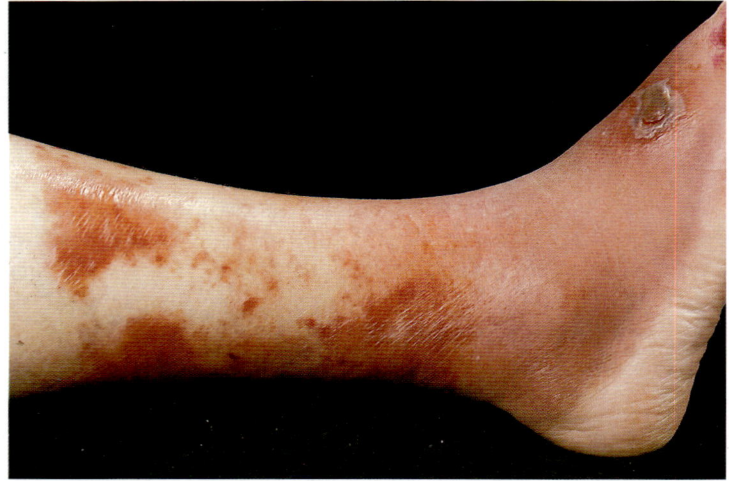

Figure 109 Erysipelas. Acute stage with erythema, edema and even blistering.

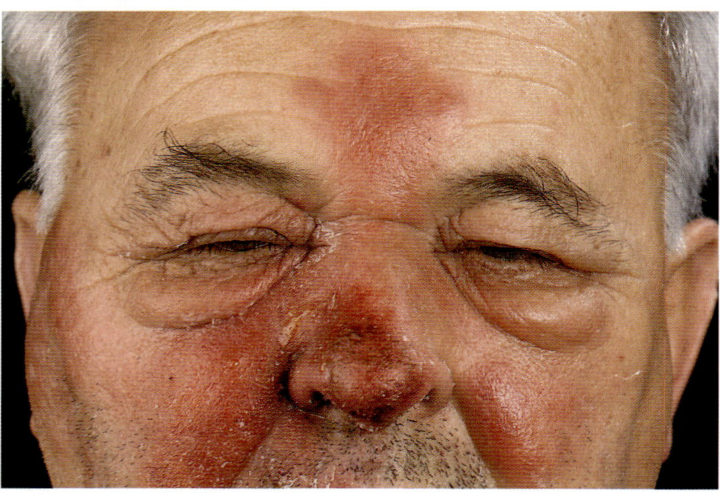

Figure 110 Erysipelas of the face. Sharply delineated erythema involving nose and cheeks.

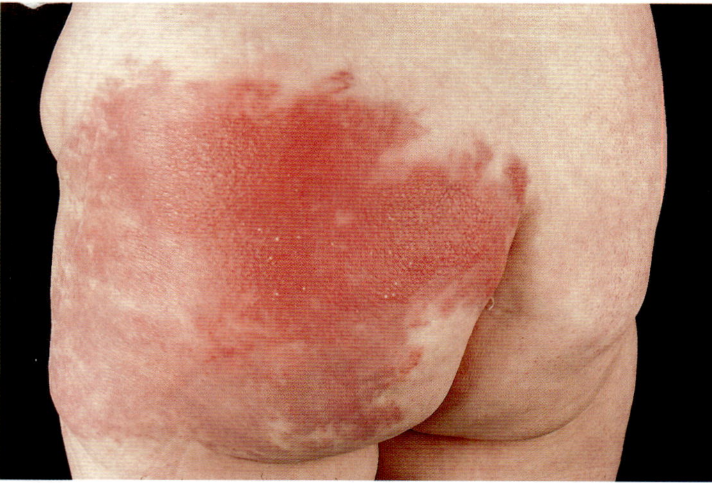

Figure 111 Erysipelas. Large erythematous area of the left gluteal region with spiked margins corresponding to the inflammation that advances along the lymph vessels.

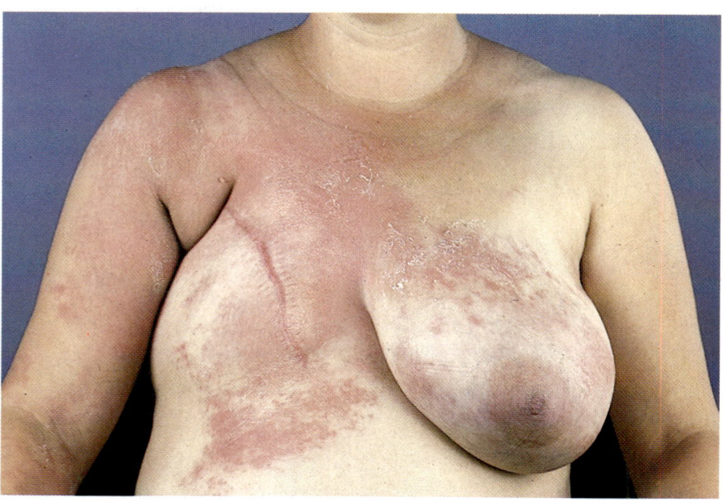

Figure 112 Erysipelas following mastectomy. Extensive involvement including the right arm, caused by postoperative lymphatic stasis.

Erysipelas

Erysipelas is a dermal streptococcal infection that progresses along the superficial lymphatics. The disease affects mainly older adults. Recurrent flare-ups with subsequent chronic persistent lymphedema are possible (see page 103). "Erysipelatoid" thrombophlebitis can produce similar symptoms but more frequently involves the lower legs without enlargement of the lymph nodes and without generalized symptoms, and the erythema stops below the knees, like knee socks. So-called necrotizing fasciitis can lead to extensive necroses of the skin and subcutaneous fatty tissue as a result of the erysipelas, depending on the pathogenicity of the microorganisms and the adequacy of blood supply (arterial occlusive disease, diabetes mellitus). The most severe and life-threatening form of necrotizing fasciitis occurs when the causative organisms spread subcutaneously along the fascia.

Clinical Features

1. The disease is characterized by intense redness with an acute onset. The erythema is irregular and has extensions like "fiery tongues" (along the lymph vessels).
2. The disorder is usually unilateral, but bilateral involvement is seen occasionally, especially in the face.
3. The lower legs and the face are affected most frequently.
4. Cutaneous symptoms are accompanied by chills, fever, and swelling of the regional lymph nodes.
5. Local complications are vesiculations, hemorrhagic infarction, ulceration and necrosis of the inflamed area. Severe sepsis is a rare complication.
6. Frequent recurrences can occasionally cause occlusion of the lymph vessels with subsequent edema that can be extremely severe in some cases (elephantiasis) (see page 103).
7. Necrotizing fasciitis with deep fascia involvement almost always appears as an increasing, localized edema of the skin, occasionally with tension blisters, in combination with the general symptoms of sepsis.

Therapy

Systemic antibiotic therapy is crucial, but general measures and topical therapy are also necessary.

General

1. Bedrest is the most important general therapeutic measure.
2. Elevation of the lower extremity, if it is affected, helps to reduce swelling and pain.

Systemic

1. Antibiotic therapy takes precedence. Penicillin is the drug of choice, either orally or, more effectively, by intramuscular injection, e.g., 1 ampule clemizole penicillin i.m. **(R. 47)** daily for 8 days. Erythromycin **(R. 51)** or quinolones **(R. 54)** can be used in patients with hypersensitivity to penicillin.
2. Analgesics such as acetylsalicylic acid or paracetamol are sometimes required.
3. Patients with recurrent erysipelas should receive long-term prophylaxis with penicillin G benzathine (Bicillin L-A), e.g., 1.2 to 2.4 million units i.m. once every 3 weeks for at least several months.
4. Necrotizing fasciitis with its life-threatening course requires immediate treatment with high doses of parenteral penicillin as well as early surgical intervention.

External

Local therapy depends on the severity of the dermatological findings. As long as only redness is present, local therapy can be omitted.

1. Wet dressings **(R. 1, 2)** are soothing and always helpful.
2. Antibiotic ointments are widely used, but their effectiveness is questionable.
3. Skin lesions, such as small wounds, rhagades, interdigital mycosis, or eczema of the ear can serve as entry sites for organisms and should be treated with appropriate local therapy to prevent recurrence.

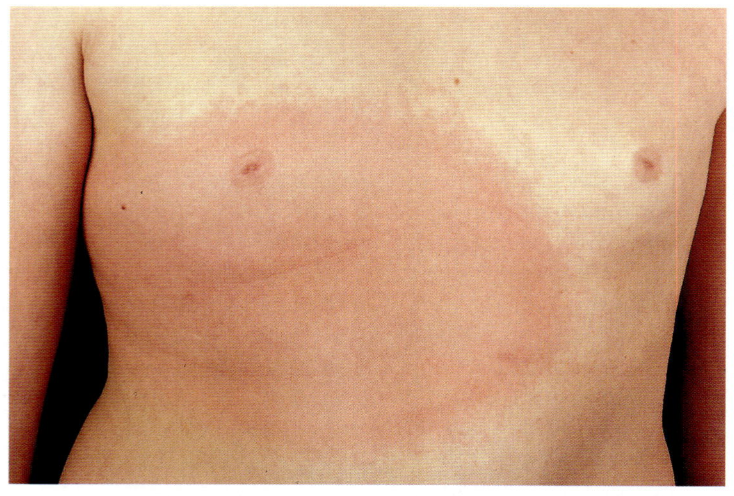

Figure 113 Erythema chronicum migrans. Round or polycyclical erythema with distinct margins.

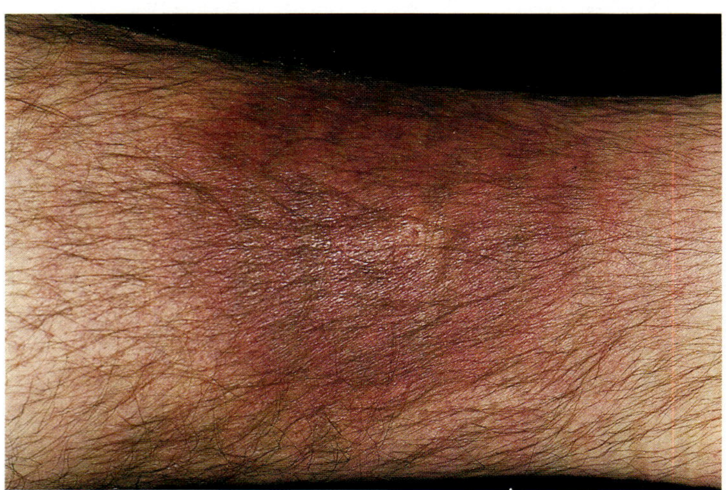

Figure 114 Hemorrhagic erythema chronicum migrans. Purpuric round erythema without distinct margins.

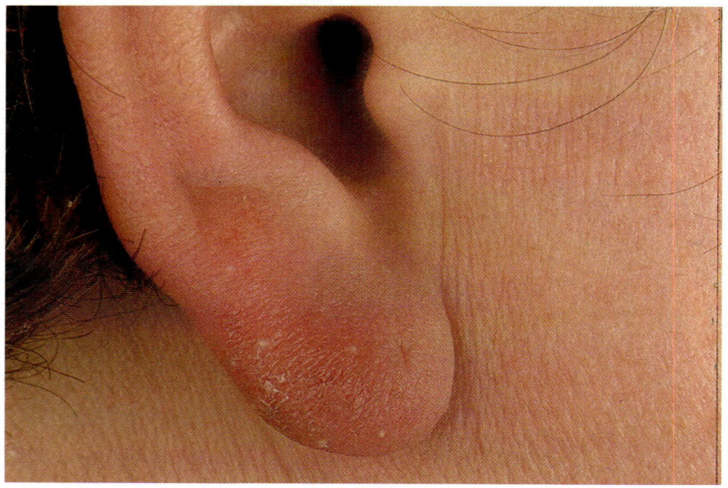

Figure 115 Lymphocytoma. Burgundy to bluish-red colored, tumor-like infiltrate of the right ear lobe.

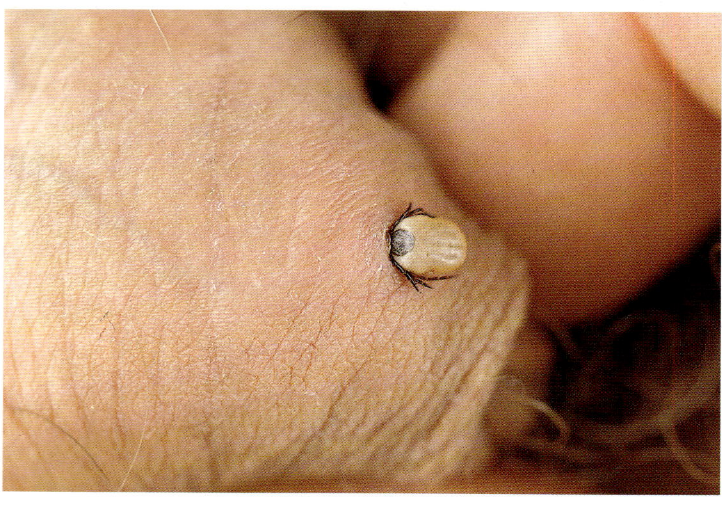

Figure 116 Tick, *Ixodes ricinus*, with enlarged abdomen from sucking blood.

Erythema Chronicum Migrans and Other Skin Disorders Transmitted by Ticks

Erythema chronicum migrans and acrodermatitis chronica atrophicans are superficial infectious diseases of the skin. They are caused by Borrelia burgdorferi and possibly other spirochetes, which are transmitted by ticks, in particular the species Ixodes ricinus. The ticks are acquired when the patient walks through woods and brush. Lymphocytoma is also often caused by Borrelia, but there can be other causes of the disease.

A. Erythema Chronicum Migrans

Clinical Features

1. Erythema chronicum migrans is a slowly expanding, circular erythema with an accentuated border. Hemorrhagic changes in the lesion can obliterate the accentuated margin.
2. The lesion expands slowly within several days or weeks. Multiple foci are rare.
3. Not only the areas of the body directly exposed to the ticks, such as the trunk and extremities, are involved, but also parts of the body covered by clothing, because the ticks can crawl underneath.
4. Erythema chronicum migrans can be one symptom of Lyme disease (Lyme borreliosis), which is characterized by mono- or polyarticular arthritis, especially of the large joints, and neurologic symptoms, such as meningitis, encephalitis, radicular neuritis, and occasionally cardiac involvement.

Therapy

Systemic antibiotic therapy is the most important part of treatment.

1. Under systemic antibiotic therapy with tetracyclines **(R. 49)** orally for 2 weeks, penicillin **(R. 47)** or erythromycin **(R. 51)**, the lesions rapidly disappear.
2. Local therapy is not necessary.

B. Acrodermatitis Chronica Atrophicans

This disease occurs much less frequently than erythema chronicum migrans, but is transmitted in the same manner. Clinical symptoms are different from those of erythema chronicum migrans.

Clinical Features

1. Clinical symptoms develop slowly over the course of months and include erythema and swelling of large areas of the skin, usually of an entire extremity.
2. The disease eventually leads to atrophy of the skin. The skin is thin and can be finely folded. Underlying blood vessels, especially veins, can be seen startlingly well through the skin.

Therapy

Treatment is the same as that for erythema chronicum migrans but must be given over a period of several weeks. The skin atrophy is permanent and cannot be altered by treatment.

C. Lymphocytoma

Clinical Features

1. This disease occurs as solitary or rarely, disseminated multiple, bluish-red, round or oval-shaped tumors up to 3 cm in size. It can also occur in the center of an erythema chronicum migrans at the site of the tick bite.
2. The most frequent localization is in the face, especially the ear lobe and the tip of the nose. Scrotum and mamillae are also often affected.
3. There are no subjective complaints.

Therapy

Treatment is the same as that for erythema chronicum migrans.

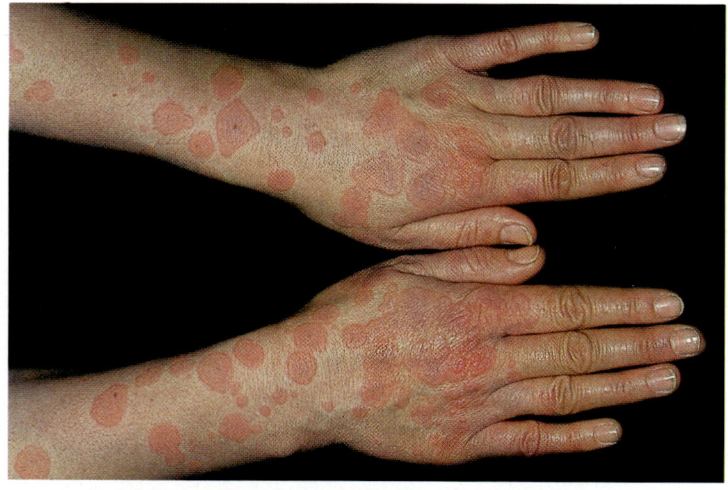

Figure 117 Erythema multiforme. Typical raised erythematous, nummular lesions with central dusky discoloration caused by stasis. Typical location.

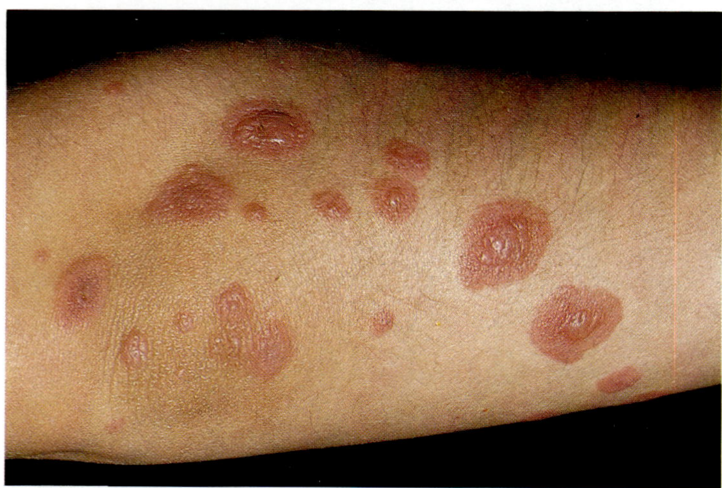

Figure 118 Erythema multiforme. Blister formation in the center of the lesions.

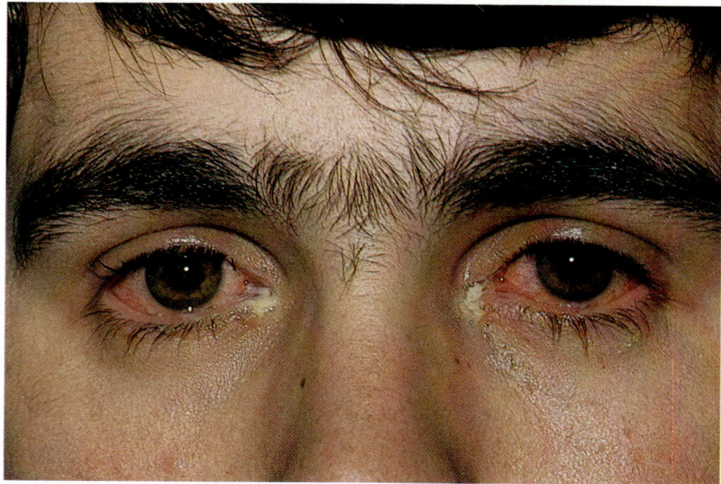

Figure 119 Erythema multiforme. Involvement of the eyes as indicated by conjunctival injection and purulent secretion into the conjunctival sac.

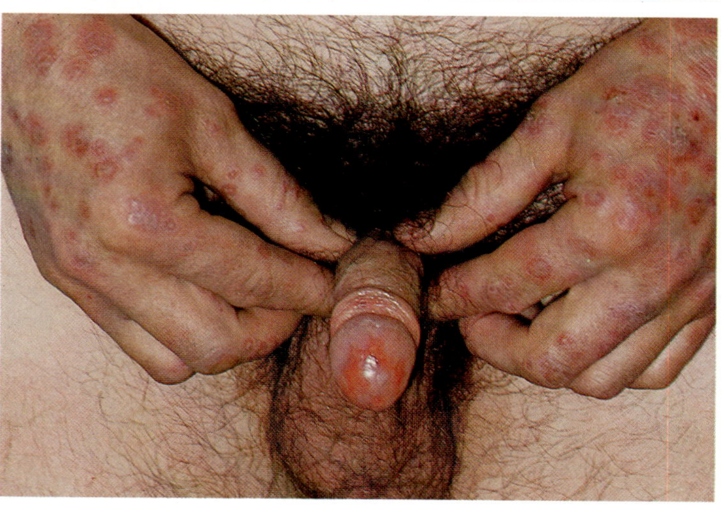

Figure 120 Erythema multiforme. Typical lesions on the dorsum of both hands, as well as involvement of the genitals.

Erythema Multiforme

Erythema multiforme is a special type of skin reaction to various causative agents. In many cases these agents cannot be identified. In others, erythema multiforme can accompany or follow a bacterial or virus infection.
Less commonly, it can be caused by drugs, x-rays or sarcoidosis. The disorder usually affects young people and heals within a few weeks, depending on initial involvement. It is important to identify the causative agents or diseases (e.g., recurrent herpes simplex or mycoplasma pneumonia). The extent of the disease is quite variable. There can be typical individual target lesions on hands or arms without involvement of the oral mucosa, or there can be extensive involvement with typical and atypical target lesions on hands or arms with massive involvement of the oral mucosa and severe general symptoms (Stevens-Johnson syndrome). Transitional forms into toxic epidermal necrolysis (see page 19) can occur. Involvement of only the mucous membranes is rare in erythema multiforme and is known as Fuchs' syndrome.

Clinical Features

1. The disease is characterized by target or iris-shaped, concentric round foci which are usually about the size of pennies. With more extensive involvement, the formation of central blisters and symmetry of lesions are characteristic. Old and new lesions can be found side by side.
2. Involvement of the dorsum of the hands and forearms, sometimes also of the palms of the hands and the soles of the feet, is typical. Extensive involvement of the entire integument is also possible.
3. The mucous membranes adjacent to the skin can also be involved, especially when the disease is widespread. The conjunctivae are reddened ("teary eyes"). In some patients, the oral mucous membranes can have severe erosions (stomatitis) with conspicuous hemorrhagic crusts on the lips. The stomatitis is found particularly in the anterior parts of the oral mucosa with erosions, ulcerations and fibrinous coatings. The patients often have halitosis, and many times it is painful to open the mouth. The genital mucous membranes can also be affected.
4. Moderate to severe pruritus is usually present.
5. In the beginning, the patients often complain of malaise, joint pain (especially of the large joints) and fever.

Therapy

Systemic

1. In severe cases (major type with mucous membrane involvement), a short-term, early systemic corticosteroid may be indicated, e.g., 100 mg prednisolone for 3 days followed by gradual reduction of the dose as clinical symptoms improve. The value of systemic corticosteroid therapy is debatable, however, because the phase of cellular damage is over by the time symptoms appear, and the subsequent clinical course of the disease represents the repair phase.
2. Analgesics may be required for severe stomatitis.
3. For severe pruritus, oral antihistamines may be required (**R. 61, 62**).

External

1. Local therapy is not necessary for mild involvement without bullae.
2. Bullae should be treated by evacuation and local disinfection (**R. 17**); otherwise a shake mixture (**R. 20a**) is sufficient.
3. Stomatitis may require frequent mouthwashes with lukewarm water, possibly with the addition of antiseptics (e.g., 0.1–0.3% H_2O_2 solution = one teaspoon of a 3% H_2O_2 solution in one glass of water).
4. Topical application of corticosteroids does not influence the course of the disease significantly.

General Measures

Bedrest is recommended. Patients with severe and extensive involvement of the mucous membranes should have a liquid or soft diet. Hospitalization may be required in severe cases.

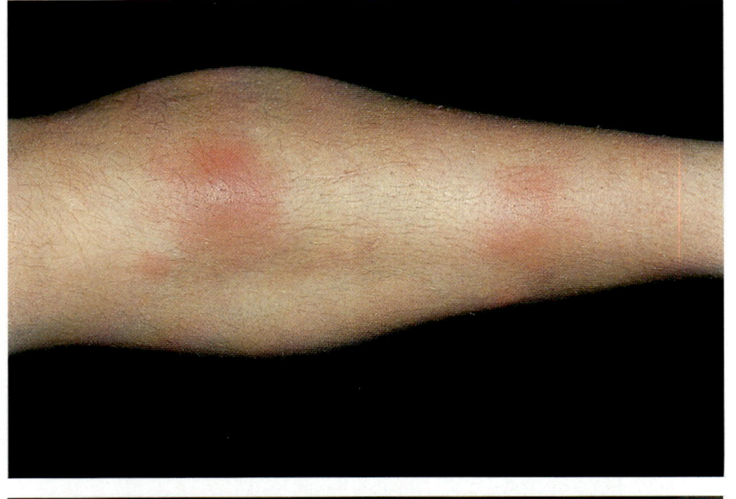

Figure 121 Erythema nodosum. Painful nodular infiltrates in the pretibial area.

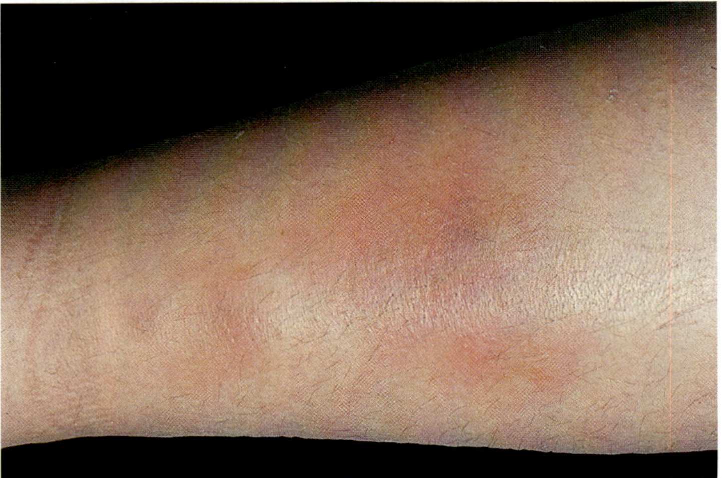

Figure 122 Erythema nodosum. Tight, shiny skin over an acute, inflammatory infiltrate.

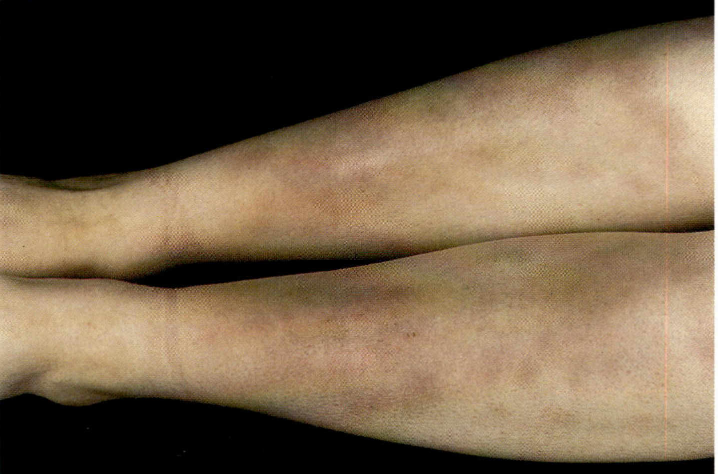

Figure 123 Contusion-like erythema nodosum. Brownish discoloration of infiltrates, resembling hematoma.

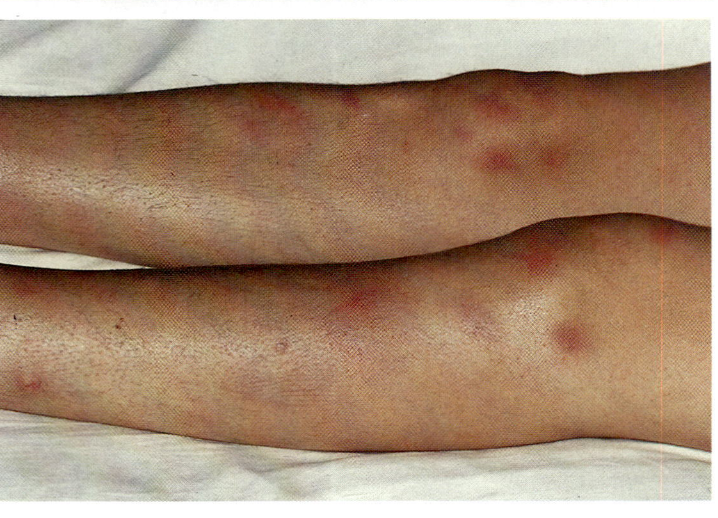

Figure 124 Erythema nodosum. Multiple nodular lesions on both lower legs and knees.

Erythema Nodosum

Erythema nodosum is a special form of skin reaction that can be due to a variety of factors. It may accompany or follow bacterial or viral infections such as angina tonsillaris, pharyngitis, yersiniosis, BCG vaccination or tuberculosis. It can also be associated with sarcoidosis (Löfgren's syndrome), Crohn's disease or colitis ulcerosa, or it can be induced by drugs (e.g., sulfonamides, phenacetin, penicillin). In most patients, however, an internal or external cause cannot be identified. The disease mainly affects young women. Erythema nodosum in old age or in men is a rare occurrence.

Clinical Features

1. The typical eruption consists of painful, nodular infiltrates on the lower legs, especially in the pretibial area. They are reddened and can develop a hematoma-like brown or green discoloration after they have been present for some time (contusion-like appearance).
2. The extreme pain is a characteristic symptom. Even the weight of a blanket can cause pain.
3. Multiple lesions are present.
4. Erythema nodosum occurs on the extensor sides of the lower legs and occasionally on the thighs. It rarely appears anywhere else on the body.
5. Constitutional symptoms consist of joint pains (knee and ankle joints, occasionally other joints), initially also fever, malaise and headaches.
6. Isolated attacks are often the case, which resolve completely within a few weeks. However, many times new infiltrates can also appear over longer periods of time; erythema nodosum can last for several months.

Therapy

After possible causative diseases have been excluded or treated, therapy of the skin condition is usually symptomatic.

1. The most important local measure is bedrest with elevation of the legs. A tunnel can minimize the pain from the blanket.
2. Corticosteroid ointments **(R. 38c)** can be used, even with an occlusive foil, but the pathologic changes are deep in the skin, so that topical therapy usually cannot reach the lesions. Cooling with wet dressings often has a soothing effect.
3. Nonsteroidal anti-inflammatory agents such as acetylsalicylic acid are occasionally helpful.
4. Systemic corticosteroid therapy with medium-range doses (see page 260) should be used only in severe cases. Corticosteroids should not be given when infection is present.

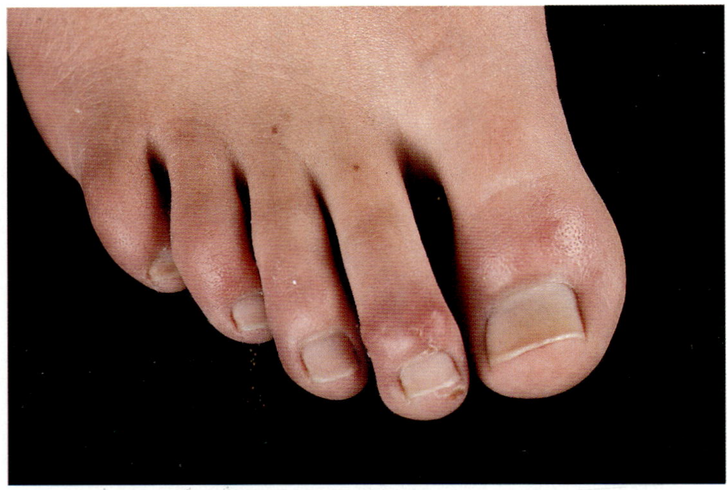

Figure 125 Chilblains. Bluish-red, mildly painful infiltrates with pruritus on the dorsum of the toes.

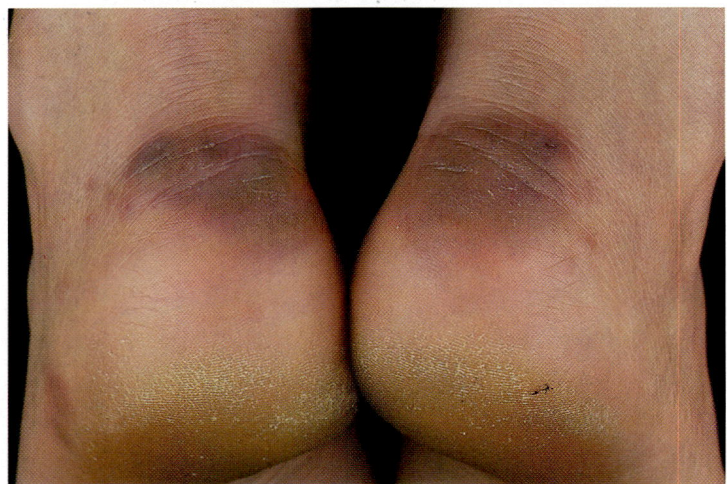

Figure 126 Chilblains. Symmetric, blue-red infiltrates in areas exposed to the cold.

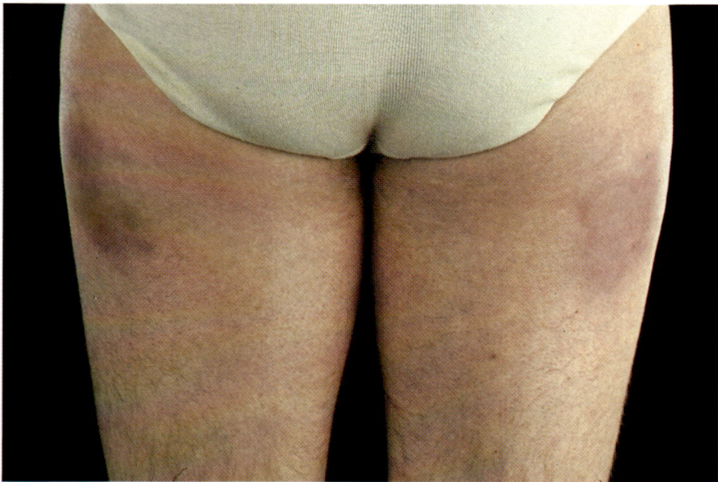

Figure 127 Chilblains can develop in areas covered by tight clothing (jeans). Characteristic location on the outside of both thighs in young women, frequently acquired during cycling or horseback riding (cold panniculitis).

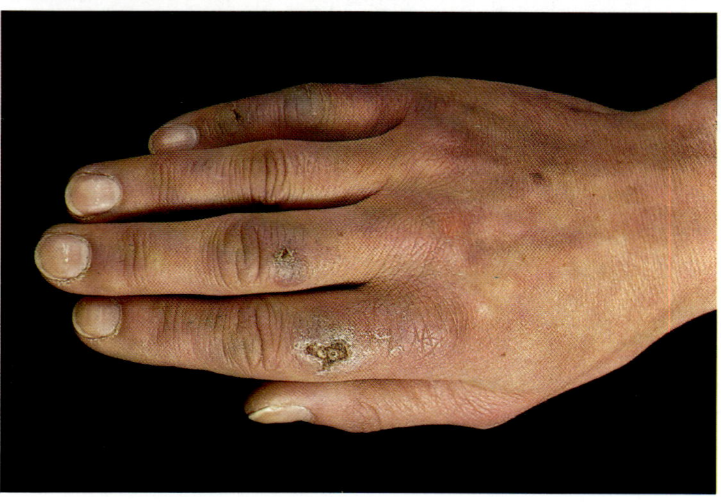

Figure 128 Chilblains can occasionally be seen with ulceration.

Chilblains, Perniosis

Chilblains are circumscribed, inflammatory changes that occur in predisposed patients after exposure to moderate cold. Genetic disposition and functional disturbance of the circulation often exist, with acrocyanosis and cold, clammy fingers and toes. Other factors, such as diet, clothing and atmospheric humidity also seem to play a role. Chilblains usually occur in damp, cold weather. They are rare in countries with cold and dry winters, because the dry air conducts temperature poorly, and people usually wear appropriate clothing for the cold weather there. Girls and young women are predominantly affected.

Areas of nodular infiltrates, especially on the lateral and posterolateral aspects of the thighs, are a special form of perniosis; they are called cold panniculitis. They are frequently seen in young, sometimes tall women after horseback riding, bicycling or winter sports. In these situations, clothing is too close to the skin (clothing is either too tight or it is pressed onto the skin) and does not insulate properly. Areas with ample amounts of subcutaneous fat are especially involved.

In infants, extensive infiltrates are frequently seen as a reaction to cold exposure following long rides in a baby carriage, especially during the winter.

Clinical Features

1. Bluish-red, circumscribed nodular swellings are typical findings. In severe cases with continued exposure to cold, blister formation and ulceration can occur.
2. Areas of predilection are the dorsal aspects of the fingers and toes, the heels and the lower legs. The hips can be involved when tight clothing is worn.
3. The so-called cold panniculitis has a characteristic appearance with red to bluish-red infiltrates on the thighs.
4. Rewarming leads to marked itching and occasionally severe pain.

Therapy

After exposure to cold has ceased, the pathologic changes heal spontaneously within 7–14 days. When deep nodules or the so-called cold panniculitis is present, healing can take several months. Care must be taken to prevent recurrent attacks. The patient must be advised to wear dry, well insulated shoes and to avoid tight-fitting clothes. Athletic activities are important for vascular training.

Internal

Vasodilatory drugs can enhance the blood supply. Antihistamines **(R. 61, 62)** are recommended for severe itching.

External

Baths can be supplemented with substances to induce hyperemia, such as benzylnicotinate. For severe inflammation, a short course of corticosteroids **(R. 38b)** may be indicated.

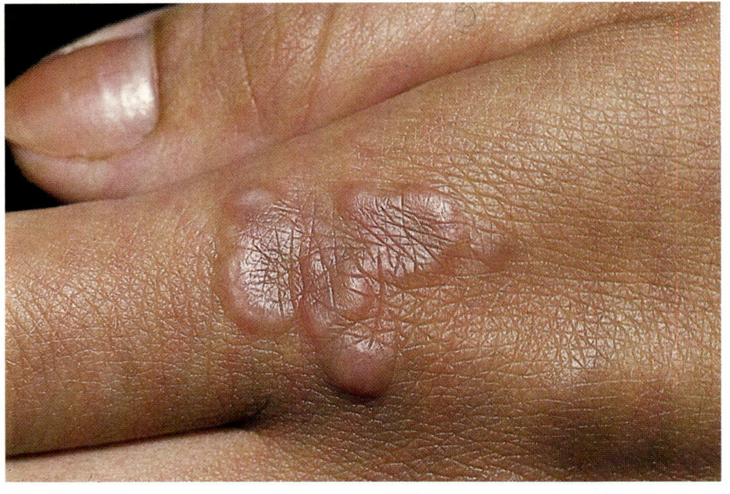

Figure 129 Granuloma annulare. Lesion with scalloped borders and small nodules in the margin.

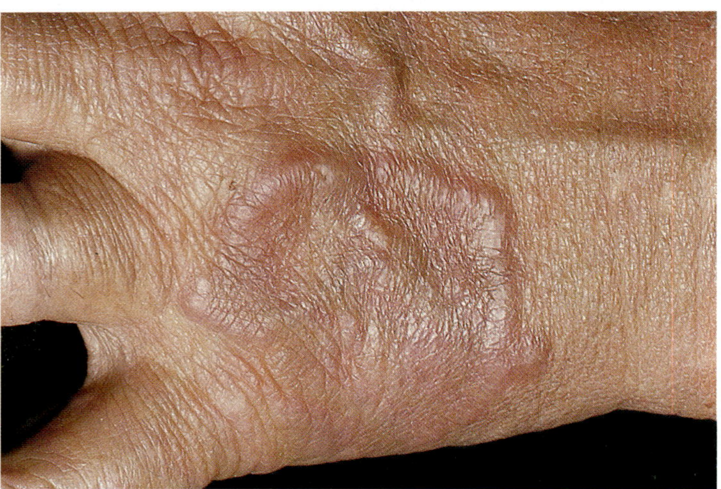

Figure 130 Granuloma annulare. Typical lesion over the knuckles with mild pitting of the center.

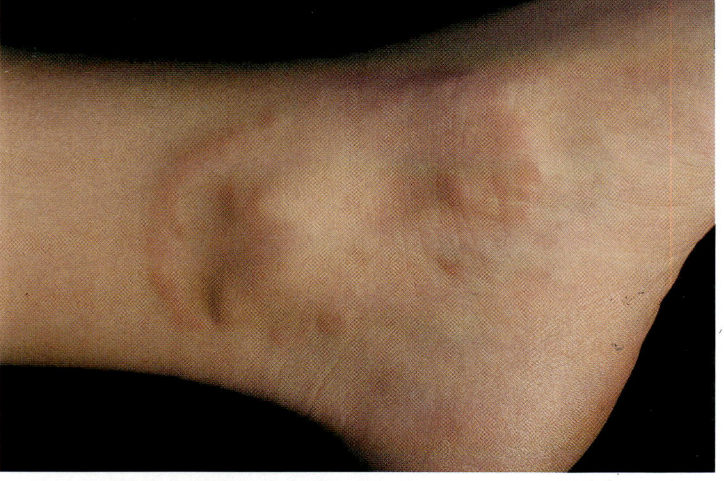

Figure 131 Granuloma annulare. The lateral malleolar region is frequently involved. Brownish discoloration of the affected area.

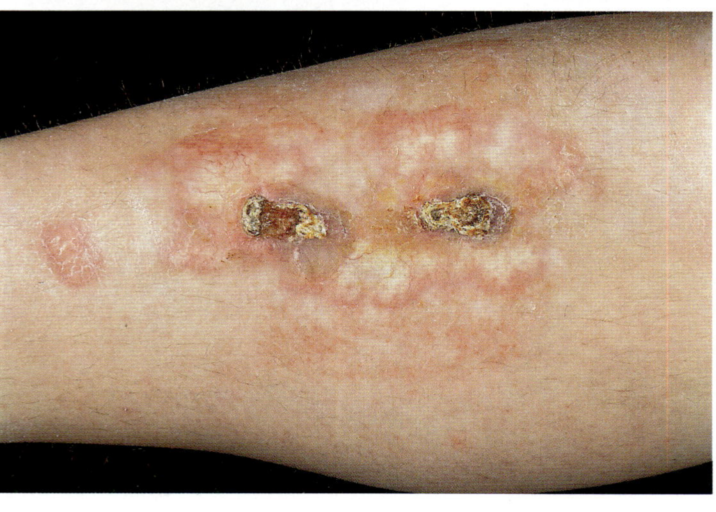

Figure 132 Necrobiosis lipoidica. Red infiltrates with yellow center and enlarged blood vessels. The center is ulcerated.

Granuloma Annulare, Necrobiosis Lipoidica

A. Granuloma Annulare

This chronic inflammatory disease mainly affects children, but can also affect adults. The cause is unknown. In adults, it is occasionally associated with diabetes mellitus, yet less often than with a related disorder, necrobiosis lipoidica. Granuloma annulare can exist for months or even years and then involute spontaneously. The lesions consist of individual nodules that can be demonstrated histologically. If in doubt, the diagnosis should be confirmed microscopically.

Clinical Features

1. Usually there are several round or annular lesions with a marginal rim of skin-colored to erythematous, slightly raised nodules. Initially, the center of the lesion is skin-colored, later changing to a livid to brownish-red color. In older lesions the nodular rim may not be distinctly visible. These lesions can appear as sharply delineated, round, persistent pale or dusky brown discolorations. The epidermis is always unchanged.
2. Areas of predilection are the dorsal surfaces of the finger and toe joints, but granuloma annulare can also appear on other parts of the body.
3. Usually there are no subjective symptoms, except for occasional mild itching.

Therapy

Therapeutic results are not satisfactory. Treatment should be carried out in consultation with a dermatologist. In patients with diabetes, the blood sugar must be kept within normal limits.

Local

1. These patients are often worried by the persistent and slowly spreading eruptions and should be informed that the disease is harmless.
2. Treatment with corticosteroid ointments **(R. 38c)** under an occlusive foil is sometimes effective.
3. Intralesional injections of a corticosteroid crystal suspension **(R. 46)** is indicated only for extensive individual lesions.
4. Occasionally, the lesions disappear spontaneously or after biopsy.
5. The disease is harmless, and systemic therapy is not necessary.

B. Necrobiosis Lipoidica

Necrobiosis lipoidica affects mainly young and middle-aged adults. Its cause is unknown. It occurs frequently in diabetics, but a latent or manifest diabetes or a diabetic disposition cannot be found in all patients. Women are affected three times more often than men. The lesions develop and spread slowly over a period of many years.

Clinical Features

1. Typical lesions are red to light-brown reddish, flat plaques that develop central atrophy with yellow discoloration and enlarged blood vessels. In approximately 25% of all patients the granuloma ulcerates. There may be individual or multiple foci.
2. Frequently the lesions are located on the anterior aspect of the lower leg.
3. The lesions are usually not painful, not even those with ulcers.

Therapy

1. Confirmation or exclusion of diabetes mellitus is important. An existing diabetes mellitus must be brought under optimal control.
2. An effective local or systemic treatment is not known. Intralesional injections of a corticosteroid crystal suspension **(R. 46)**, either with a hypodermic needle or a Dermojet, can improve the symptoms. Occasionally, triple therapy (a strong corticosteroid ointment on top of a steroid solution, covered by an occlusive dressing, e.g., plastic wrap) can help.

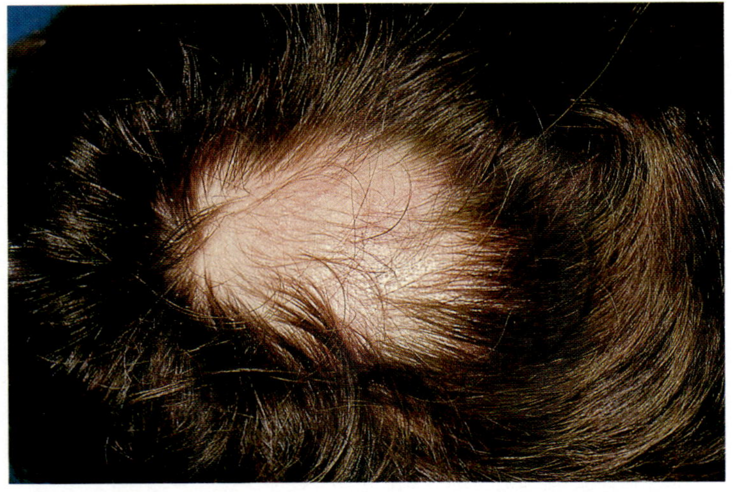

Figure 133 Alopecia areata. Circumscribed round area of baldness without visible inflammatory changes.

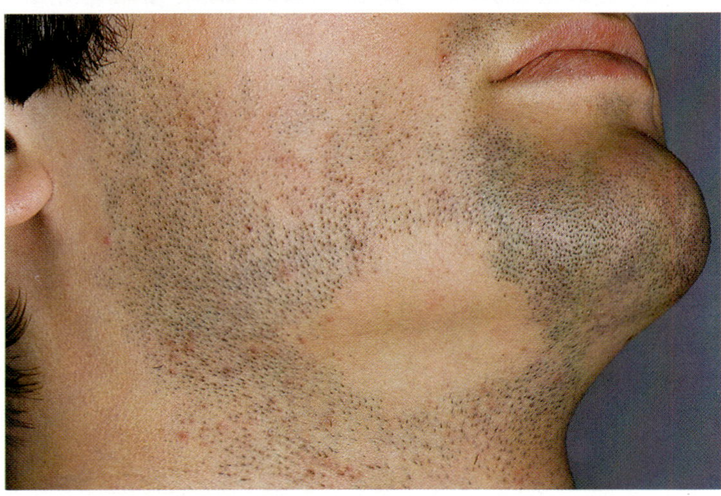

Figure 134 Alopecia areata. Circumscribed round area of baldness in the region of the beard.

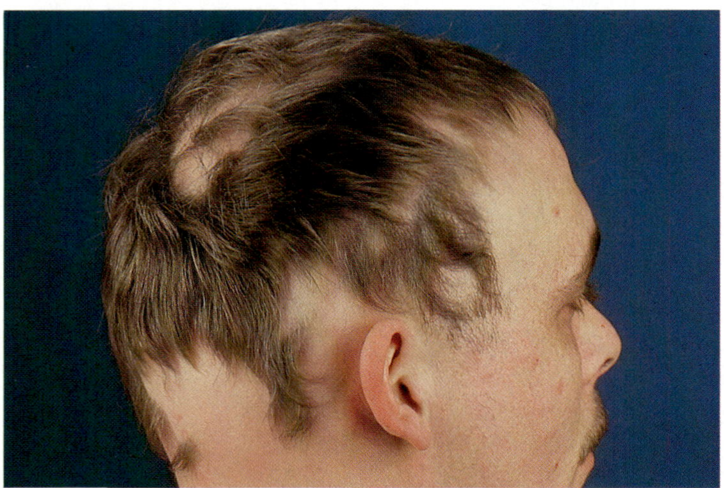

Figure 135 Alopecia areata. Numerous, partly coalescing alopecia lesions of varying sizes.

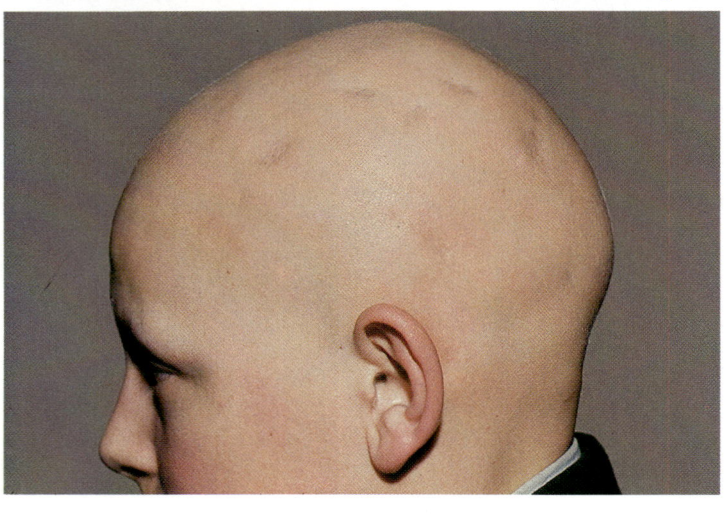

Figure 136 Alopecia areata totalis with absence of eyelids and eyelashes. The pitted, atrophic areas were caused by subcutaneous injections of a corticosteroid crystal suspension.

Diseases of the Hair

In addition to the rare congenital anomalies of the hair, premature loss of the hair is often felt to be a sign of bad health. The condition can be due to a simultaneous disease of the scalp, as in psoriasis, in fungal diseases or as part of a seborrheic dermatitis (see page 49). More frequently, it is seen without visible involvement of the scalp, as diffuse alopecia or as alopecia areata. It can be transient or permanent, irrespective of the presence of scars on the scalp.
Diffuse alopecia in women without any underlying disease is especially common and significant for the practicing physician. The hair becomes intermittently (in phases or "waves") thinner all over the scalp. This is not only a cosmetic problem, but is also often psychologically relevant. In some patients hair loss, whether substantiated or not, may cause massive complaints, though in reality the complaints are an expression of an inner conflict situation.

A. Alopecia Areata

The disease affects men and women equally and occurs in attacks. It is often already manifest in childhood; it rarely begins after age 40. The cause of the disease is still unknown. Different factors, such as genetic disposition or immunologic disturbances play a role. For some individuals with susceptible personalities, emotional stress (accidents, exams, mourning) can be identified as predisposing causes. Sometimes the patient suffers from atopic dermatitis (see page 41) or vitiligo (see page 109). The course of the disease varies. Complete recovery can take place after a few weeks, but in extreme cases, there can be total or permanent loss of all body hair.

Clinical Features

1. Complete loss of hair in round patches without signs of pathologic changes in the underlying scalp, such as scaling, inflammation or atrophy, is characteristic. At first, the hairs that regrow are thin and without pigment (downy hair).
2. Alopecia areata affects mainly the scalp, but the lesions can occur on any other part of the body with hair, especially the eyebrows and beard. In the most severe form, alopecia universalis, there is complete loss of all bodily hair.
3. Other symptoms, such as itching, are absent.

Therapy

The course of the disease is unpredictable, so that many of the so-called "cures" following a specific treatment must be regarded merely as spontaneous recoveries. The patients should be informed about the nature of the disease to keep them from seeking help from "mystical" or expensive and dubious treatments.
Sometimes a wig is the only possible treatment. Surgical procedures (hair transplants) are not advisable because of the unpredictable nature of the disease.

Internal

1. An effective systemic treatment of the disease is not known. No successful therapeutic attempts have been confirmed thus far.
2. Amino acids which contain sulfur, vitamins and trace elements, especially zinc, have been recommended, but their effectiveness has not been confirmed.

External

1. Substances producing hyperemia, sometimes in combination with corticosteroids or cignolin, lead to new hair growth in some patients.
2. Intralesional injection of a corticosteroid crystal suspension can be tried for small foci of alopecia areata (caution: This can produce skin atrophy).
3. Creation of an allergic contact dermatitis with diphencyprone appears promising. The procedure is still in the experimental stage and cannot be recommended for general use at this time.

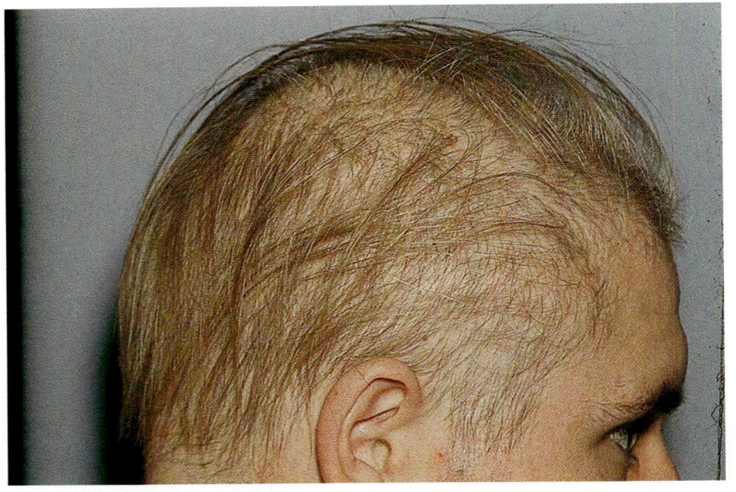

Figure 137 Diffuse alopecia following thallium poisoning.

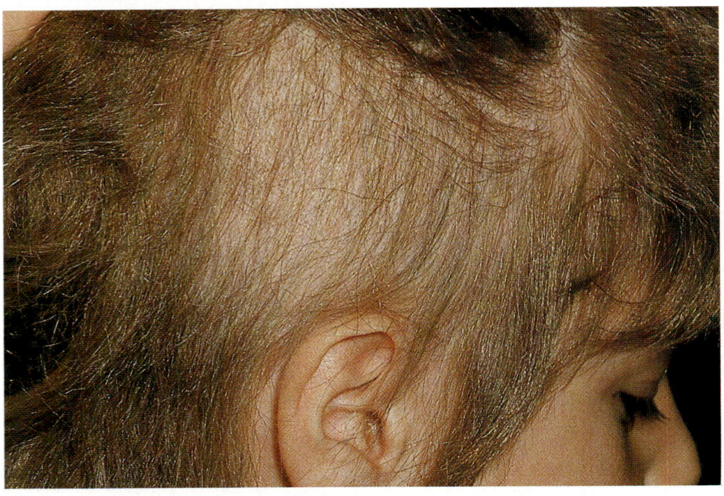

Figure 138 Trichotillomania. Habitual pulling of hair in a circumscribed area.

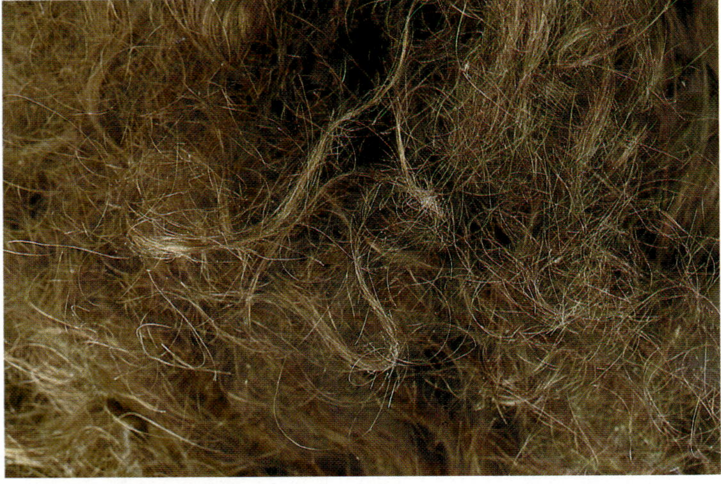

Figure 139 Toxic damage to the hair caused by permanent wave solution. The hair is severely matted and cannot be combed.

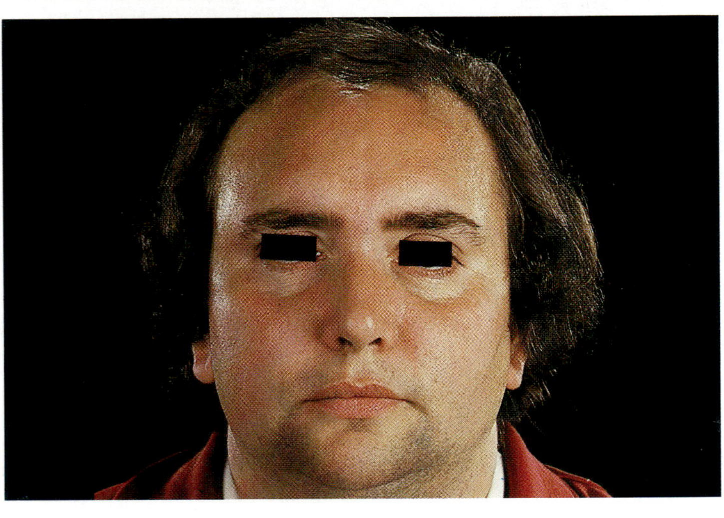

Figure 140 Hirsutism. Androgenetic alopecia and beard development in a 28-year-old woman.

B. Diffuse Alopecia

In women, androgenetic alopecia of the male type is usually a sign of hormonal disturbance (androgen-producing tumors). In men, early onset and rapid progression can lead to significant psychological impairment, especially in patients with a vulnerable emotional structure. There may also be transient diffuse alopecia following severe, acute generalized disorders, infectious diseases, operations, as well as delivery. Other causes can be drugs, such as cytostatic, anti-coagulant and thyrostatic agents, or acute (e.g., thallium) and chronic (e.g., pentachlorphenol, lindane) intoxications.

Clinical Features

1. Androgenetic alopecia of the male type begins with a receding hairline, followed by a circumscribed bald area on the occiput (tonsure). The area where the hair is parted becomes thinner. Eventually, only a fringe of hair remains over the ears and the occiput.
2. In contrast to this, androgenetic alopecia of the female type initially shows a thinning of the hair over the entire parietal area, whereas the hairline remains unchanged.
3. In diffuse alopecia caused by intoxication, the entire scalp is evenly affected.

Therapy

In androgenetic alopecia in women, the underlying hormonal disturbance must be evaluated and treated. In men, appropriate treatment is determined largely by the psychological structure of the patient. In transient diffuse alopecia, specific therapy is not necessary.

Systemic

At present there is no totally effective drug therapy for androgenetic alopecia. In androgenetic alopecia of women, antiandrogen therapy with cyproterone acetate has been tried.

External

1. Hair lotion containing estrogen in combination with corticosteroids (**R. 18**).
2. Antiseborrheic shampoos (**R. 10**) for oily, scaling scalp.
3. Other topical remedies, trace elements, vitamins or scalp massage are not promising. Hair transplants or other plastic surgical procedures rarely lead to acceptable results. It is better to prescribe a wig.

C. Trichotillomania

This disorder, seen mainly in children, is characterized by habitually pulling out hair. It is usually caused by emotional problems (familial conflict situations, school stress). A serious psychiatric disease is rarely found.

Constantly pulling hair out of the same spot gradually leads to a bald spot with hair of varying lengths. The hair that regrows is normal. Usually the hair of the scalp and less frequently the eyebrows and eyelashes are pulled. The nature of the underlying disorder should be clarified in discussions with the patient and the parents.

D. External Damage to the Hair

These disorders are generally of a cosmetic nature, such as excessive combing and brushing, excessive washing, dyeing, bleaching, permanent waves or straightening of curly hair.

Clinical Features

The appearance depends on the causative factors and can include increased fragility, split ends, or even matted, uncombable hair.

Therapy

The damage is usually limited to the hair shaft. Removal of the causative factors will lead to regrowth of healthy, normal hair in most cases.

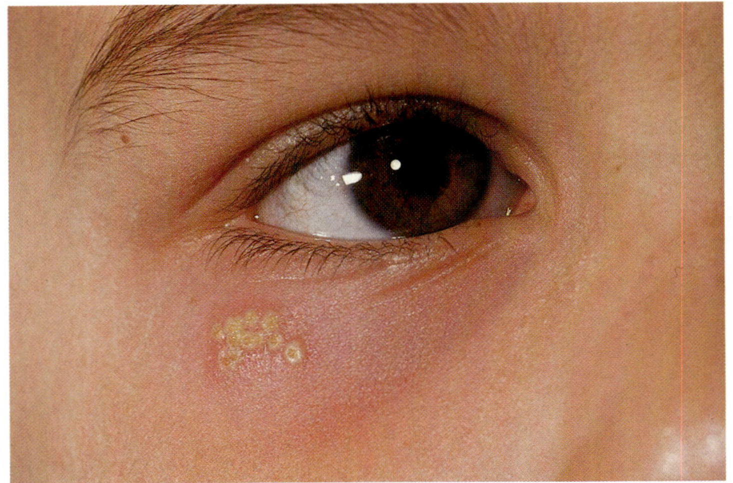

Figure 141 Herpes simplex. Groups of pitted vesicles on inflammatory erythema, here already partly converted into pustules.

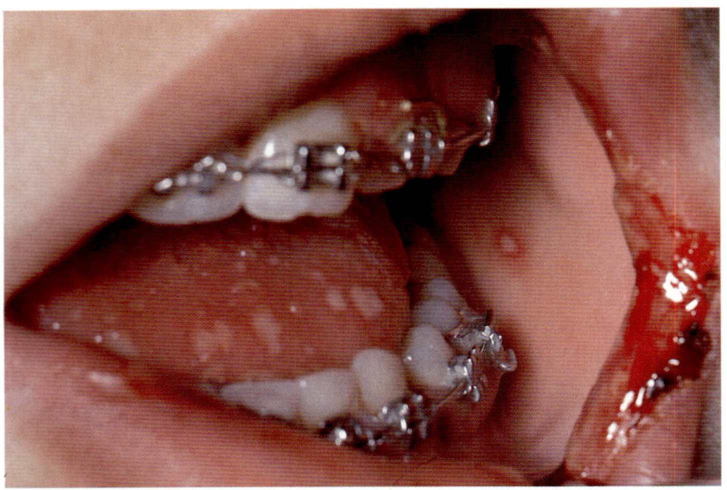

Figure 142 Herpetic gingivostomatitis. Multiple, painful, small erosions of the gingiva covered with fibrin.

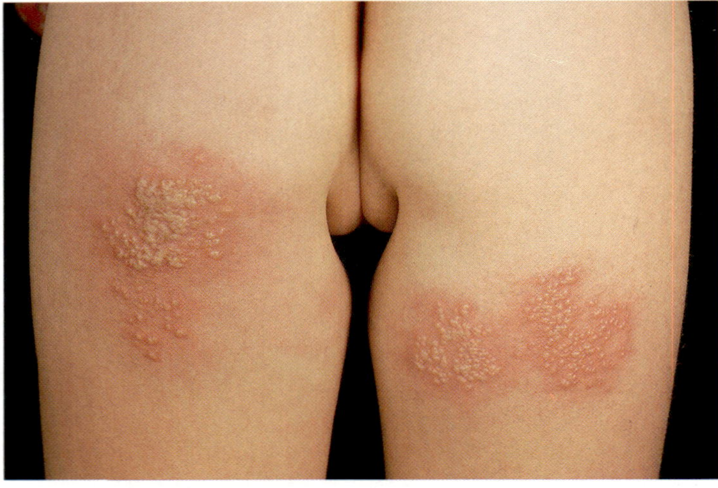

Figure 143 Herpes simplex multilocularis. Extensive recurrent herpes simplex lesions which always recur at the same site.

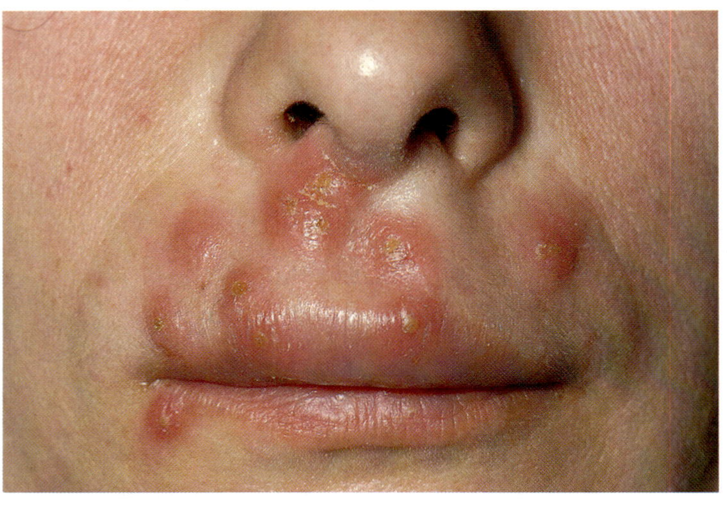

Figure 144 Recurrent herpes simplex of the lips extending to the nostrils.

Herpes Simplex

Diseases caused by the herpes simplex virus are among the most frequent infectious diseases of the skin. The primary and recurrent infections differ in their clinical appearance and their course. Due to its prevalence, primary infections usually occur during childhood and are often completely asymptomatic. The incubation period of genital herpes simplex is 11–49 days. Since recurrences develop in some patients in intervals of a few weeks, they are seen much more frequently by the practicing physician. Two serotypes of the herpes simplex virus (HSV) can be distinguished. HSV-1 is responsible for herpes lesions in all areas of the body except the genital and anal infections, which are caused by HSV-2. The herpesvirus is transmitted by direct contact or by droplet infection. Primary and recurrent eruptions remain infectious for approximately 4 days. Chronic infections are due primarily to immune defects (AIDS, leukemia). Recurrences are caused by reactivation of latent organisms that have remained dormant in the body after a primary infection. Reactivation can be triggered by menses, trauma, UV-radiation or febrile infections, as demonstrated by such terms as "flu blisters" or "fever blisters". The incidence of recurrent attacks varies considerably among individuals; they become less with advancing age.

A severe form of herpes simplex infection occurs in patients with atopic dermatitis, the so-called eczema herpeticum. These patients have a deficiency in cell-mediated immunity, and the herpesvirus spreads rapidly over large areas of the skin.

Clinical Features

a) Primary manifestations

1. Primary infection with herpes simplex virus becomes manifest as an acute gingivostomatitis, vulvovaginitis, or balanitis and urethritis. The clinical manifestations consist of densely grouped blisters, erosions, and purulent, malodorous crusts. Skin eruptions like those in extensive recurrent herpes simplex are also possible.
2. Hypersensitivity and pain in the affected area shortly before eruption of the lesion are the earliest symptoms.
3. The lesions are quite painful and are accompanied by swelling of the regional lymph nodes. There can be high fever, especially with extensive involvement of the oral mucosa.

b) Recurrent manifestations

1. The patients often complain of a feeling of tension and itching in the affected area before eruptions occur.
2. The typical eruption consists of grouped, centrally pitted, clear vesicles that later change into pustules. After a short time, erosions with polycyclic borders develop, often covered with hemorrhagic fibrinous, occasionally purulent, crusts.
3. The most frequently involved site is the face, especially the lips and the nares. The genital region may also be involved: in women the vulva, in men the glans penis and the foreskin (transmission by intercourse). Herpes simplex infections can appear in any region of the body; recurrent attacks usually occur in the previously involved site.
4. The lesions are often accompanied by painful swelling of the lymph nodes. With recurrent attacks, the course of the disease is much less dramatic than it is with primary infections.
5. Involvement of the eye, with development of herpes keratitis, is a serious complication that can lead to scarring and impaired vision. Ophthalmologic consultation is necessary in these cases. Occasionally, herpes simplex infection can be complicated by erythema multiforme (see page 61).
6. Herpes simplex of the birth canal can be an indication for cesarean section to avoid infection of the child (herpes sepsis in the newborn has a high mortality rate).

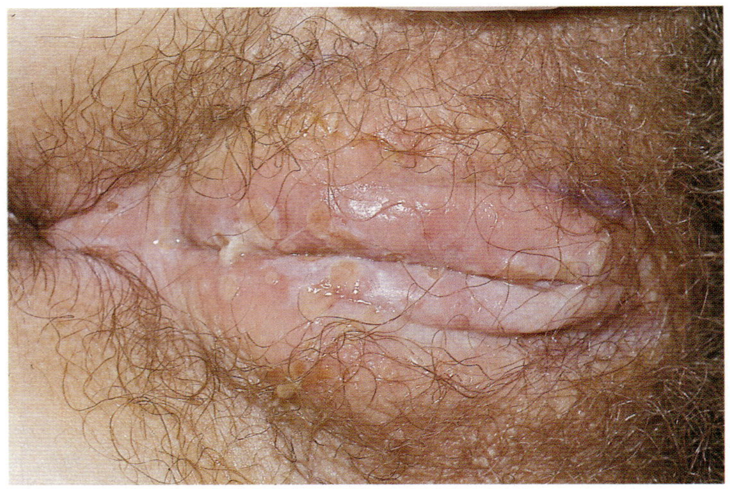

Figure 145 Herpes simplex of the vulva. Multiple painful erosions.

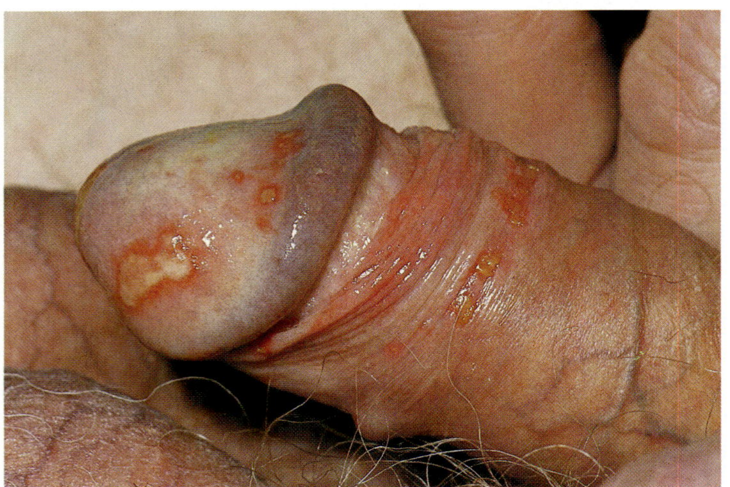

Figure 146 Genital herpes simplex. Round or polycyclic (through confluence of lesions) erosions on the glans penis and foreskin that are coated with fibrin.

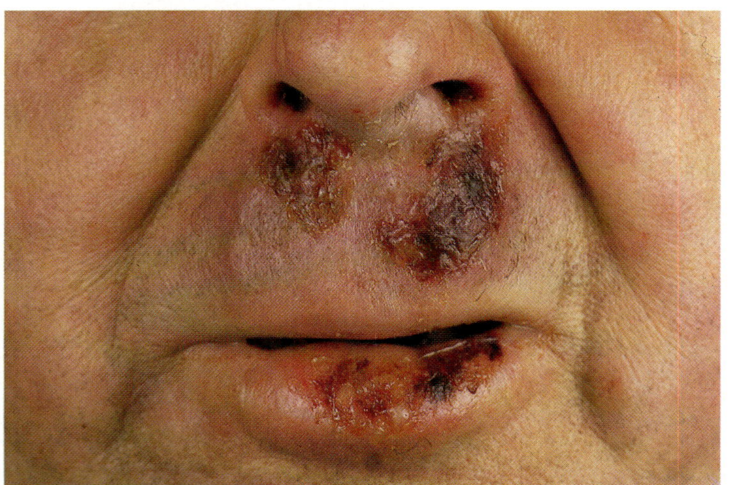

Figure 147 Recurrent herpes simplex in a patient with chronic lymphatic leukemia. Crusty infiltrates of the lips in varying stages of development. The lesions have persisted over a period of months.

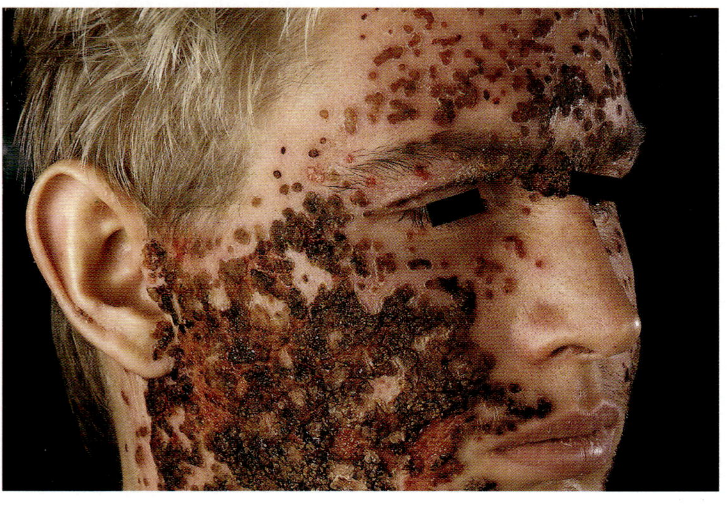

Figure 148 Eczema herpeticum. Development of pitted vesicles and hemorrhagic crusty erosions on the face.

c) Eczema herpeticum

1. Dense patches of pitted vesicles rupture after a short time and develop into small and larger erosions.
2. Areas of predilection are the face and neck; occasionally the entire skin can be involved.
3. The patients are very ill with high fever and life-threatening complications, such as meningitis, encephalitis and herpes sepsis. Primary infections are usually more severe than recurrent manifestations.

Therapy

Treatment of recurrent herpes infections is still unsatisfactory; most "treatment results" are usually placebo effects or spontaneous recoveries. At the present, it is not possible to eliminate the dormant virus from the human organism, which would be the only way to truly prevent recurrent attacks.

Systemic

1. For severe cases of acute herpes infection, high-risk patients, and eczema herpeticum, we recommend intravenous acyclovir **(R. 60)**; for less severe cases, acyclovir can be given orally.
2. For frequent recurrences and for persistent skin symptoms as a result of HIV infection or leukemia, long-time oral therapy with acyclovir is recommended.
3. Several immunomodulating or immunostimulating substances, such as Isoprinosine have been recommended. Their effectiveness in recurrent herpes simplex has not been confirmed, however.
4. Immunoglobulins to boost the patient's immune system are controversial.

External

1. External forms of acyclovir and other antiviral drugs **(R. 36)** are available. It is important to apply these substances during the phase of eruption, preferrably when premonitory symptoms appear. Once the lesions are a day old, these preparations are practically useless.
2. Crusts of pyoderma are best removed with a fatty ointment, such as vaseline or an antibiotic ointment **(R. 34)**.
3. The patients must be advised not to rub their eyes to avoid auto-inoculation. When acute genital herpes is present, condoms must be used for protection.

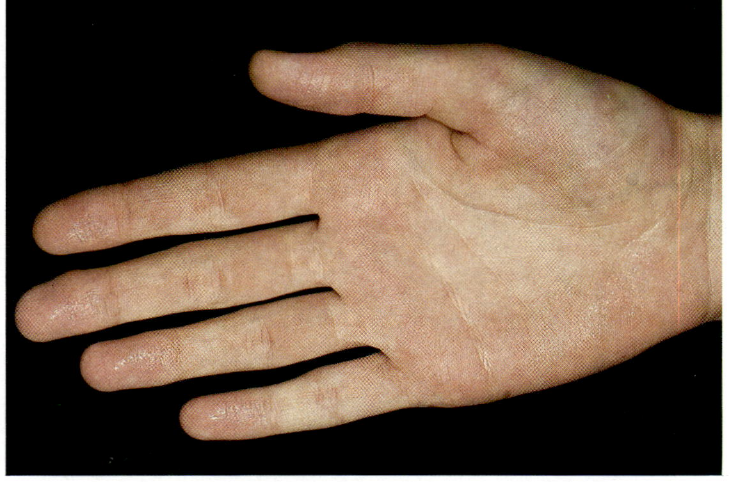

Figure 149 Hyperhidrosis of the palm, most pronounced on the tips of the fingers.

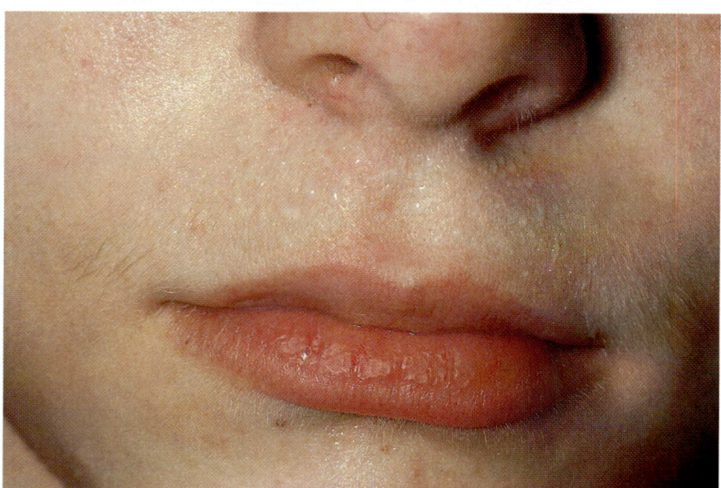

Figure 150 Hyperhidrosis of the lips in a patient with chronic mercury poisoning.

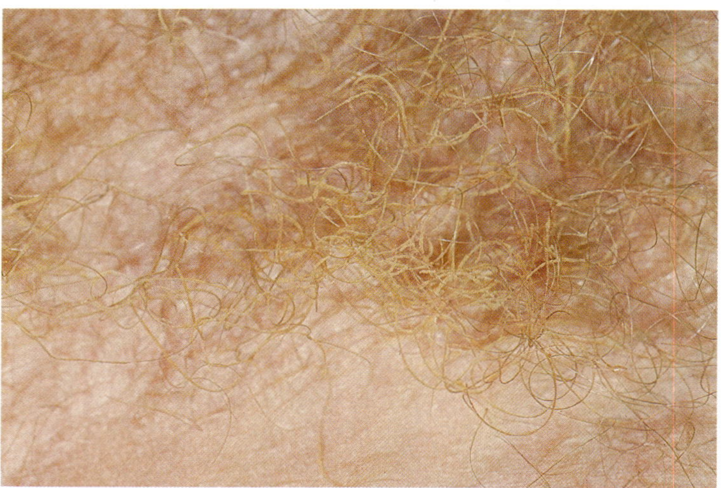

Figure 151 Trichomycosis palmellina. Yellow sheaths on axillary hair.

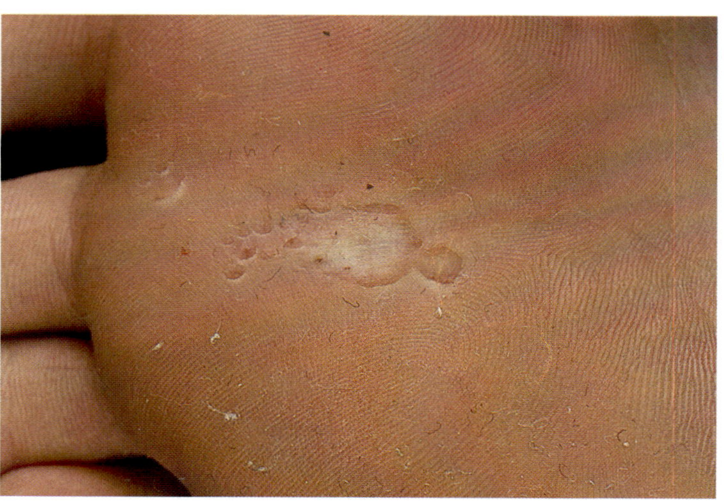

Figure 152 Keratoma plantare sulcatum. "Punched out" appearance of superficial keratin defects on the ball of the right foot.

Hyperhidrosis and Sequelae

A. Hyperhidrosis

For practical purposes we distinguish a generalized or symmetric form from an asymmetric form that is usually due to a neurologic disorder. Generalized sweating is seen in disorders of thermoregulation (infectious diseases, such as malaria or tuberculosis), in metabolic diseases such as diabetes mellitus and hyperthyroidism, in menopause, with malignant tumors (pheochromocytoma, Hodgkin's disease), in alcoholism, from certain drugs, such as tricyclic or tetracyclic antidepressants, caffeine, theophylline, from cholinergic and sympathomimetic drugs and from chronic mercury intoxication. Emotional factors (anxiety, stress) can also lead to increased sweating, especially on the palms, soles, axillae, inguinal region, and face. Some people have a tendency to sweat excessively (genuine hyperhidrosis), which can be severe enough that it must be regarded as pathologic. Constant excessive sweating can result in unpleasant sequelae such as bromhidrosis (malodorous sweating due to bacterial decomposition) or diseases like miliaria (see page 105), pityriasis versicolor (see page 119), trichomycosis palmellina (see below) or pitted keratolysis (keratoma plantare sulcatum) (see below).

Therapy
Systemic

1. Anticholinergic drugs for excessive pathological emotional sweating, if necessary with the addition of mild sedatives. Habit-forming components should be avoided because this is usually long-term therapy.
2. Extract of tea of sage may occasionally bring improvement.

External

1. Aluminum chloride in aqueous solution once a day **(R. 19)**.
2. Iontophoresis with tap water is effective for hyperhidrosis of the palms and soles.
3. For sweaty feet, daily foot baths with potassium permanganate solution (1:10,000 for 10 to 20 minutes) can be helpful.
4. In severe cases that are resistant to therapy, surgical sympathectomy can be considered, or surgical removal of most of the axillary sweat glands. It must be kept in mind these are irreversible procedures. Since sweat production diminishes with advancing age, excessive dryness of the skin may result in later years and may be much more distressing.

B. Trichomycosis Palmellina (Trichomycosis Axillaris)

This is a dense bacterial colonization of the axillary hair with *Corynebacterium* due to hyperhidrosis.

Clinical Features There are yellowish-white, firmly attached deposits on the axillary hair.

Therapy If the condition is severe, the axillary hair may have to be shaved. Treatment of the underlying hyperhidrosis is important. Frequent use of antiseptic soap or detergents **(R. 5)** is advisable. Local application of imidazole preparations **(R. 35a)** is usually effective.

C. Pitted Keratolysis (Keratoma Plantare Sulcatum)

This is a superficial infection of the skin with *Corynebacterium*.

Clinical Features There are multiple superficial, round defects of the stratum corneum of the soles and the underside of the toes associated with hyperhidrosis, maceration and bromhidrosis. Subjective symptoms are usually minimal. However, prolonged mechanical stress (marching) can produce significant pain.

Therapy Treatment of the underlying hyperhidrosis is important. Severe cases may require a short course of topical antimicrobial therapy (dye solutions, 5% benzoyl peroxide gel).

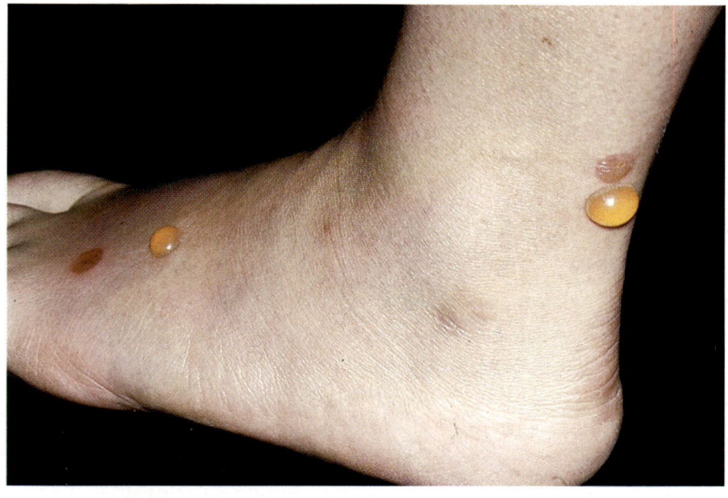

Figure 153 Culicosis bullosa. Bullous reaction to mosquito bites.

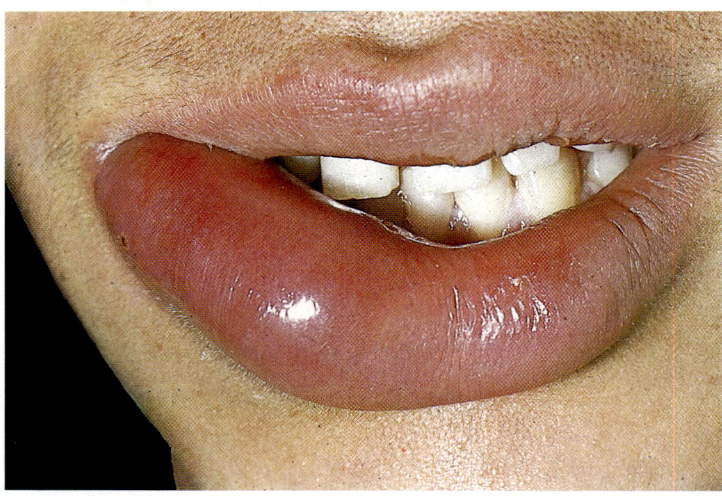

Figure 154 Inflammatory edema of the lips from a bee sting.

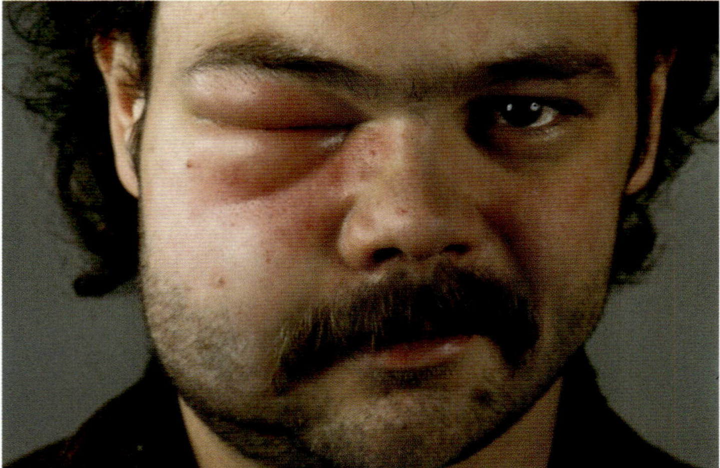

Figure 155 Extreme local reaction to a bee sting.

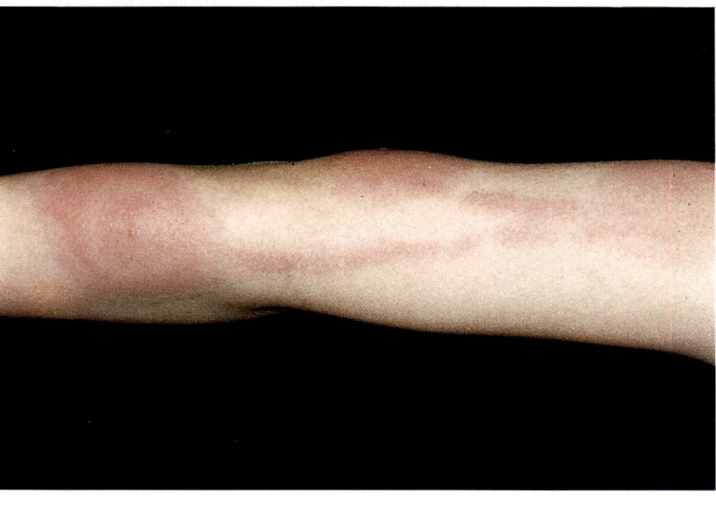

Figure 156 Reaction to an insect bite with lymphangitis. This is usually due to an exaggerated local reaction to the venom (as in this case), and only rarely due to an infection.

Insect Bites

A. Mosquito Bites

Clinical Features

Mosquito bites are usually manifest as pruritic wheals, or in some patients, as vesicular reactions, especially on the lower legs.

Therapy

Urticarial reactions do not require treatment. Vesicular reactions can be evacuated. Antibiotic ointment can be applied to prevent superinfection.

Prophylaxis

1. The patient should try to avoid future mosquito bites (no walks near lakes or ponds, no vacations in mosquito-infested countries, use of a mosquito net at night, no perfumes or cosmetics containing them, frequent washing to reduce body odor). Mosquitoes are attracted by dark clothing and increased skin temperature and moisture.

2. Topical repellents afford protection for a few hours (even for trips to tropical countries).

B. Wasp and Bee Stings

Clinical Features

These stings produce swelling of varying degrees at the puncture site. Generalized reactions are possible, such as urticaria, or even anaphylactic shock if there is a corresponding allergy. An insect sting in the oral mucosa can lead to a life-threatening edema of the glottis. The clinical appearance following bee and wasp stings varies, and treatment must be administered according to the clinical symptoms.

Therapy

1. *For local reactions:* Cooling with wet dressings, dabbing with diluted alcohol (evaporating alcohol has a cooling effect), application of a corticosteroid cream or lotion, and elevation of the involved extremity are helpful. Following a bee sting, the stinger must be carefully removed from the skin without squeezing out the poison sac (remove with a fingernail or a knife, not with tweezers!).

2. *For mild systemic reactions* (generalized itching, urticaria): Application of a tourniquet proximal to the sting (in extremities), removal of the stinger, and if necessary also injection of 0.3 ml epinephrine solution (1:1000 in 1 to 2 ml saline) under and around the puncture site. Histamine receptor blocker (H_1 and H_2 blocker) and steroids are given intravenously.

3. *For severe systemic reactions* (anaphylactic shock), treatment is determined according to the symptoms: Maintain vital functions, positioning, respirator, and cardiac massage. If necessary, use a slow intravenous injection of a diluted epinephrine solution (0.5 ml, 1:1000 in 20 ml 0.9% saline). Histamine receptor blocker (H_1 and H_2 blocker) and steroids are given intravenously.

4. *For stings into the posterior oral cavity* with impending edema of the glottis, the symptoms may be relieved by spraying the oral mucosa with adrenaline aerosol; in severe cases, intubation or tracheostomy may be necessary.

Prophylaxis

1. Later, it must be determined whether an allergy is present (identification of specific IgE antibodies with RAST). The patient should be warned to avoid bee stings in the future and should be instructed what to do if stung again.

2. Persons with an allergy should be advised to have an emergency treatment kit with them at all times, which includes antihistamines and steroids in water-soluble form for drinking or injection, adrenaline aerosol, a tourniquet, and an epinephrine injection kit. The patient must be given exact instructions of what to do in an emergency (these instructions are best obtained in an allergy outpatient clinic).

3. The indication for hyposensitization (immunotherapy) should be determined by an experienced allergy specialist following appropriate diagnostic tests (RAST, threshold testing).

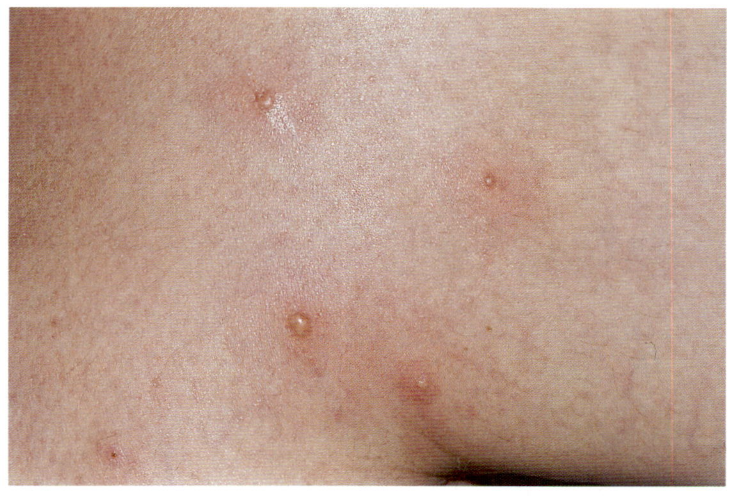

Figure 157 Flea bites.

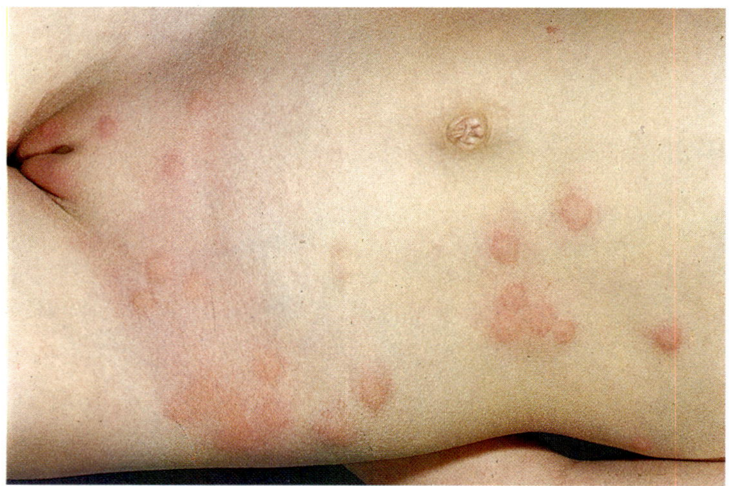

Figure 158 Bedbug bites. Multiple wheals, most pronounced where clothes are tight.

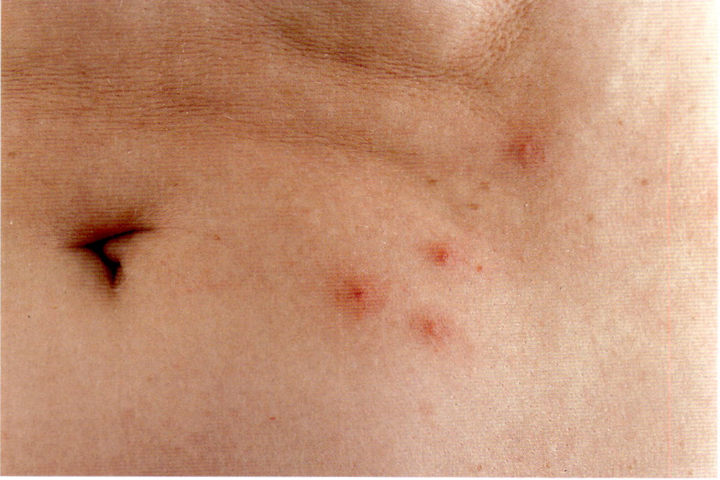

Figure 159 Trombidiosis. Severely itching papules surrounded by erythema.

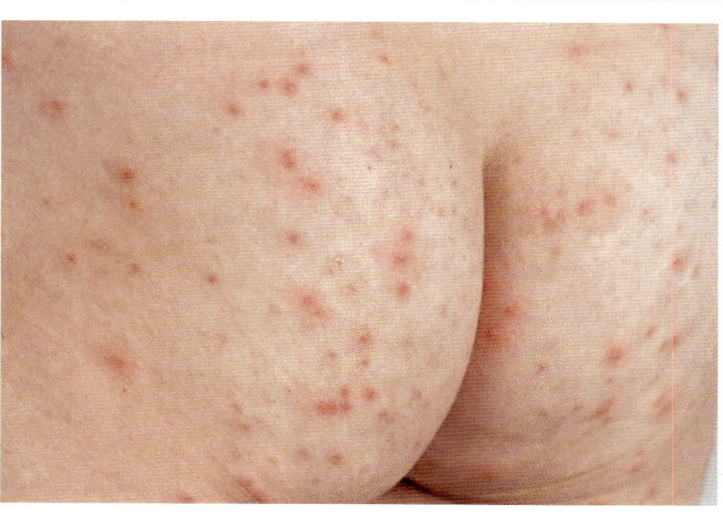

Figure 160 Trombidiosis. Fresh and older lesions.

C. Flea Bites

Usually only individual persons are affected in our areas, whereas flea epidemics occur mainly in mass lodgings if dogs and cats are kept. They are also seen in places where stray cats live in large numbers; e.g., in basements or ducts in the cities. Determination of the causative organism is often difficult in patients with flea bites. In many cases, fleas can only be suspected as the cause of the bite, but they are not easily found or caught. In most cases, flea bites are caused by dog fleas, *Ctenocephalides canis*, or by cat fleas, *Ctenocephalides felis*. Human fleas, *Pulex irritans*, are practically extinct.

Clinical Features Papules and lentil-sized erythemas with or without a reddened center (the bite wound) are characteristic. A central bloody spot ("purpura pulicosa") is often found there. Lentil-sized to larger wheals with or without a central hemorrhage are also found frequently. The lesions are often grouped or arranged in rows. They are usually found on the legs and on the trunk. Severe itching is a typical symptom.

Therapy Reactions to flea bites heal within a short time spontaneously. Aqueous zinc lotion **(R. 20)** or steroid lotion or cream **(R. 38)** are helpful to relieve itching. The flea stays on the human skin for only a short time. Thorough vacuuming of the residence is usually sufficient for the control of fleas. When only a few fleas are present, the services of an exterminator are not necessary.

Prophylaxis Fleas are often found on hedgehogs, badgers, bats, chickens or pigeons. From there, they frequently migrate to cats and dogs. The involvement of cats and dogs can be demonstrated by combing the fur over a light-colored surface (red flea excrements), especially on the belly, the legs, the tail and behind the ears.

D. Bedbug Bites

The bedbug (*Cimex lectularius*) has a flat, broad body and is found almost everywhere in the world. At night, it leaves its hiding place (cracks in the woodwork, metal, or stone, behind wallpaper, in electrical fuse boxes, behind the mouldings of older houses) and drops from the ceiling onto the sleeper. The reactions from the bites of these blood suckers can be found on the uncovered parts of the body. Clinically, bedbug bites appear as wheals or purple dots. Frequently, a significant number of bedbugs must be present before the bites are discovered. Application of an aqueous zinc shake mixture **(R. 20)** is usually sufficient.

E. Trombidiosis

Trombidiosis is a common disease caused by mites. It frequently occurs in the fall or in the late summer ("harvest mite"). *Trombicula autumnalis* is a mite that lives in herbs, grass, brush, and often in gardens. The mites get on uncovered regions of the skin (ankles, lower legs, etc.) and move to other parts of the body under the patient's clothing. The itchy reactions to the bite are found especially in areas where the clothing fits tightly. The mites liquefy epidermis material with their saliva, eat it, and then fall off the skin when they are finished.

Clinical Features The clinical appearance consists of multiple itching papules or erythemas with central, often hemorrhagic blisters. These foci are often grouped or arranged in a row. The legs and trunk are affected most often, as well as the skin of the abdomen and occasionally the waist. The reactions often last several weeks; there appears to be an individual disposition to them. It is possible that the clinical symptoms are the result of an allergic reaction to the mites or their excrements, similar to scabies.

Therapy Anti-eczematous, desiccating therapy is sufficient, e.g., application of an aqueous zinc shake mixture **(R. 20)**. A full bath is recommended to kill the mites.

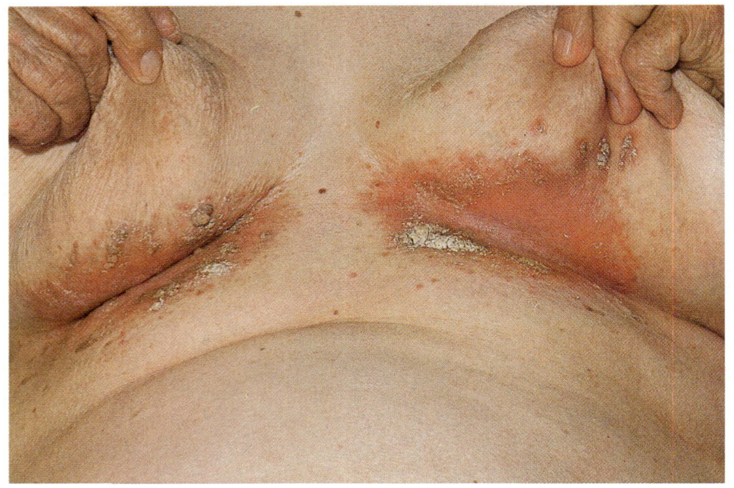

Figure 161 Intertrigo. Relatively sharply delineated, symmetric erythema with weeping and crust formation in the submammary region.

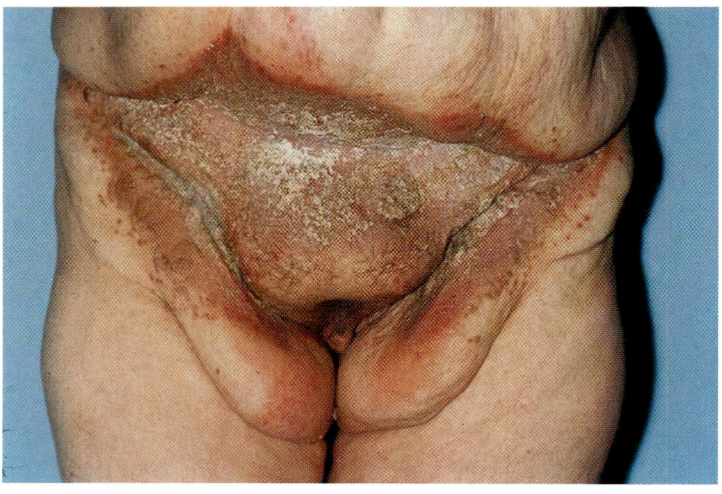

Figure 162 Intertrigo. Extensive involvement in an obese patient.

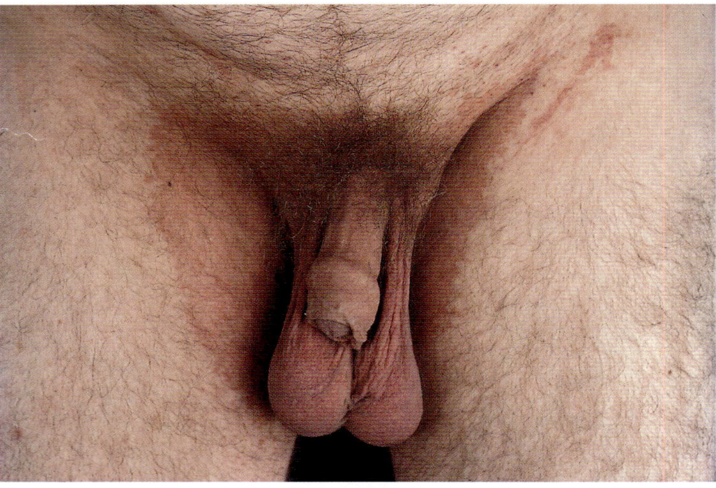

Figure 163 Erythrasma. Symmetrical erythema of long duration in the inguinal region and thighs.

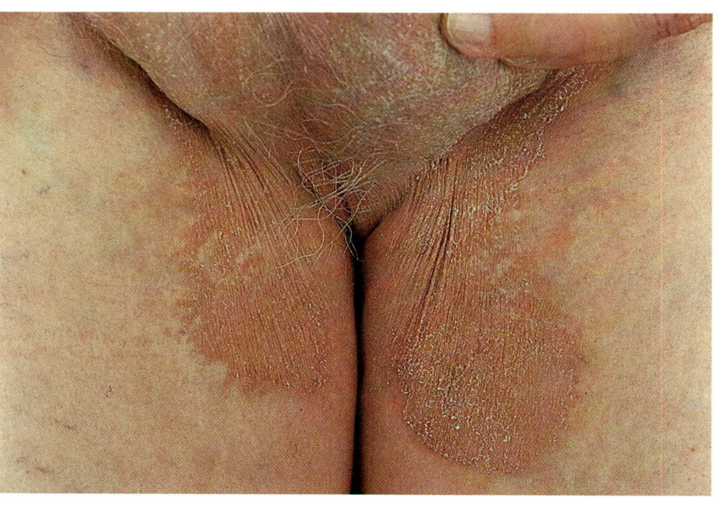

Figure 164 Erythrasma. Sharply delineated, slightly scaling erythema in the inguinal region.

Intertrigo, Erythrasma

A. Intertrigo

Intertrigo is an inflammation of the skin in areas where two skin surfaces are in apposition, especially in obese individuals. Infection with *Candida albicans* (thrush) occurs in practically all long-standing cases (see page 117). Increased sweating, e.g., with fever and in hot weather, encourages intertrigo.

Clinical Features

1. Sharply delineated areas of shiny erythema are characteristic. In advanced cases, the erythema can be weeping and itching. It is often covered with scratch marks and crusts.
2. Areas of predilection are the submammary, inguinal and intergluteal regions.
3. Secondary candidal infection may lead to "satellite lesions", which are disseminated, round, erythematous foci with scaling margins surrounding the main lesion.

Therapy

Symptomatic treatment is rapidly successful in most cases. For small areas, zinc lotion 2 to 3 times daily is helpful. More pronounced inflammation may require pastes **(R. 29)**. For infections with *Candida albicans* which are so common, appropriate local therapy should be used (see page 117).

Prophylaxis

A bland powder should be used to keep the involved areas dry after intertrigo has healed **(R. 11)**. Insertion of linen gauze strips helps to keep the skin surfaces separated. The skin should always be dried thoroughly after washing. A hair dryer can be used for the intertriginous areas. Weight reduction is necessary for obese patients.

B. Erythrasma

This is a common, chronic superficial bacterial infection of the skin with *Corynebacterium minutissimum* and affects mainly adults. Diagnostic criteria are the clinical features and a coral-red fluorescence of the lesions when exposed to Wood's light. The disease is harmless and may not require treatment. Complications have not been reported.

Clinical Features

1. The initially reddish, later brownish, sharply delineated lesions are smooth at first. Later, they show fine plications with mild scaling. Normally, there is no pruritus. Itching may indicate eczematization of long-standing lesions, sometimes in the axillae.
2. Erythrasma is often seen particularly in the inguinal and axillary regions, but also in the interdigital spaces of the toes. Typical are symmetric, sharply delineated patches on the thighs close to the scrotum. There are no satellite lesions.

Therapy

1. Treatment of this harmless disease consists of topical application of imidazole derivatives which are also effective against gram-positive bacteria. They can be applied as creams **(R. 35a)** or as solutions **(R. 14c)**. Prophylactic measures are the same as for intertrigo.
2. Treatment with erythromycin or tetracyclines, which is also effective, is not necessary for this disease, since it is harmless and does not produce subjective symptoms.

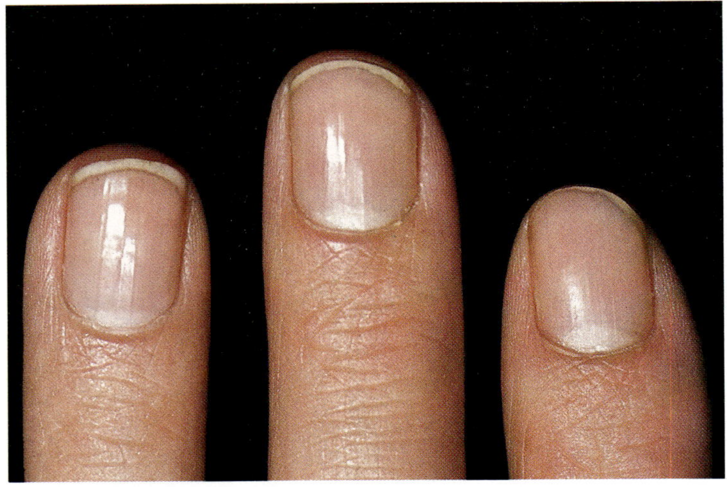

Figure 165 Smoothly polished fingernails from continuous rubbing of the skin to relieve itching.

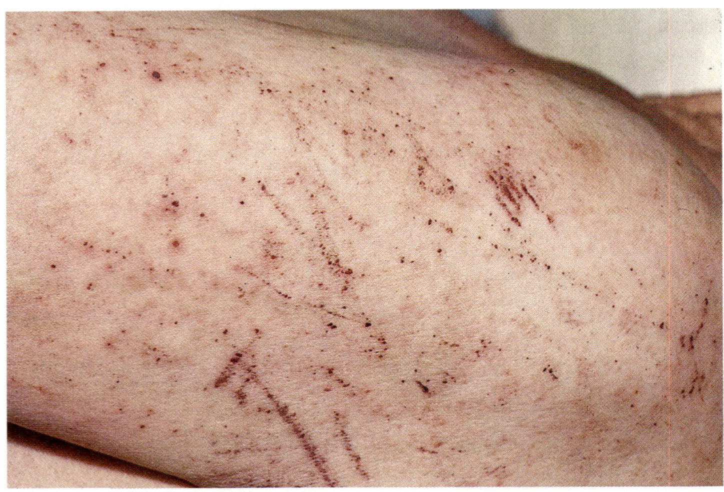

Figure 166 Hemorrhagic scratch marks in a patient with universal pruritus.

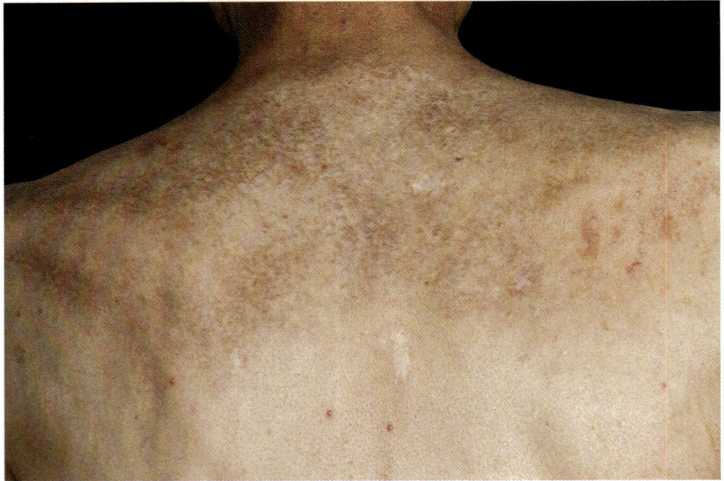

Figure 167 Scratch marks with hyper- and depigmentation, secondary to chronic scratching in a patient with generalized pruritus.

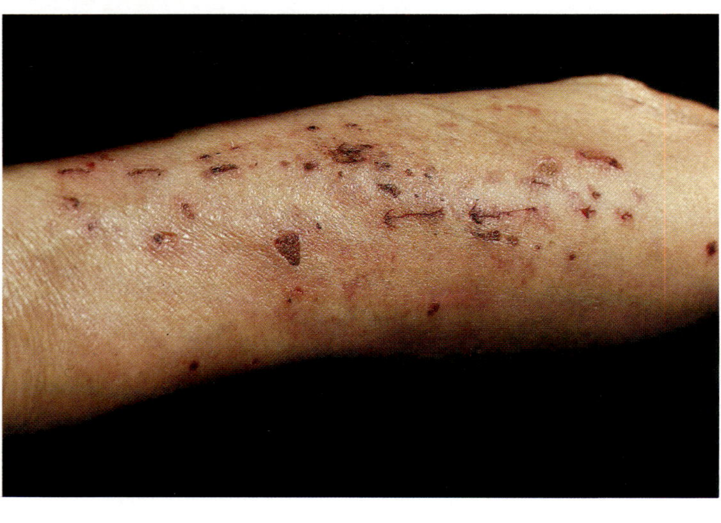

Figure 168 Generalized pruritus in a patient with icterus. Deep scratch marks on the forearm.

Pruritus

A. Generalized Pruritus

Many skin diseases are accompanied by pruritus. Pruritus can also occur as an independent disorder. Its causes can be harmless, such as cold weather, especially in combination with low humidity (central heating), dry skin in the elderly (see page 149), and exaggerated hygiene with excessive bathing and use of alkaline soaps and detergents. On the other hand, there are many serious internal diseases that may be accompanied by generalized pruritus. These include diabetes mellitus, liver and kidney diseases, leukemia, malignant lymphomas, malignant visceral tumors, as well as psychiatric diseases (such as delusions of skin parasitosis and drug abuse). Massive pruritus can also occur during pregnancy. Pruritus can be an adverse side effect of certain medications. Severe pruritus which lasted many months was reported following repeated infusions of hydroxyethylene starch. This makes a thorough medical evaluation necessary in all patients with generalized pruritus, unless a trivial cause is evident. Constant scratching can eventually lead to significant skin damage. Clinically, one may see an eczema, a prurigo or artifacts (see the appropriate chapters).

Clinical Features

1. Scratch marks, usually from several fingers simultaneously and running parallel to each other, are characteristic. The involved skin is otherwise inconspicuous except for occasional erythema or dryness.
2. Shiny, polished fingernails are an obvious indication of habitual scratching.
3. The scratch marks are usually found in areas easily accessible to the hands. Older, less flexible patients often use mechanical aids to scratch other parts of the body.

Therapy

A thorough work-up to find and treat an underlying disease is necessary.

Systemic

1. Antihistamines **(R. 61, 62)**, preferably those with a sedative component, are helpful. In these conditions, the advantages of sedation must be weighed against the disadvantages (reduced responsiveness, driving ability, etc.).
2. Sleeplessness may require the addition of a hypnotic (e.g., chloral hydrate).
3. For severe pruritus, antihistamines with a neuroleptic component (promethazine) are helpful.
4. For delusions of skin parasitosis, neuroleptic drugs, e.g., haloperidol (Haldol) or sedatives, e.g., levomepromazine (Levoprome) can be used. These disorders usually respond to much lower doses than those used for psychiatric diseases (e.g., Haldol 3x 5 drops a day).

External

1. Dehydration of the skin must be avoided by regular skin care with lubricants and emollients **(R. 33b)**, and lubricants may be added to the bath water (**R. 7**).
2. Topical steroid preparations should be used for short periods of time only for marked irritation of the skin.

General

1. Excessive washing may have to be reduced.
2. The room climate should be improved (lower temperature, adequate humidity).
3. Stimulating or hot beverages (coffee, coke, alcohol) should be avoided, especially in the evening.

B. Localized Pruritus

Several regions of the body are sites of predilection for diseases mainly accompanied by pruritus.

Scalp: Seborrheic dermatitis, psoriasis, head lice, acne necroticans.

Periorbital Region: Contact dermatitis caused by cosmetics and airborne allergens.

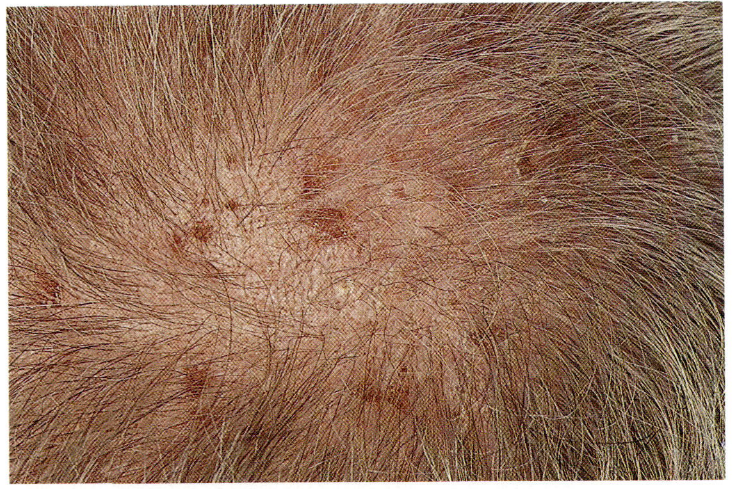

Figure 169 Localized pruritus with round excoriations and impetiguous changes of the scalp. Clinical appearance of “acne necroticans”.

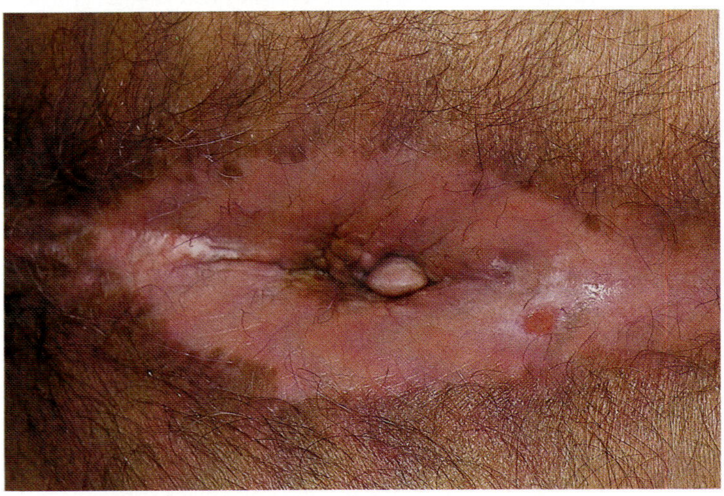

Figure 170 Pruritus ani. Chronic anal eczema with erythema, erosions, hyper- and depigmentation.

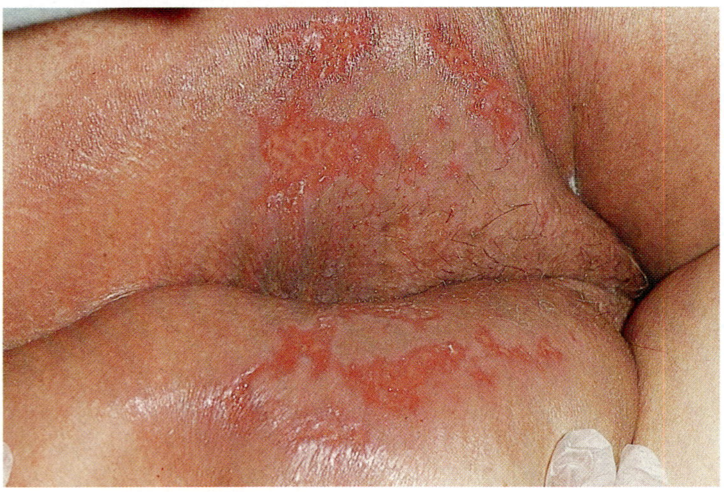

Figure 171 Pruritus ani with extensive erosions as a result of maceration and excoriation.

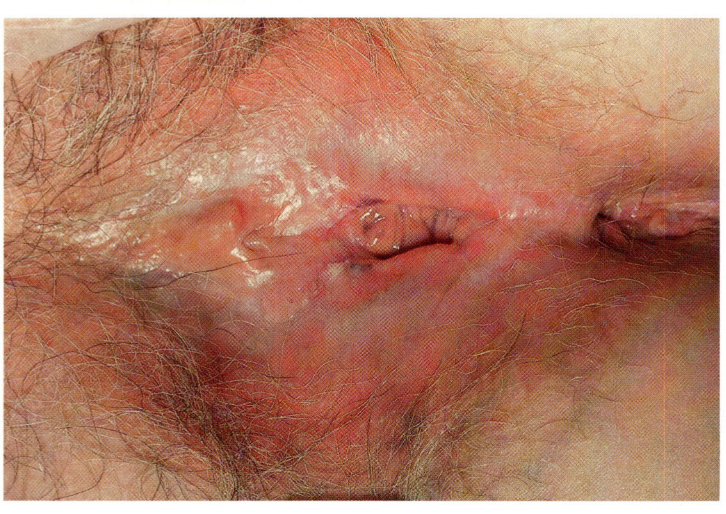

Figure 172 Vulvar pruritus as the main symptom of genital atrophy from lichen sclerosus.

Nose: Hayfever, intestinal parasites in children.

Perianal Region: Oxyures (pinworms), dermatomycoses, *Candida* infection, abuse of laxatives, exaggerated anal hygiene, contact allergies to drugs, hemorrhoids, anal fissures, anal or rectal carcinoma, neuroses or psychoses.

Vulvar Region: Vaginal discharge (*Candida* infection, trichomoniasis, chlamydial infection, mycoplasma infection (genital carcinoma must be excluded!), atopic dermatitis, eczema due to contact allergy, urinary incontinence, pubic lice, mental disorders.

Scrotum: Candida infection, dermatomycoses, contact dermatitis.

Legs: Chronic venous insufficiency.

In individual cases, those causes mentioned above for generalized pruritus can also be responsible for localized pruritus. Dermatoses that cause pruritus can be masked by secondary changes induced by constant scratching, especially in the perianal region, the scrotum, and the vulva, and may not be readily identifiable in the beginning.

Clinical Features

Erythema, scaling, and scratch marks, or when scratching is pronounced, even weeping, crusty lesions covered with thick yellowish crusts as a result of bacterial infection. The constant irritation from prolonged scratching due to persistent pruritus may eventually lead to thickening of the skin and even to "elephant skin".

Therapy

As in generalized pruritus, evaluation of possible etiologies, followed by causal therapy is the treatment of choice. Recommendations for systemic therapy are the same as those for generalized pruritus (see above).

External

1. In acute cases, cold wet dressings should be applied for periods of 60 minutes. The dressings should be changed every 20 minutes.
2. Bland lotions, or creams or ointments **(R. 33b, c, d)** for chronically dry skin are recommended. In exceptional cases, steroids **(R. 38a, b)** may be used for short periods of time.
3. For pruritus in the anogenital region, sitz baths with tar-containing additions 1 to 2 times daily are helpful.
4. Anesthetic substances (with the exception of pramoxine hydrochloride 1%) should not be used for local therapy, since they can cause contact allergies.
5. The skin should be carefully cleansed with warm water and should only be dabbed or blow dried so that it is not rubbed.

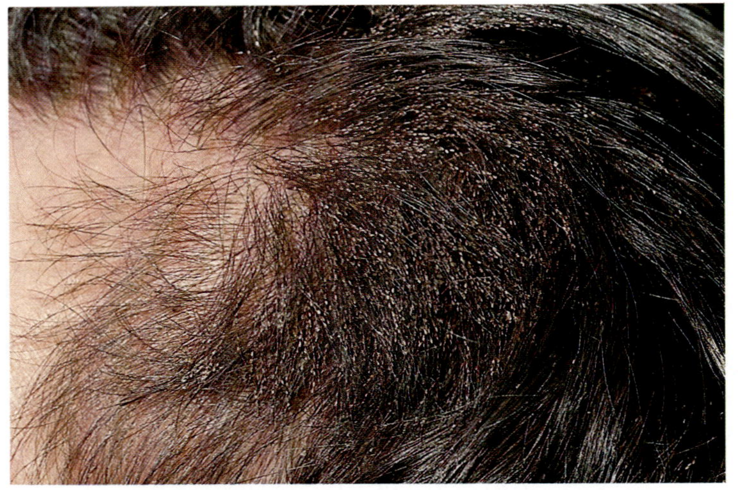

Figure 173 Head lice. Nits attached to the hair like strings of pearls.

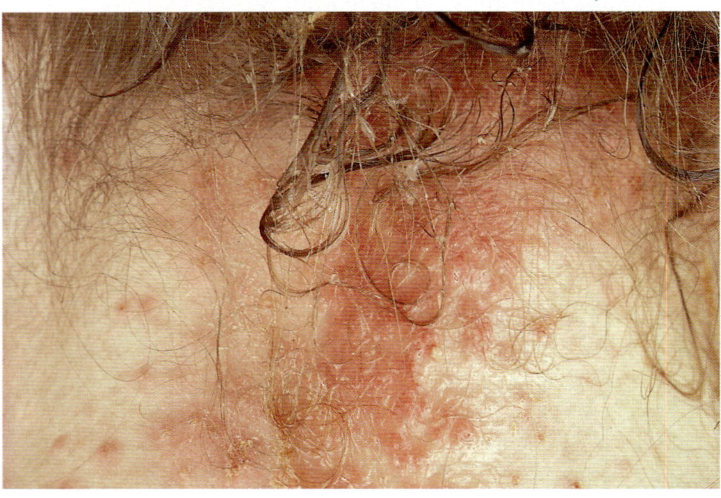

Figure 174 Head lice. Eczema of the neck as a diagnostic sign.

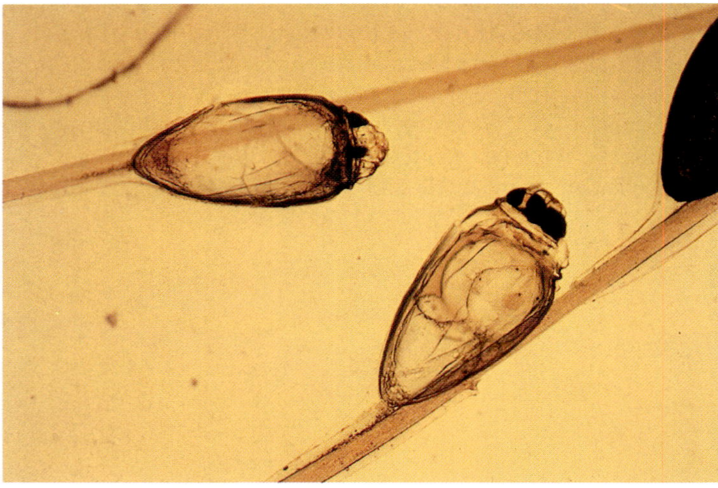

Figure 175 Nits of head lice.

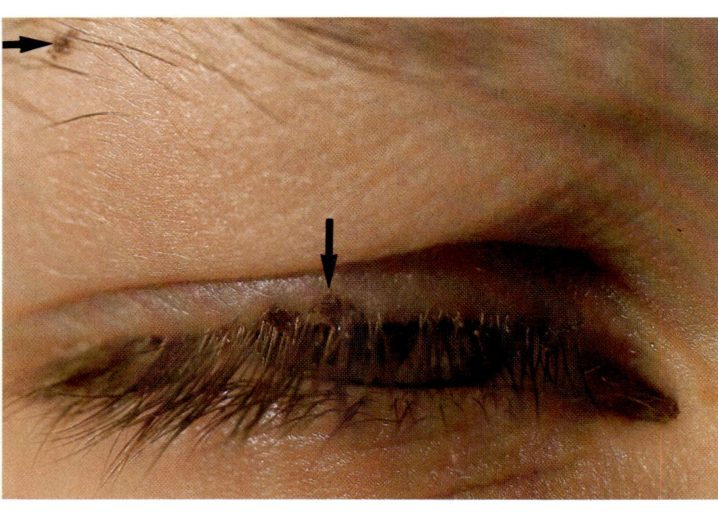

Figure 176 Pubic lice (arrows). Involvement of upper lid and eyebrow.

Lice

Three types of lice have pathogenetic significance in humans: head lice (Pediculus humanus capitis), body lice (Pediculus humanus corporis), and pubic lice (Pediculus pubis).

A. Pediculosis Capitis

Head lice are still found fairly frequently today, especially in children. Despite hygienic conditions, epidemic outbreaks occur from time to time, especially in schools and kindergartens. Adults can be affected as contact persons. Head lice are otherwise rare in adults and are usually found only in neglected patients.

Clinical Features

1. Clinical signs are yellow crusty excoriations with moderate or severe pruritus. Close inspection with a magnifying glass reveals rows of nits attached to the hairs. The nits are approximately 1 mm in diameter. Lice are found less frequently; they are seen in large numbers only in neglected patients.
2. Head lice are found almost exclusively on the scalp, especially behind the ears and in the occipital region. They are approximately 2 to 3 mm long.
3. In patients with long-lasting infestation, there is marked yellowish-purulent eczematization, especially in the occipital and ear regions.

Therapy

1. An antiparasitic preparation **(R. 28)** is recommended. This medication is best used as a gel. The medication should be rubbed thoroughly into the scalp and left for 12 hours.
2. The hair is then washed thoroughly.
3. This treatment is repeated daily for several days.
4. Following this therapy, there is no risk of infection for contact persons. Children can now return to school or kindergarten, even if nits are still visible.
5. Nits are killed by this treatment but continue to adhere to the hair. The following procedure is recommended for removal of the nits: The hair is thoroughly rinsed with diluted vinegar (ordinary cooking vinegar diluted with water 1:1). The hair should be wrapped in a towel soaked in the diluted vinegar for 30 minutes. The nits can then be removed from the drip-wet hair with a fine-tooth comb, and the hair is then washed with a regular shampoo. This procedure is repeated daily until all nits have been removed.
6. Combs, hairbrushes, hats, and bed sheets are washed or cleaned chemically to avoid reinfection.
7. Contact persons (family, kindergarten, school) must be examined and treated if necessary to avoid epidemic spread of the infestation.

B. Pediculosis Corporis

Body lice are on the body only when they suck blood. One must search for them in the clothing. In today's hygienic conditions, they are found almost only on neglected persons. The 3–4.5 mm long body louse is significant from an epidemiologic point of view because it transmits rickettsiae and relapsing fever.

Clinical Features

1. The bite of the body louse causes marked itching. Deep scratch marks and excoriated papules, at times with pyoderma and hyper- and depigmentation, represent the clinical picture of "vagabond's skin" or cutis vagantium.
2. The abnormal changes are found primarily on the trunk, the shoulders and the gluteal area.

Therapy

1. All infested clothing and bedding must be disinfected.
2. Cleansing soap baths and treatment of an existing pyoderma are helpful (see page 131).

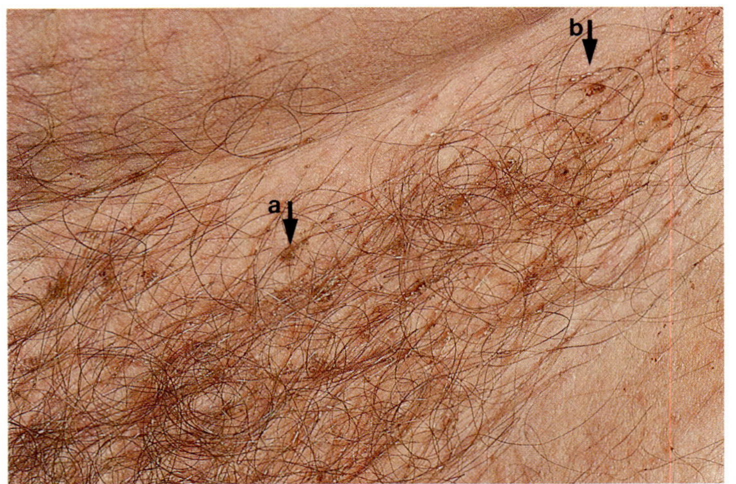

Figure 177 Pediculosis pubis. Pubic lice. Brownish changes (a) that can only be recognized clearly as lice with a magnifying glass, and nits attached to the hairs (b). Lateral pubic hair.

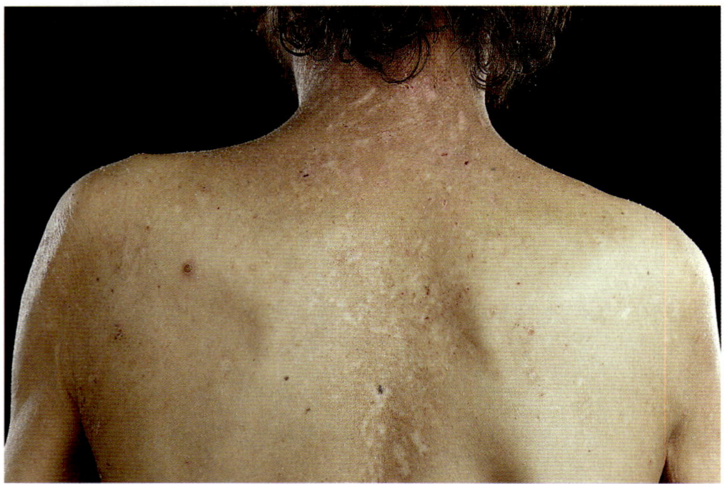

Figure 178 Appearance of the skin in a patient with lice. Scratch marks and postinflammatory pigmentation after long-standing infestation with lice (so-called cutis vagantium).

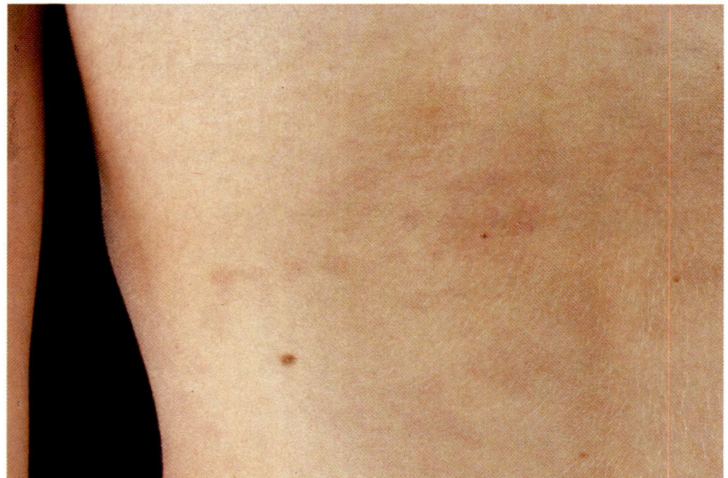

Figure 179 Maculae caeruleae. Pale bluish spots caused by lice bites.

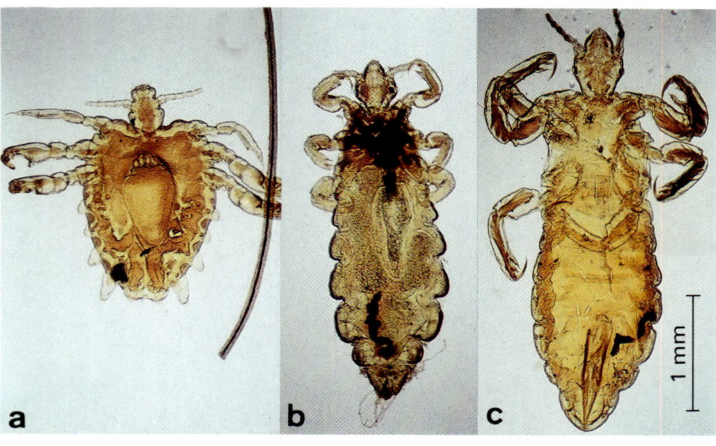

Figure 180 a) Pubic louse, b) head louse, c) body louse. Relative sizes. Magnification 15x.

3. Itching should be treated (see page 85).
4. Body lice are not found on the body, and treatment with contact insecticides is not necessary.

C. Pediculosis Pubis

Pubic lice are found in all hairy body regions with apocrine glands, especially in the anogenital region, the axillae, and occasionally on the eyebrows and eyelashes. Pubic lice are transmitted by close physical contact, mostly during sexual intercourse. They survive outside the human skin for only 1 or 2 days; indirect transmission is extremely rare.

Clinical Features

Maculae caeruleae, pale blue spots of up to fingernail size due to bites, are indicative of pubic lice. They cause moderate to severe itching. The 2 mm long lice and the 1 mm long nits attached to the hairs are easily overlooked on superficial inspection. The lice are normally firmly attached to the hairs and are immobile. They can be stimulated to move by careful scratching and are then readily identified even without a magnifying glass.

Therapy

1. Cleansing bath.
2. Antiparasitic gel **(R. 28)** is applied to all infested areas of the body, except the eyelashes, for 12 hours. This treatment should be carried out on 3 subsequent days. The eyelashes and eyebrows are cleaned mechanically with tweezers after suffocation with vaseline (2x daily for 1 week).
3. Examination and treatment of contact persons.

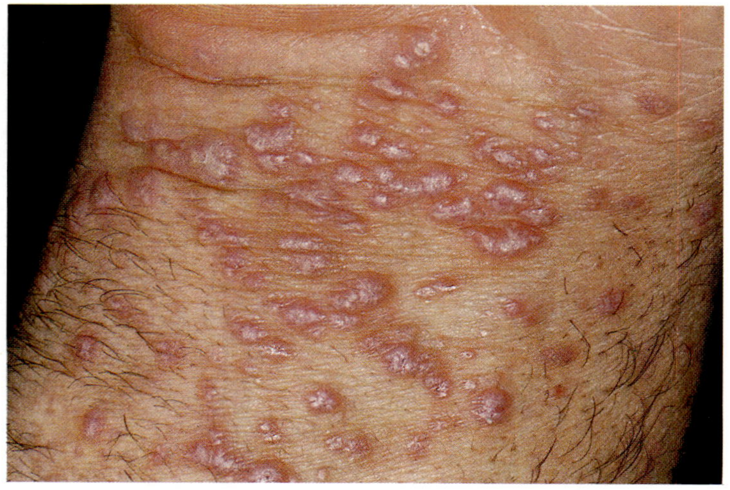

Figure 181 Lichen planus. Polygonal, firm, blue-red papules with slightly shiny surface on the wrist. Reticulated white lines (Wickham's striae) on the papules.

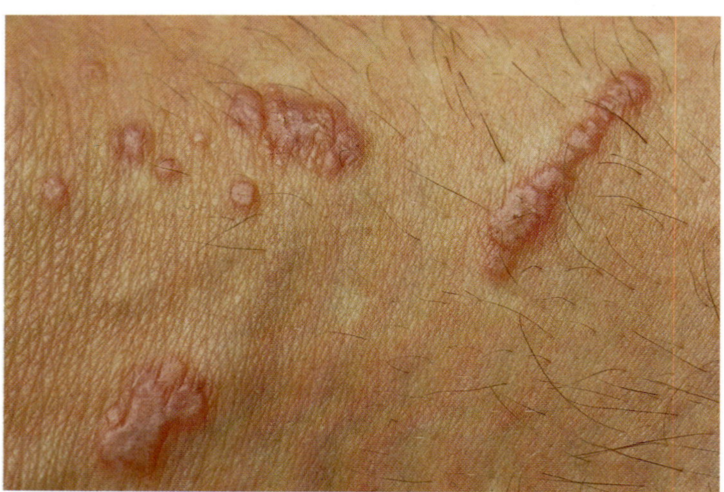

Figure 182 Lichen planus. Koebner's phenomenon: Development of lichen planus papules along a scratch mark.

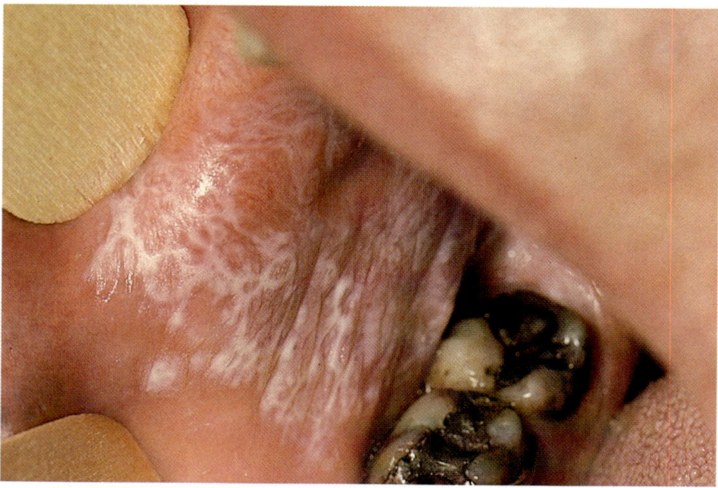

Figure 183 Lichen planus. Pronounced reticulated white coloring of the buccal mucosa.

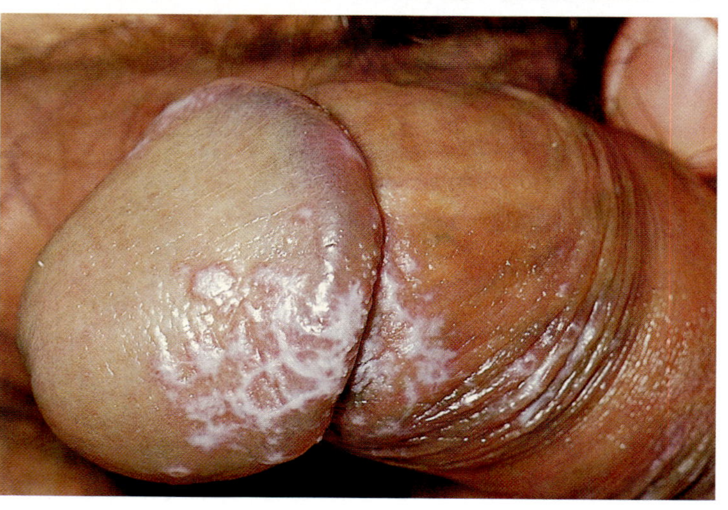

Figure 184 Lichen planus. The same reticular markings on penis and foreskin.

Lichen Planus

Lichen planus is a skin disorder that lasts several weeks or months and occasionally several years. It is characterized by widespread eruption of individual papules that can coalesce to form larger lesions. The etiology is unknown. In rare cases, the disease can be evoked by drugs (such as gold, pyritinol or penicillamine), or by transplantation of immune-competent stem cells (graft-versus-host reaction). Lichen planus lesions can develop at the site of a skin injury (Koebner's phenomenon).

Clinical Features

1. The individual lesion of the disease is a flat, smooth, polygonal papule of dark red, or often bluish-red color (violaceous).
2. The individual lesions often coalesce to form larger lesions. Dabbing the papules with oil makes a network of white lines visible (Wickham's striae). Other lesions are ring-shaped (ca. 1 cm in diameter) with a raised margin and depressed, often pigmented, center. Some lesions are hyperkeratotic.
3. Pruritus is practically always present and is mostly severe, especially in the initial stage.
4. Areas of predilection are the flexor sides of the hand, but lichen planus can affect almost any area of the skin. The lesions often appear as individual papules in a rash-like distribution, especially on the trunk.
5. Involvement of the oral mucosa can be an isolated observation; it is very characteristic and confirms the diagnosis. The buccal mucosa shows a network of prominent white lines with occasional erosions. The tongue, gingiva and lips can also be affected.
6. The genital mucosa is involved less frequently with a network of white lines that may be raised or appear ring-shaped.
7. The lesions often heal with a residual melanin pigmentation as result of damage to the melanocytes.

Therapy

Causal therapy is rarely possible. The goal of treatment is to diminish itching and expedite involution of the lesions. Consultation with a dermatologist is recommended. Topical treatment takes precedence; systemic treatment should only be considered if local treatment is unsuccessful. Erosive changes of the oral mucosa (precancerous) require treatment and regular follow-up until they are completely healed.

Systemic

1. Treatment is antipruritic; if necessary, antihistamines with a sedative component **(R. 62)** should be given.
2. Acitretin **(R. 64)** is effective, especially for mucosal involvement. Skin changes do not respond quite as well to this medication.
3. Systemic steroids are effective, but their use is generally not recommended since the lesions promptly recur after the drug is discontinued.

External

1. Topical therapy can be tried with steroid ointments **(R. 38c)** or with tar preparations.
2. Lichen planus lesions of the oral mucosa that are closed do not require treatment and are hardly accessible. Topical treatment can be tried with a corticosteroid preparation **(R. 38e)**.
3. For erosive foci of the oral mucosa, topical corticosteroids as well as topical vitamin A acid preparations are helpful. Good results have been reported with Retin-A gel 0.025–0.01%. In severe cases, systemic acitretin has been used with good results. For long-term therapy, advantages and disadvantages should be considered carefully because of the possible side effects of this medication.

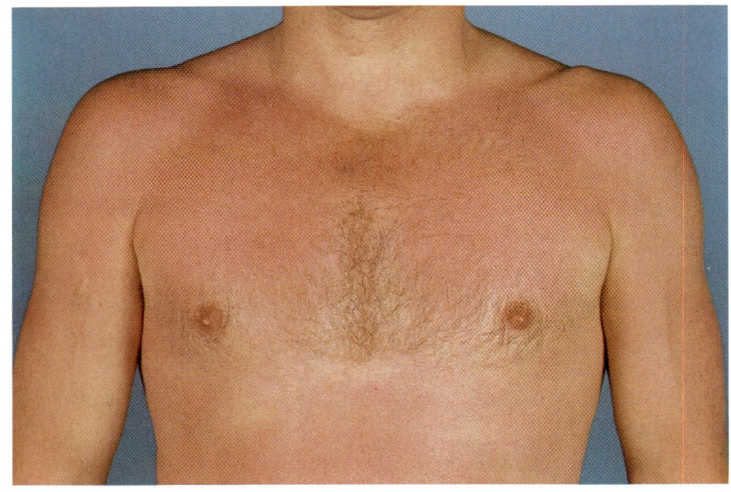

Figure 185 Sunburn. Dermatitis solaris.

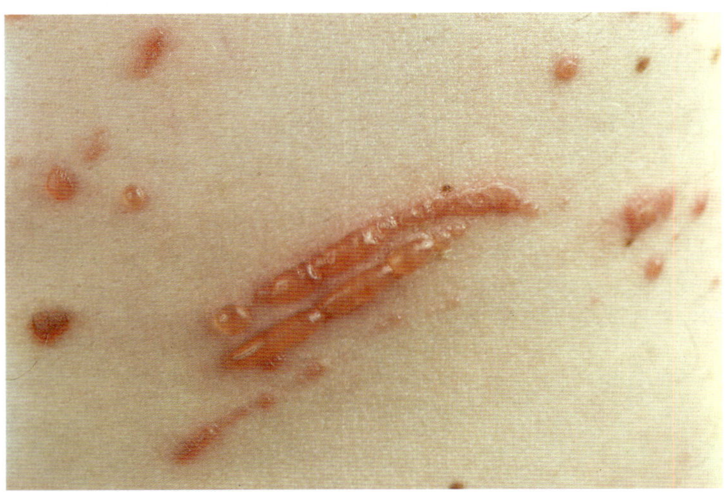

Figure 186 So-called grass dermatitis. Phototoxic reaction with typical vesicular and erythematous streaks caused by furocoumarins from acanthus plants.

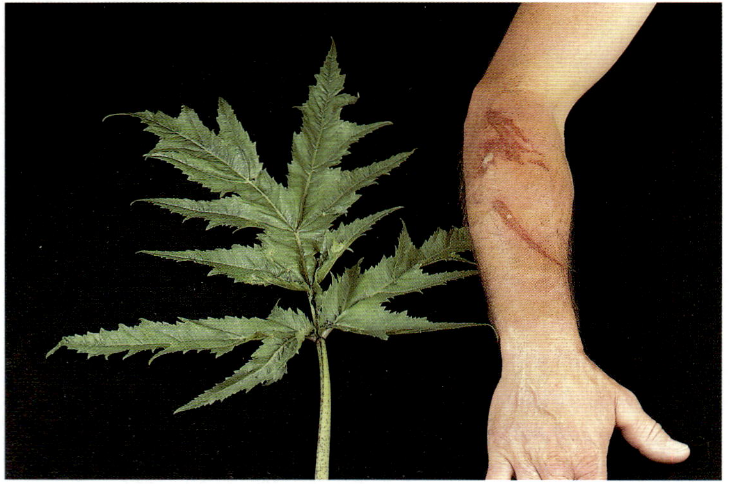

Figure 187 Phototoxic dermatitis with linear blisters caused by contact with acanthus (Heracleum).

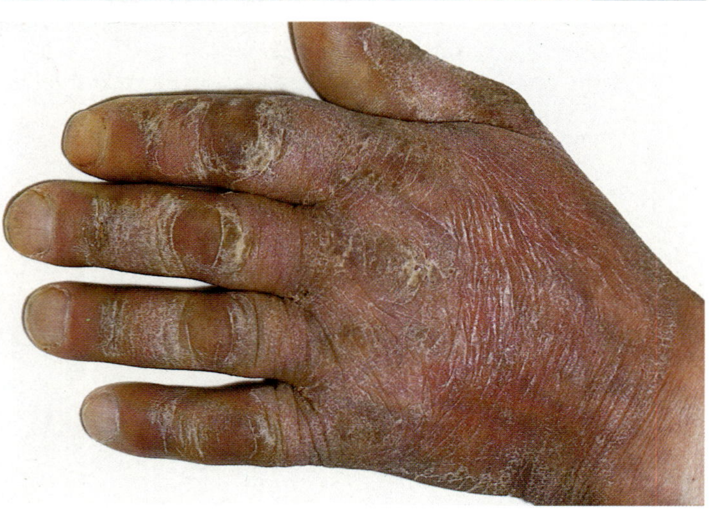

Figure 188 Phototoxic dermatitis. Sharply delineated erythema with scaling.

Sun Reactions

An overdose of natural or artificial light (UV) causes a radiation reaction of the skin to varying degrees – sunburn – depending on the individual's pigmentation. Sensitivity to light is determined genetically; it is high in persons with blond hair and light skin and very low in blacks and people of Asian origin. Internal or external use of various substances can also increase sensitivity to light to a point where a dose of UV radiation that would otherwise be tolerated can cause an undesirable UV reaction. In addition to these phototoxic reactions, which can be produced in any person, there are certain substances that can cause photoallergic reactions. Furthermore, some skin diseases, such as lupus erythematosus, herpes simplex, porphyria cutanea tarda and rosacea can be provoked or aggravated by UV radiation. Finally, there are long-term injuries from prolonged exposure to UV radiation, even doses below the erythema dose. These injuries include damage to the connective tissue of the skin and induction of actinic keratoses, squamous cell carcinoma, basal cell carcinoma and melanoma.

A. Sunburn (Dermatitis Solaris)

Clinical Features

1. A mild erythema appears approximately 30 minutes after UV exposure (sunlight, sunlamp). This reaction is followed by a long-lasting pigmentation. Excessive exposure leads to edema and blister formation after several hours, depending on the intensity of the radiation. The maximal reaction is reached after 24 hours and then disappears rapidly. This is followed by desquamation of the skin and later by a long-lasting, occasionally spotty pigmentation, depending on the extent of the damage.
2. Only the exposed areas are affected.
3. Pruritus and burning, which can disturb the patient's sleep, occur frequently. Severe and extensive sunburn can cause generalized symptoms, such as headache, fever and even shock.

Therapy

1. Wet, cool dressings are of great relief **(R. 1)**.
2. For more severe symptoms, steroid lotions or creams are helpful **(R. 38a, b, c)**.
3. Patients who are particularly sensitive to light should use a sunscreen with a high protective factor **(R. 45)** as a prophylactic measure.
4. In cases of severe sunburn, early administration of aspirin or indomethacin can alleviate the symptoms caused by the release of inflammation mediators. Systemic steroids are less effective in these cases.

B. Phototoxic Reactions

These are sunburn-like reactions of the skin to a dose of UV radiation (UVA) that would normally be tolerated. The skin reaction is caused by simultaneous external or internal use of a substance that increases sensitivity to light (photosensitizer). These substances include medications, such as tetracyclines, vegetable substances, such as furocoumarins (contained in plants of the acanthus family or in bergamot oil) or in coal tar.

Clinical Features

1. An acute dermatitis with erythema, edema and blister or bulla formation appears a few hours after exposure to UV light.
2. The skin changes are limited strictly to the body regions exposed to the light.

Therapy

Treatment is the same as that for sunburn (see above).

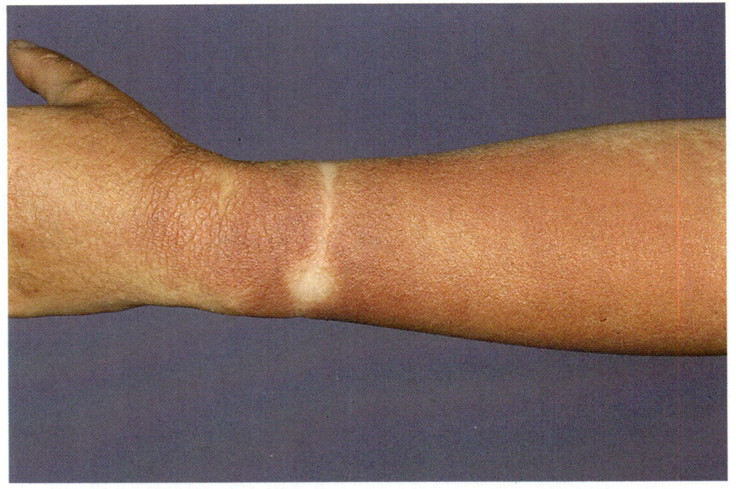

Figure 189 Phototoxic drug reaction. Increased sensitivity to light in a patient treated with carbutamide. The area covered by the wristwatch is distinctly unaffected.

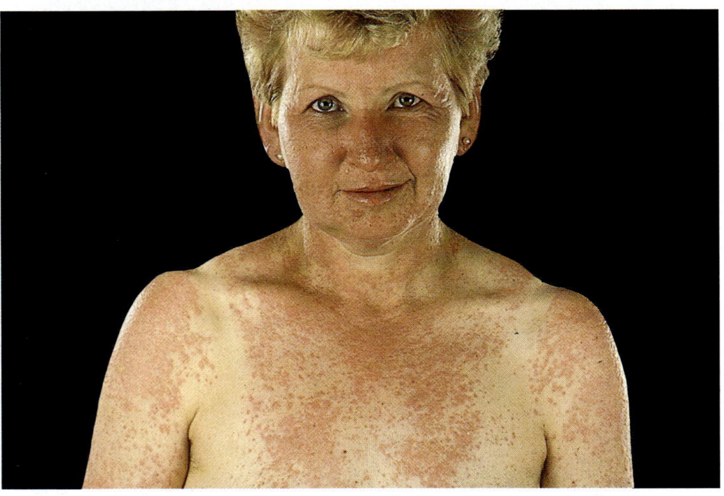

Figure 190 Photoallergic drug reaction from pyrimethamine-sulfadoxine (Fansidar).

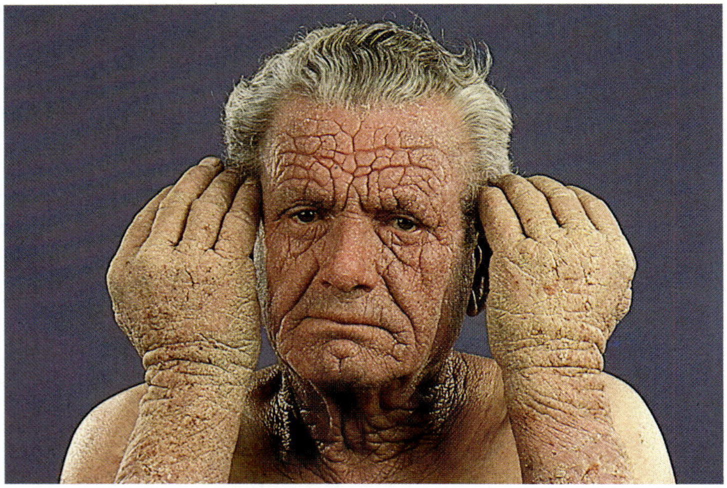

Figure 191 Chronic light reaction; so-called actinic reticuloid. Appearance of chronic eczema with massive thickening of the skin and furrowing on the light-exposed areas of the body.

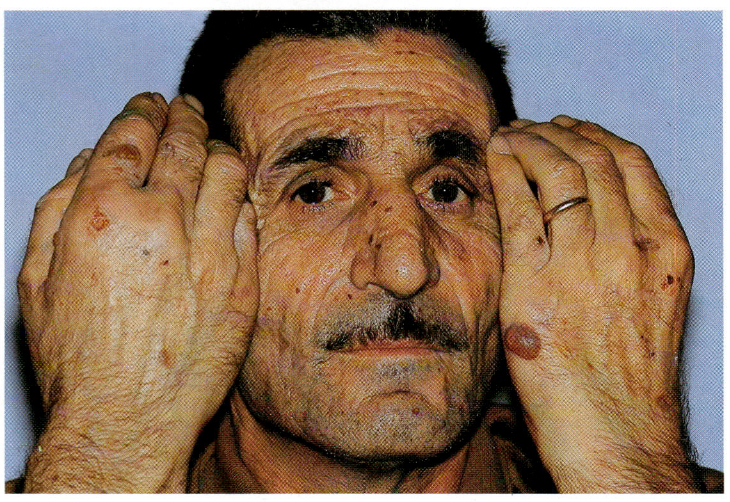

Figure 192 Porphyria cutanea tarda. Blisters and erosions on skin areas exposed to light, especially dorsum of the hand, forehead and nose.

C. Photoallergic Reactions

These reactions occur only in sensitized individuals upon exposure to light (UVA). Frequent photoallergens are salicylanilides, sulfonamides and phenothiazine derivatives.

Clinical Features

1. The clinical appearance is that of an allergic contact dermatitis (see page 37). Occasionally, the photoallergic reaction is manifest as an urticaria.
2. The skin changes are most pronounced in the exposed areas but are not as sharply delineated as those of a phototoxic reaction. Occasionally, there can be disseminated lesions in the unexposed skin.
3. There is marked pruritus that subsides very slowly.
4. The clinical course is protracted, contrary to that of a phototoxic reaction. It can last several weeks.

Therapy

1. Detection and elimination of the photoallergen is of primary importance, if necessary through special tests (photo patch test) performed by a dermatologist.
2. A sunscreen that will protect against UVA radiation must be used. One must keep in mind that UVA radiation penetrates window glass.
3. Topical therapy is the same as that for acute contact dermatitis (see page 39).
4. Sunlight must be avoided (broad-brimmed hat, long sleeves, gloves).

D. Persistent Light Reaction, Actinic Reticuloid

Clinical Features

If a photoallergy is not recognized early enough, it can result in a persistent light reaction after several years. This means that the symptoms of the disease (the morphology corresponds to a chronic dermatitis) can be provoked and maintained by light exposure alone, without an allergen. Actinic reticuloid is the most severe form of a persistent light reaction that is elicited not only by UV light but also by visible light.

Therapy

Thorough light protection with opaque sunscreen preparations (Reflecta, UV-Paque, zinc oxide cream) and clothing impermeable to light. Chronic light dermatitis can be severe enough that systemic administration of immunosuppressive drugs may become necessary. These patients should be referred to a dermatologist.

E. Porphyria Cutanea Tarda

The symptoms of porphyria cutanea tarda are a special form of phototoxic reaction of the skin. The disease is caused by a disorder in the porphyrin metabolism with elevation of the uroporphyrins stored in several organs, including the skin. The disorder is often hereditary. The disease itself is frequently evoked by chronic liver disorders (alcohol, post-hepatitis, drug-induced, toxic).

Clinical Features

Dense bullae, followed by poorly healing erosions, appear after minimal trauma. The patient develops dark skin color and hypertrichosis, especially on the upper, lateral parts of the face.

Therapy

Internal

1. Chloroquine, 125 mg two times per week.
2. Phlebotomy to reduce the markedly elevated serum iron.
3. Alkalinization of the urine and regular monitoring of the urinary pH (7.2–7.5). This enhances elimination of the porphyrins.
4. Substances toxic to the liver (alcohol, drugs) must be avoided.

External

Sunscreening with pastes or lotions is necessary because maximum absorption of porphyrins takes place in the spectrum of visible light.

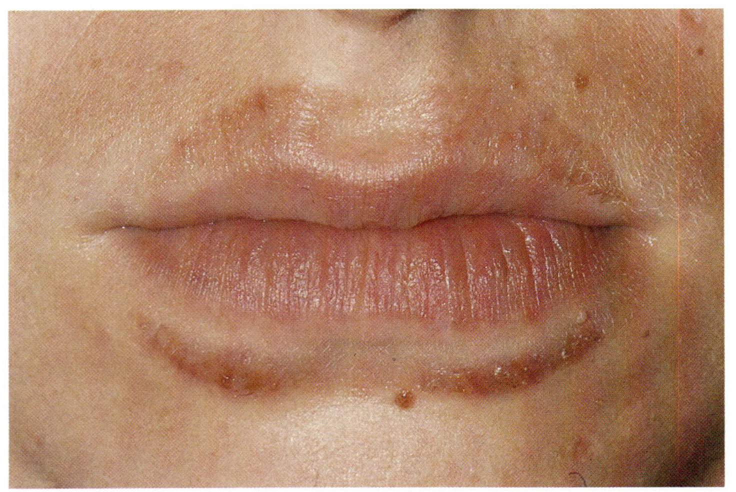

Figure 193 Cheilitis caused by lip-licking. Inflammatory erythema and crusts caused by habitual licking of the perioral area.

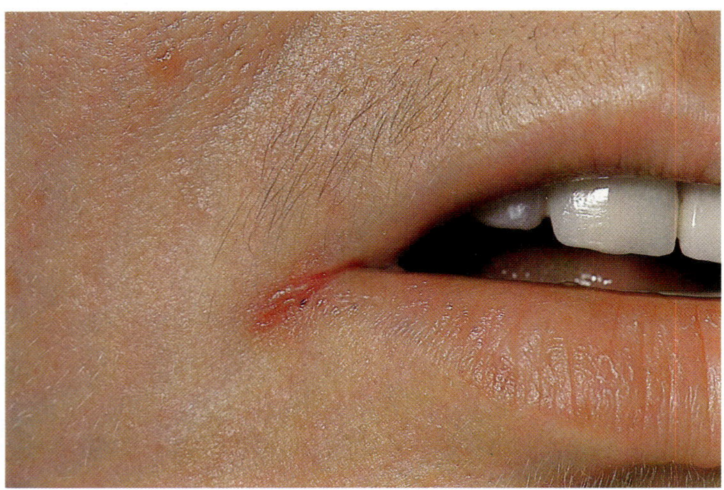

Figure 194 Perlèche. Inflammatory rhagade in the corner of the mouth.

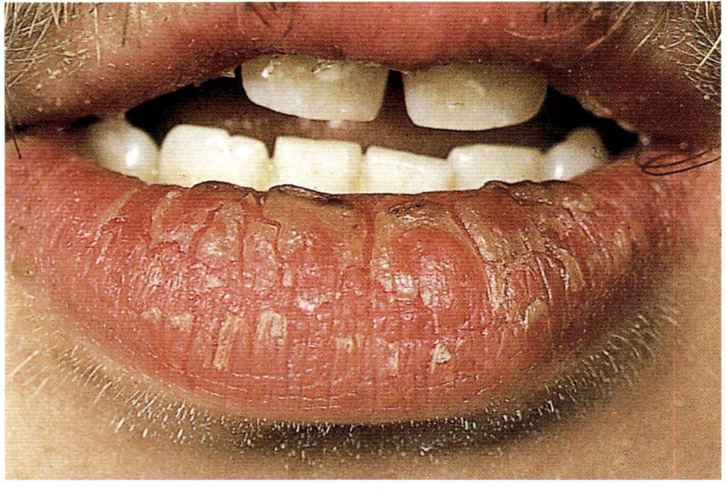

Figure 195 Cheilitis simplex chronica. Scaling and crust formation with radial tears.

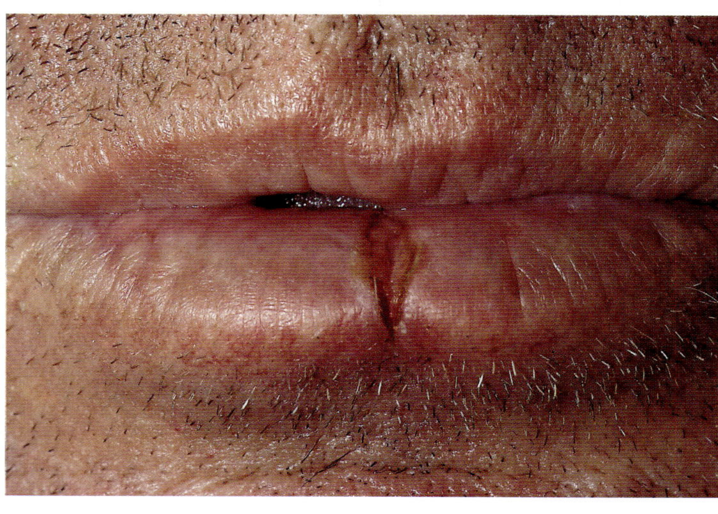

Figure 196 Rhagade of the lower lip.

Inflammations of the Lips

A. Lip-Licking Cheilitis

This disorder is seen frequently in children (almost always patients with atopic dermatitis) and is the result of habitual licking of the upper or lower lip, or both, with the tongue, or constant moistening with the other lip.

Clinical Features The typical appearance is a sickle-shaped erythema with a raised margin in that area of the lip that can be reached by the tongue or the other lip. Crust formation with secondary infection by bacterial or mycotic organisms (*Candida albicans*) is a frequent finding.

Therapy Topical treatment with imidazole derivatives is effective (also effective against gram-positive bacteria) **(R. 35a)**. Treatment has lasting success, provided the child's habit can be broken.

B. Perlèche, Angular Cheilitis

This is a symptom that can have many causes: Atopic dermatitis, staphylococcal infections (in children), increased skin creases, hypersalivation, generalized diseases, and poorly fitting dentures. Secondary infection with *Candida albicans* occurs frequently.

Clinical Features Rhagades can be found in the corners of the mouth, at times with eczematization. Pruritus is minimal.

Therapy The causative factors must be eliminated. Topical treatment of *Candida albicans* infection with imidazole derivatives **(R. 35a)** or nystatin **(R. 35c)** for 1 to 2 weeks.

C. Chronic Actinic Cheilitis, Chronic Light-Induced Inflammation of the Lips

Chronic light-induced inflammation of the lower lip is often seen in persons who work outdoors. Chronic actinic cheilitis must be regarded as a facultatively precancerous lesion.

Clinical Features The red of the lips becomes paler through thickening of the epithelium. The borders between lips and skin become less distinct. The lip is thickened and may be covered with painful erosions or crusts. The lower lip is most often involved, rarely the upper lip. Wind and cold make the condition worse and occasionally produce rhagades.

Therapy Sunlight should be avoided as much as possible. Topical treatment consists of lubricating, bland ointment bases **(R. 33a, b)**, and prophylaxis with sunscreen preparations **(R. 45)**.

D. Thrush Cheilitis, Candidiasis of the Lips

Extensive thrush infection of the oral mucosa can involve the lips.

Clinical Features There is swelling and erythema of the lips, occasionally with augmented or newly formed rhagades in the corners of the mouth.

Therapy Treatment is the same as that for other candidal infections (see pages 117 and 119).

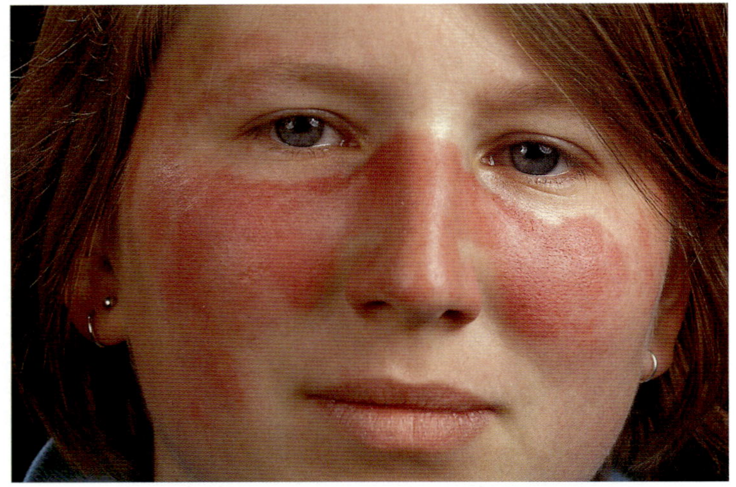

Figure 197 Systemic lupus erythematosus. Butterfly rash.

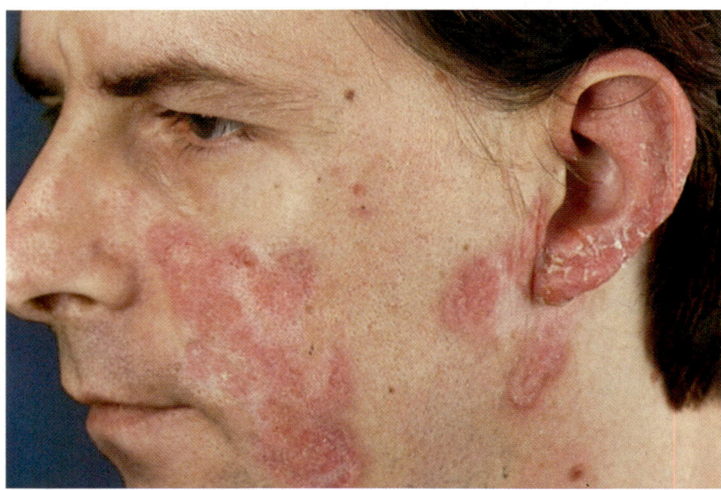

Figure 198 Discoid lupus erythematosus. Extensive infiltrates have a slight depression in the center and show markedly enlarged follicle openings. Destruction of the rim of the concha is typical of the disease.

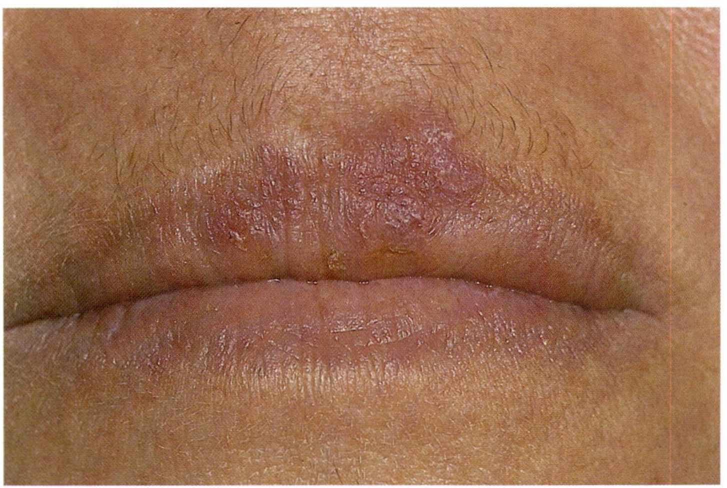

Figure 199 Discoid lupus erythematosus. Persistent infiltrates that spread to the red of the lips.

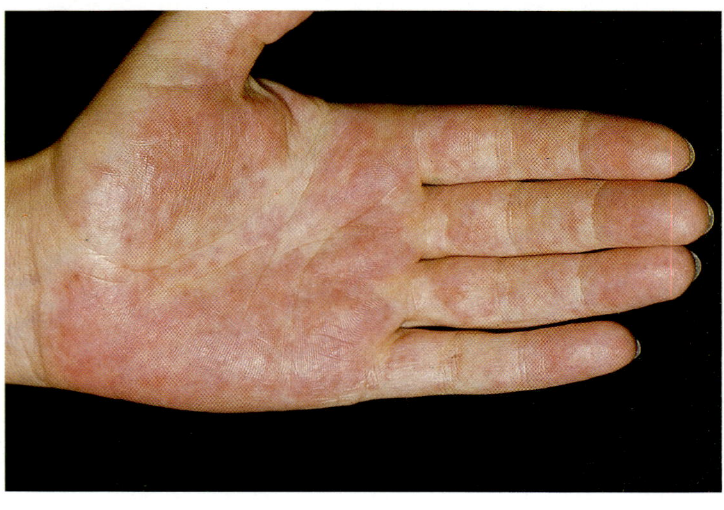

Figure 200 Systemic lupus erythematosus. Bluish-red erythemas of the palm.

Lupus Erythematosus

Two separate forms of lupus erythematosus can be distinguished that, on rare occasion, can blend into one another: Systemic lupus erythematosus (SLE) is a serious generalized disease involving mainly internal organs which predominantly affects young women. Discoid lupus erythematosus (DLE) is limited to the skin. At first glance, it is often impossible to tell which of the two disorders is present, so that a thorough examination of the entire patient is necessary. DLE is a chronic dermatologic disease that lasts for months or even years. Increased exposure to light, as well as prior liver disease promote its development. Autoantibodies that are characteristic for lupus erythematosus (anti-ds-DNA, antibodies against organs, etc.) are found in the serum of SLE patients.

A. Systemic Lupus Erythematosus

Clinical Features

1. Cutaneous symptoms are present in approximately three fourths of all patients. A butterfly-shaped, fixed erythema of the face ("butterfly rash") is typical of the disease. Long-lasting erythematous changes with hemorrhages can be found in the nail folds. The trunk can exhibit an uncharacteristic macular eruption with maculae of varying sizes. Hemorrhage and ulceration of the oral mucosa can also be found.
2. Symptoms of the generalized disease, such as polyarthritis, polymyositis, nephritis, myocarditis and pericarditis, as well as mental dysfunctions from CNS involvement, often predominate.
3. The patients complain of malaise to widely varying degrees, fatigue, lassitude and sometimes even prolonged fever attacks.

Therapy

This is a severe and even today sometimes fatal disease that almost always requires, at least in severe cases, hospitalization of the patient for diagnostic procedures and introduction of immunosuppressive therapy.

B. Discoid Lupus Erythematosus

Clinical Features

1. Discoid lupus erythematosus foci with raised borders and a depressed center that exhibits scaling, enlarged follicular openings, and occasionally small keratotic cores are characteristic. The skin is atrophic in the central zones, and a scar remains after the lesion has healed. Less chronic lesions show persistent infiltrates which look like wheals.
2. The face and neck are predominantly involved, especially in the infraorbital region, but also the nose and other parts of the face are involved.
3. The infiltrates hurt if stroked by a fingernail.

Therapy

1. Avoiding exposure to UV light is of foremost importance. In addition, the skin should be protected by appropriate clothing and sunscreen preparations **(R. 45)**.
2. Symptomatic topical therapy consists of corticosteroid ointments **(R. 38c)**, which can be additionally covered by an occlusive plastic wrap (see page 253).
3. Systemic steroids, immunosuppressive or cytostatic drugs are not necessary for discoid lupus erythematosus.
4. In severe cases, systemic hydroxychloroquine (Plaquenil), 250 mg daily is useful during the sunny season. These patients should be examined regularly by an ophthalmologist for early detection of retinopathy. Consultation with a dermatologist is recommended.

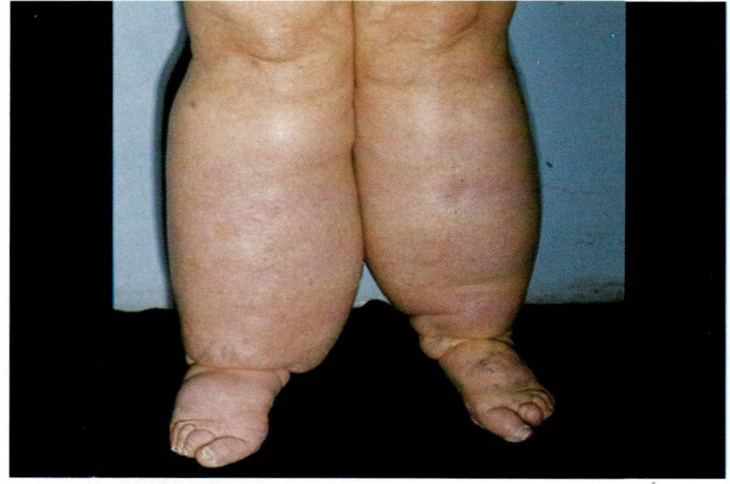

Figure 201 Chronic lymphedema. Elephantiasis. Monstrous persistent swelling following recurrent erysipelas.

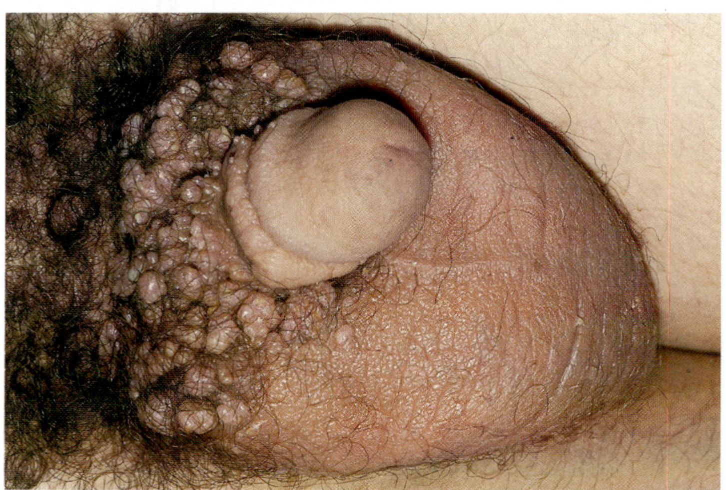

Figure 202 Chronic lymphedema of the scrotum with secondary development of tumor-like dilatations of the lymphatic vessels.

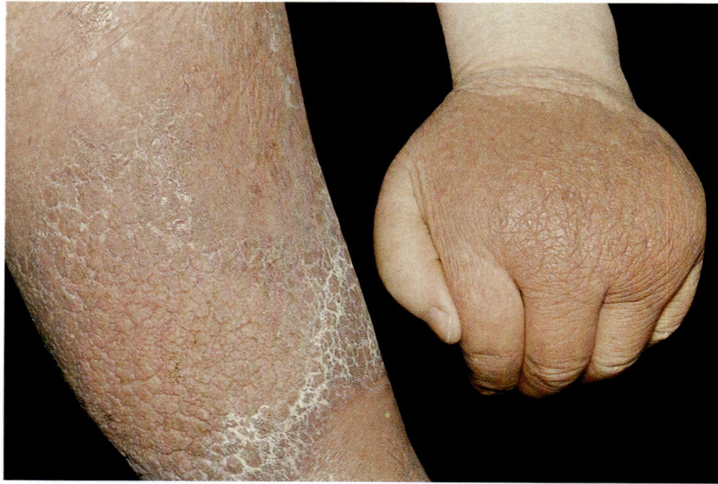

Figure 203 Chronic lymphedema with secondary thickening of the skin, papillomatosis and induration.

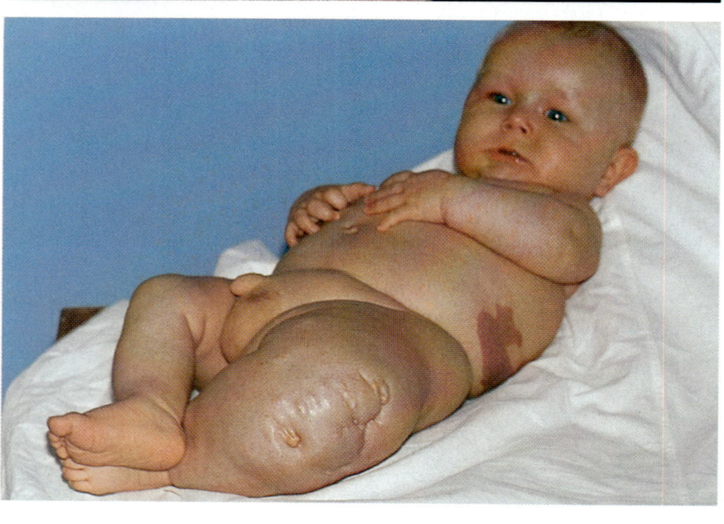

Figure 204 Massive lymphedema in a patient with congenital hematolymphangioma.

Lymphedema

Chronic persistent lymphedema develops where drainage of interstitial fluid is inadequate. The practicing physician usually sees secondary lymphedema. A primary lymphedema, generally due to congenital hypoplasia of the lymphatic vessels, is very rare. The most frequent cause of secondary lymphedema in the northern hemisphere is chronic, recurrent erysipelas (see page 57). Other causes are malignant tumors with blockage of the lymphatic vessels or obstruction of the lymph ducts secondary to operative procedures on the lymph nodes, usually in the axillary or inguinal area. A rare complication of chronic lymph stasis is the development of a lymphangiosarcoma (Stewart-Treves syndrome).

Clinical Features

1. Initially, there is pitting edema that disappears completely following elevation of the limb. In longer-standing cases, the formation of new connective tissue leads to increasing induration with warty, sulcated skin and hyperkeratoses. Continued and increasing swelling produces massive deformity of the affected body regions: "elephantiasis".
2. Lymphedema most frequently involves the legs, arms, and genitals.
3. Long-standing edema with increased pressure of the interstitial fluid leads to the formation of small, isolated, skin-colored, tumor-like enlargements of the lymphatic vessels that resemble condylomata acuminata. They emit lymphatic fluid either spontaneously or when punctured. Widespread, malodorous macerations often develop with extensive involvement.

Therapy

Before a primary lymphedema is diagnosed, a secondary lymphedema and its possible causes must be excluded and treated (see above).

Systemic

1. Erysipelas which recurs in short intervals requires long-term prophylaxis with a depot penicillin for at least several months.
2. All possible entry sites for a chronic erysipelas must be eliminated (see page 57).
3. Diuretics are not helpful in the treatment of chronic lymphedema.

External

1. Compression therapy is possible for lymphedema of the extremities, especially the legs, where it is also necessary to prevent the previously mentioned complications. This therapy must be carried out with elastic stockings of compression class III or, even better, IV. Putting these stockings on is difficult and requires strength. Treatment is effective only when it is followed regularly. It is important to elevate the legs for several hours during the day, if possible, especially before the stockings are applied.
2. These measures can be assisted by drainage of the lymphatic fluid either manually or mechanically.
3. Surgical reconstructive procedures are indicated only in exceptional cases for primary lymphedema.

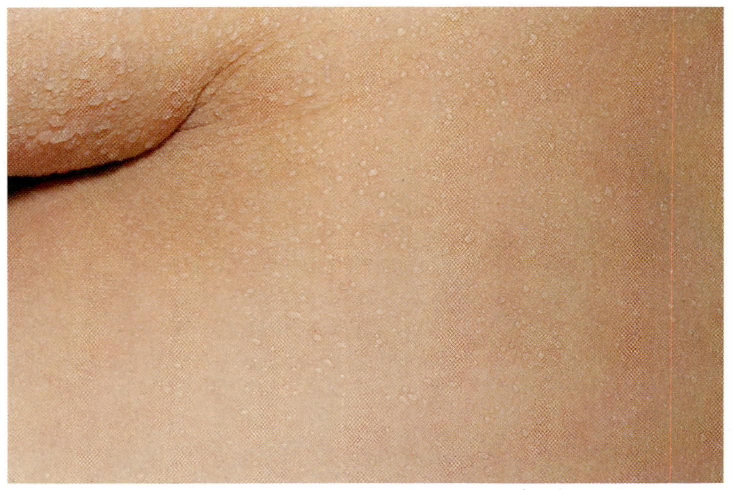

Figure 205 Miliaria cristallina. Disseminated vesicles without inflammatory reaction.

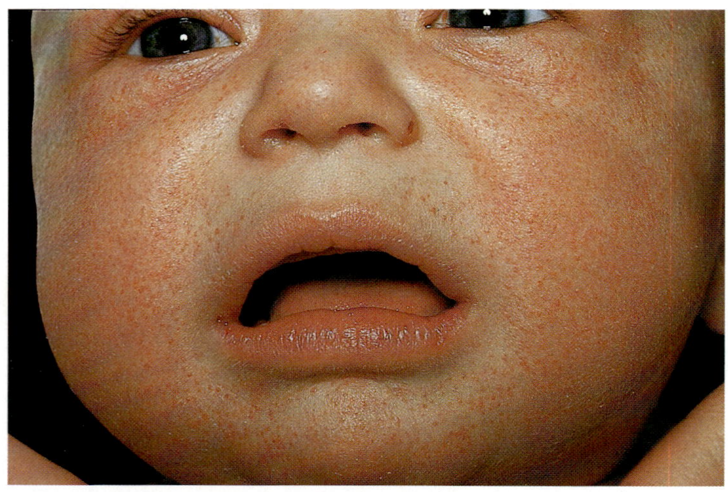

Figure 206 Miliaria rubra. Pinhead-sized, reddened, disseminated papules.

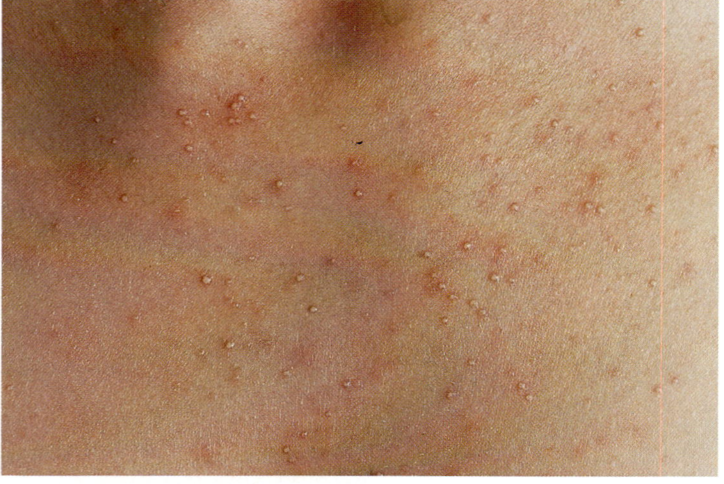

Figure 207 Pustular miliaria rubra. Disseminated reddened papules and pustules on the upper chest.

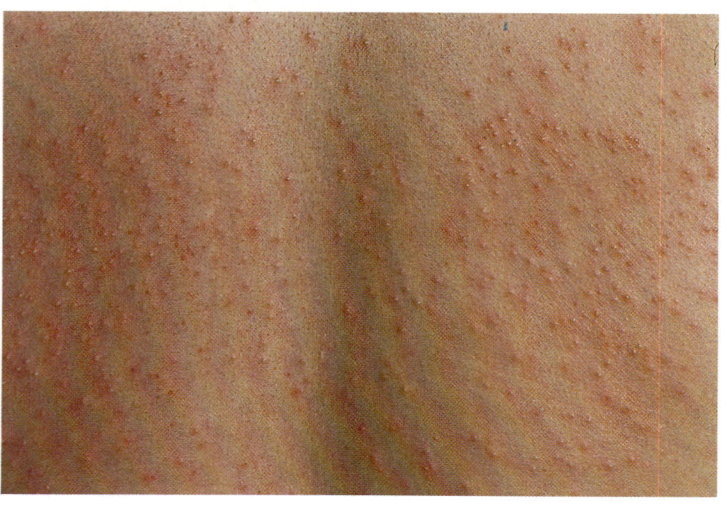

Figure 208 Pustular miliaria rubra. Dense groups of papules and pustules on the back.

Miliaria

Miliaria develops as a result of obstruction and rupture of the sweat glands and ducts in combination with excessive sweating. Sweat penetrates into the surrounding tissue and causes inflammation. Miliaria is most pronounced during travel to tropical climates with high humidity and usually heals spontaneously after a few days of acclimatization. In cooler climates, it is seen mainly after febrile infections. Clothing made of obstructive, usually synthetic material that does not absorb moisture readily promotes miliaria when the patient sweats. Infants sometimes develop miliaria when the face is moist from saliva and rests on a rubber mattress pad. Three different forms of miliaria can be distinguished, depending on the clinical symptoms and the location of the obstruction: miliaria cristallina, miliaria rubra and miliaria profunda.

Clinical Features

a) Miliaria cristallina

Clear, thin-walled, pinhead-sized vesicles are located under the stratum corneum. There is no inflammatory erythema; the vesicles are found mainly on the trunk. Long-lasting febrile diseases can lead to repeated attacks of miliaria. The vesicles rupture easily and last only a short time. They are followed by the development of fine, lamellar scales. The patients do not complain of itching.

b) Miliaria rubra

The tiny bright red spots or nodules occasionally have small vesicles or pustules embedded in them. They are usually widely disseminated. The lesions are found mainly on the trunk and on the flexor sides of elbows and knees, especially under tight clothing. The patients describe sensations of itching, burning and formication. Itching subsides when the surrounding temperature is lowered.

c) Miliaria profunda

This disorder develops as a result of recurrent attacks of miliaria rubra and is characterized by pinhead-sized, skin-colored, relatively firm nodules that are located mainly on the trunk and do not itch.

Therapy

1. Prevention of further sweating is the only effective therapeutic measure. The patients should be advised to wear light clothing and avoid hot or stimulating beverages, intense physical exercise and tropical climates. Weight reduction is important. The condition usually heals within a few days if the patient can be in fully air-conditioned surroundings for at least 8 hours a day.
2. If a tendency to develop miliaria exists, soap should be used sparingly.
3. Cooling alcohol dressings and dabbing with alcoholic zinc shake mixture **(R. 20b)** will soothe the unpleasant sensations caused by miliaria rubra eruptions. A bland powder **(R. 11)** can be used on the flexor surfaces of the elbow and knee joints. Topical use of steroid shake mixtures **(R. 22)** helps against inflammation and itching.

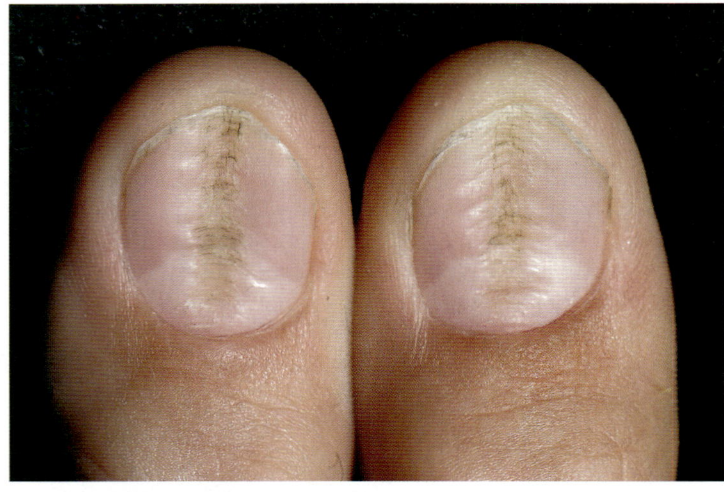

Figure 209 Median dystrophy of the nail. Typical appearance of a longitudinal groove, caused by habitual manipulation of the eponychium.

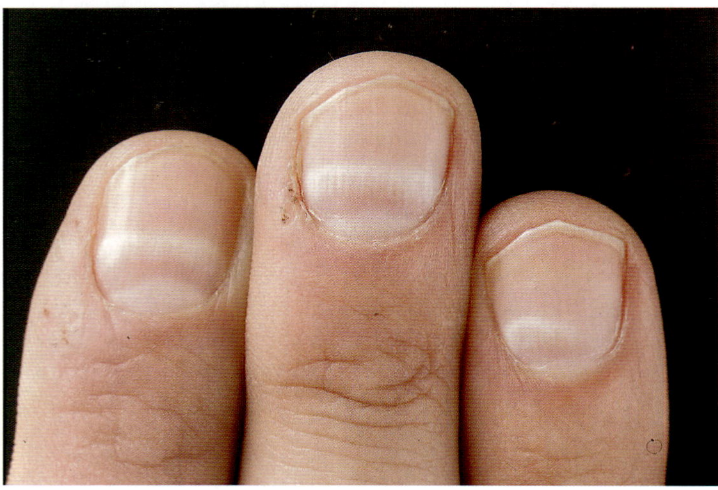

Figure 210 Mees' lines. White transverse lines on the nails following chemotherapy with several different agents.

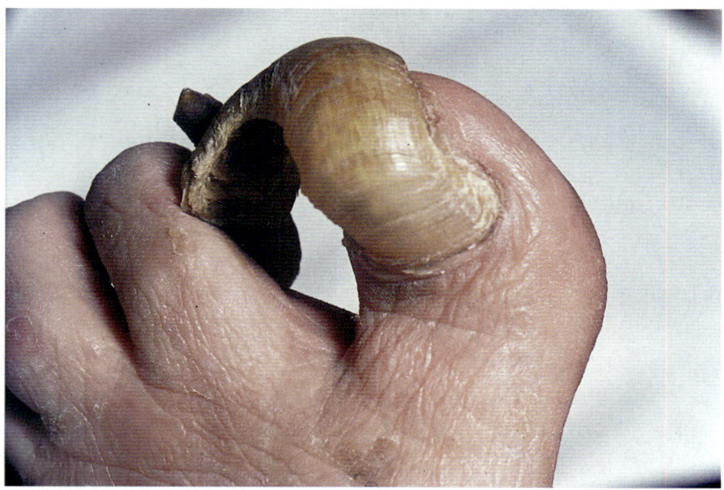

Figure 211 Onychogryphosis. Growth disturbance leading to thickening and deformity of the nail.

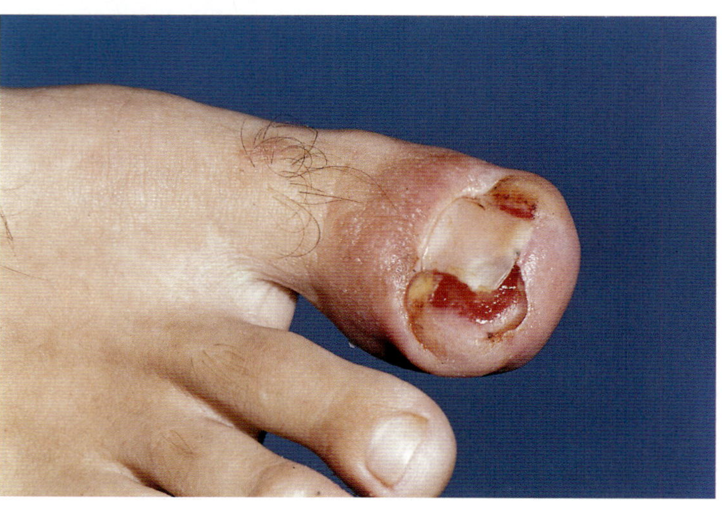

Figure 212 Ingrown nail. Unguis incarnatus. Long-standing inflammation of the nail wall.

Diseases of the Nails

Diseases of the nails involve the matrix, the nail bed, the nail plate, and the nail fold. Infections of the nail or the paronychium are seen relatively often, especially bacterial (see below) and mycotic (see pages 115 and 119) infections. Involvement of the nails is also seen in patients with psoriasis, eczemas, lichen planus, alopecia areata (see page 69), or as a result of mechanical forces, acute (hematoma of the nail) and chronic trauma, as well as from acids and lyes. Complaints about brittle finger nails are heard frequently in medical practice; however, this is a harmless and temporary condition. In most cases, the cause cannot be found. Occasionally, an outside cause can be found (frequent washing, contact with solvents), or there is an iron deficiency.

A. Ingrown Nail (Unguis Incarnatus)

Clinical Features Ingrown nails are seen almost exclusively on the big toe, either unilaterally or bilaterally. The distal corner of the nail appears to "dig" into the paronychium. In reality, there is an irritation (often not noticed by the patient) combined with a bacterial infection which leads to growth of inflammatory tissue (caro luxurians). Frequently, it has been triggered by a generalized febrile illness (with transient impairment of the defense mechanism against bacteria) or by poorly fitting shoes. The nail continues to irritate this hyperplastic inflammatory granulation tissue, especially when caro luxurians (proud flesh) surrounds the corner of the nail. The result is a painful, chronic or recurrent inflammation which can last for weeks, months or even years.

Therapy In the acute stage, an antibacterial solution (e.g., povidone-iodine solution) is applied. A small gauze strip is then placed under the corner of the nail, if possible. The involved nail should not be cut too short. The corner of the nail should not touch the skin. In chronic cases, partial resection of the lateral part of the nail bed may be necessary (Emmert plasty) to achieve complete healing. Simple extraction of the nail does not solve the problem. Systemic administration of antibiotics is not necessary. Permanent elevation of the distal-lateral corner of the nail can be achieved by application of nail clips to the big toe (additional information can be obtained from podiatrists).

B. Bacterial Paronychia

Bacterial paronychia can present with other symptoms in addition to unguis incarnatus.
Acute bacterial paronychia develops as a blister on the nail wall or as a panaritium with redness, swelling and pulsating pain. Occasionally, it can extend into the subcutis and into the deeper structures. Therapy of an acute panaritium consists of surgical incision and systemic antibiotic treatment, as well as immobilization of the involved part of the body, depending on the extent of the disease.
When involvement is chronic with erythema, thickening and tenderness of the nail wall, bacteria enter the enlarged crack between nail and skin, especially in the nail fold. Prolonged contact with water (housewives, cleaning personnel, etc.), as well as chronic eczema promote its development.
Treatment consists of elimination of the cause, avoidance of excessive contact with water and application of antibacterial and antimycotic (frequent *Candida* infections!) solutions **(R. 14)** to the paronychial space. Chronic infections of the big toe with painful hyperplastic inflammation, enlargement of the big toe, and cessation of nail growth require soap baths and antibiotic gels or ointments (**R. 34**). The patient should wear comfortable shoes with adequate room for the big toe. Elevation of the involved leg helps. It takes several weeks for the infection to heal.

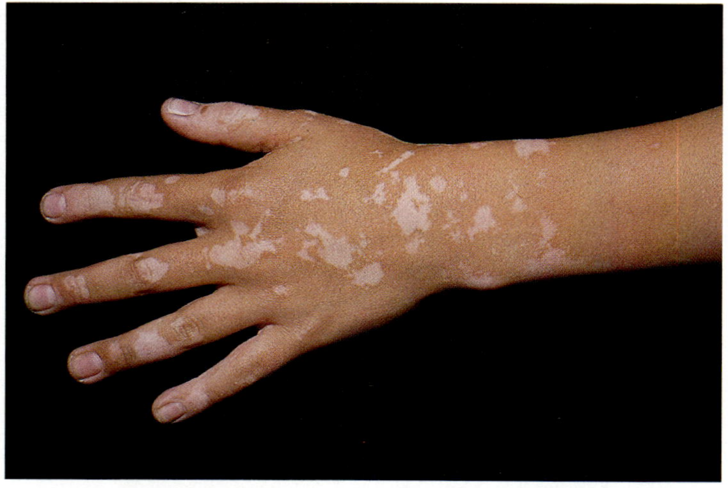

Figure 213 Vitiligo. Symmetrically arranged, depigmented areas of irregular configuration.

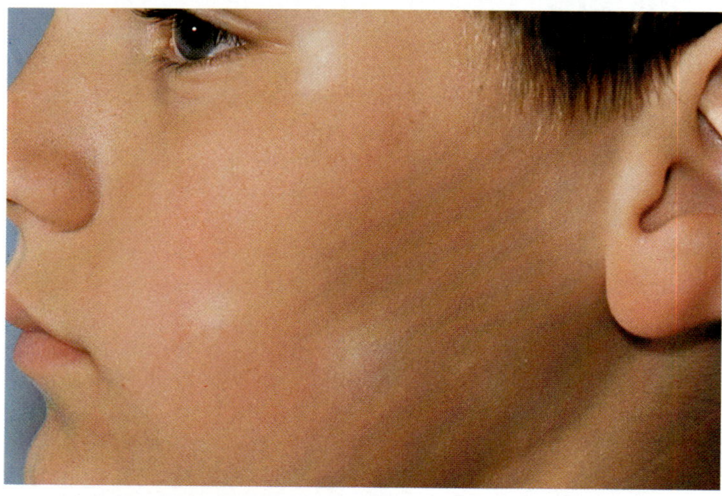

Figure 214 Pityriasis alba. Minimally scaling, round, light-colored spots on the cheeks.

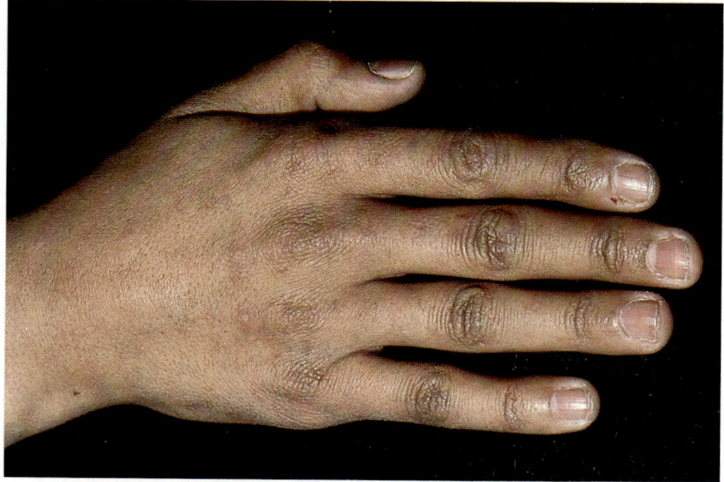

Figure 215 Addison's disease. Diffuse hyperpigmentation, increased over the joints.

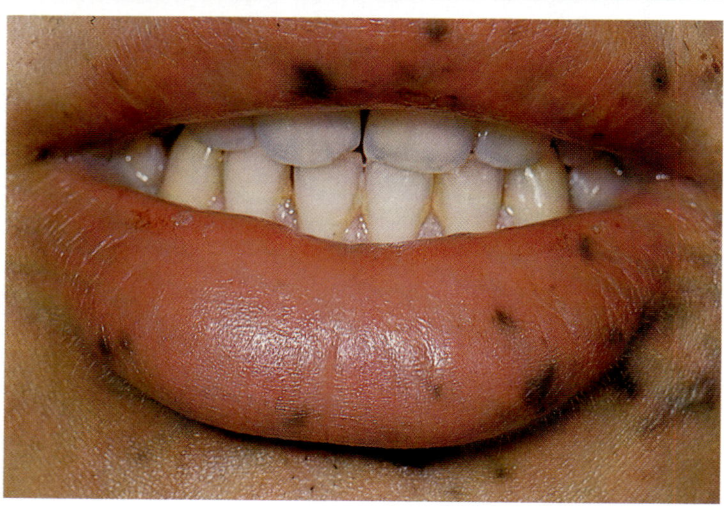

Figure 216 Artificial pigmentation produced by impregnation with silver dust.

Pigmentation Disorders

A. Vitiligo

Vitiligo is a chronic skin disease of essentially only cosmetic significance. It is caused by partial destruction of the melanocytes in the epidermis, but its exact pathogenesis is not known. Familial occurence is frequent, and it sometimes occurs in combination with alopecia areata, or other family members have alopecia areata. The disease persists for many years or even decades. In approximately 20% of the patients it disappears completely, in another 20%, partially. Repigmentation often begins at the follicles.

Clinical Features

1. Depigmented, white to pink-colored, rounded patches of skin that often coalesce into larger areas.
2. The borders are often hyperpigmented.
3. The lesions are usually symmetric and involve mainly the distal ends of fingers and toes, hands and feet. On the trunk, face and genito-anal regions, the lesions are usually found on the midline.
4. The risk of sunburn on the affected areas is great due to the lack of protection from pigment.

Therapy

To date, treatment is unsatisfactory.

1. It is beneficial in all cases to use external sunscreens **(R. 45)**, on the lesions to protect the depigmented areas from sunburn, and on the surrounding skin to avoid tanning of the healthy skin, which would exaggerate the difference in pigmentation even more.
2. For involvement of the face, application of water-resistent make-up that is matched to the tone of the healthy skin is recommended. The cosmetic results of staining the lesions with dihydroxyacetone are often unsatisfactory.
3. Photochemotherapy (PUVA) can be tried in an attempt to achieve repigmentation. This must be done by a dermatologist experienced in the procedure who has the necessary equipment at his or her disposal.

B. Pityriasis Alba

Pityriasis alba is a superficial eczema which occurs mainly on the face of children. These harmless skin changes are especially visible during the summer months when the surrounding skin is tanned. They are often associated with generally dry skin.

Clinical Features

A discrete white scaling is visible, occasionally only along the margin. The lesions are round, vary in size from a penny to a dollar, and are conspicuous because of their much lighter color. There is no erythema. The areas of predilection are the face, the cheeks and occasionally the forehead, neck, upper arms, abdomen and back. There is no itching.

Therapy

Regular skin care **(R. 33)** is usually sufficient, even when there is scaling. Repigmentation occurs after approximately 4 to 6 weeks.

C. Universal Hyperpigmentation

This disorder has many causes. Increased secretion of ACTH or of the melanocyte-stimulating hormone (MSH), as it occurs in Addison's disease, can lead to universal hyperpigmentation with accentuation of the lines of the palm. This can also be seen following a prolonged course of ACTH injections. Other drugs can also induce undesirable hyperpigmentation, e. g., bleomycin, minocycline and amiodarone. Another possibility is that melanin is secreted excessively by melanoma metastases and is deposited universally. Much more frequently we see so-called postinflammatory pigmentations, i.e., universal pigmentations following inflammatory diseases,

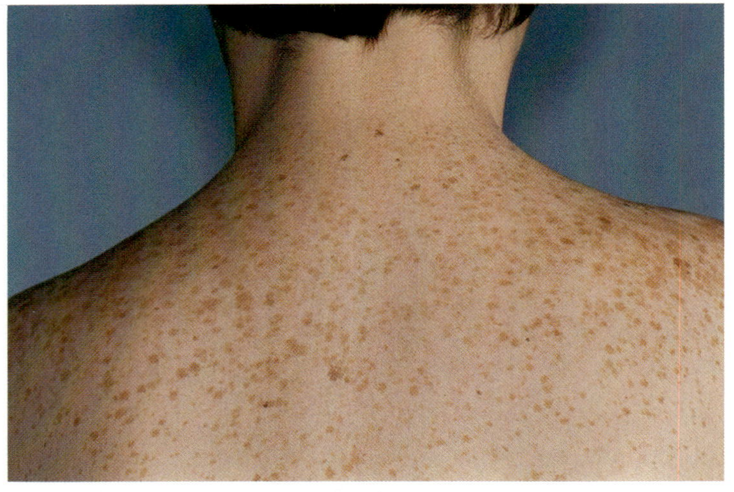

Figure 217 Ephelides (freckles).

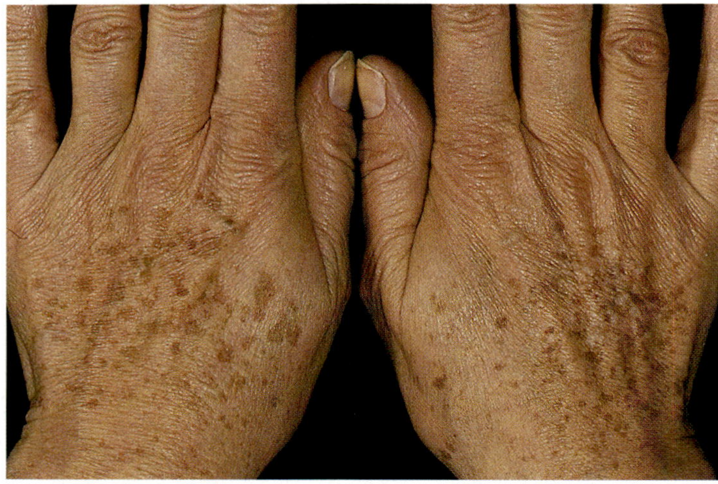

Figure 218 Solar lentigines. Sun-induced freckles. Typical location on the dorsum of the hand.

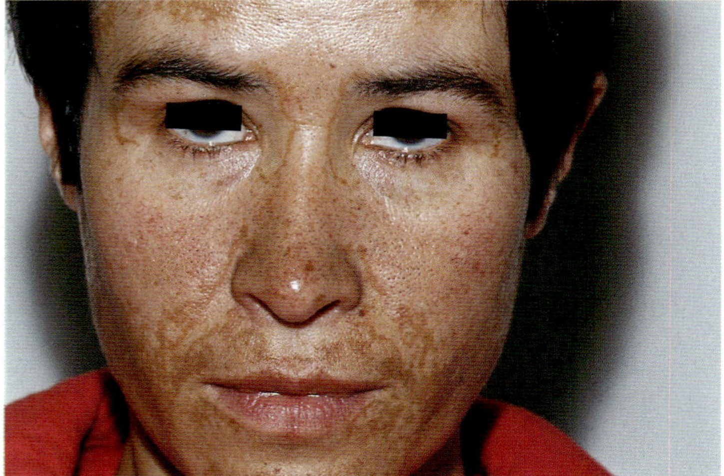

Figure 219 Melasma (chloasma). Spotty brownish discoloration in the face.

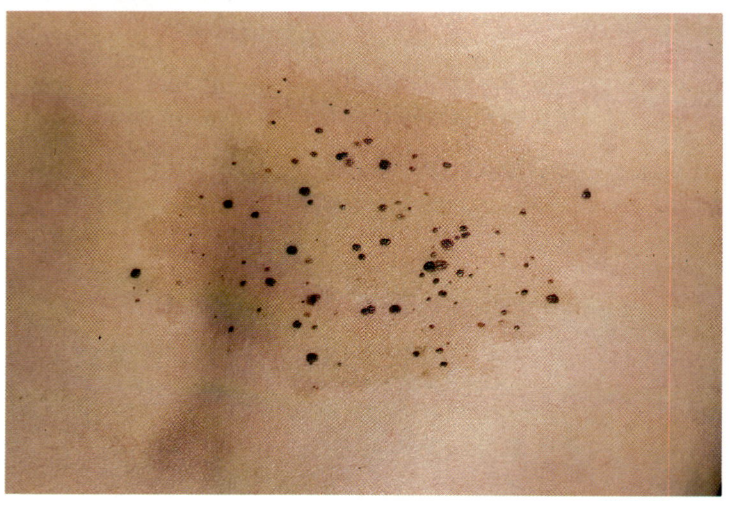

Figure 220 Nevus spilus. Light brown, sharply delineated lesion with multiple interspersed nevomelanocytic nevi.

especially erythrodermas. Finally, depositions of exogenous particles, such as metal dust or "dirt tattoos" from accidents can occur.

D. Ephelides, Freckles

Clinical Features

1. Disseminated, light brown pigmented spots with a diameter of a few millimeters are characteristic. They occur frequently on constitutionally light skin with a tendency to sunburn.
2. Areas of predilection are the face, especially the nasal region, the shoulders, and the back.

Therapy

Treatment is not necessary, since this is a harmless, normal variant. Sunscreen preparations **(R. 45)** and creams or lotions containing hydroquinone (Artra, Eldoquin, Melanex, etc.) can be applied externally if less pigmentation is desired.

E. Solar Lentigines (Sun-Induced Freckles)

These lesions occur in the elderly, predominantly on the back of the hand and in the face. They are harmless normal variants and do not require any treatment. They can be removed for cosmetic reasons with a calibrated ruby laser.

F. Melasma, Chloasma

This is a permanent hyperpigmentation of the face caused by pregnancy or estrogen drugs.

Clinical Features

1. Spotty or band-shaped, generally symmetric brown pigmentation is characteristic.
2. Chloasma is localized in the face and involves mainly the forehead, infraorbital region and upper lip.
3. The brown discoloration is intensified by UV radiation (sunlight, sun lamps).

Therapy

1. If the chloasma is caused by estrogens, a non-hormonal method of contraception should be chosen.
2. Excessive exposure to sunlight must be avoided. Application of external sunscreens should be used to protect the skin.
3. Depigmentation with a combination of tretinoin, cortisone and hydroquinone can be tried if the simple procedures above do not succeed.

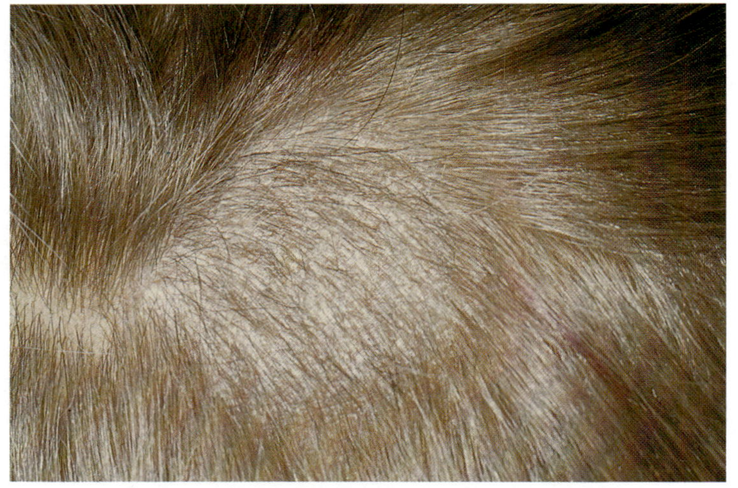

Figure 221 Tinea capitis superficialis (microsporia). Round, "bald" area with white scales. Stumps of broken hairs are visible.

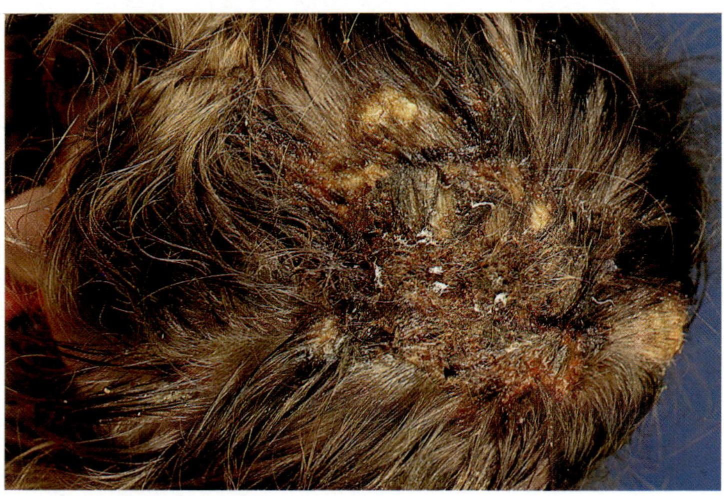

Figure 222 Tinea capitis profunda. Extensive parietal lesions covered by bloody and purulent crusts. The affected hairs have either fallen out or are stuck together.

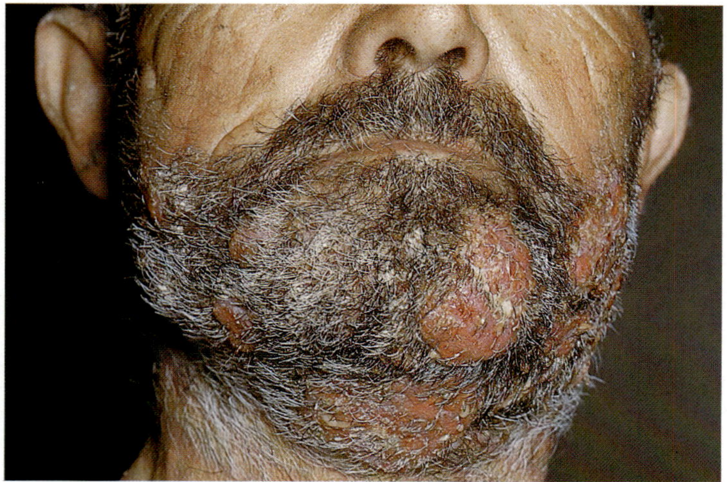

Figure 223 Tinea barbae. Vegetating nodular inflammation with formation of pustules, abscesses and crusts.

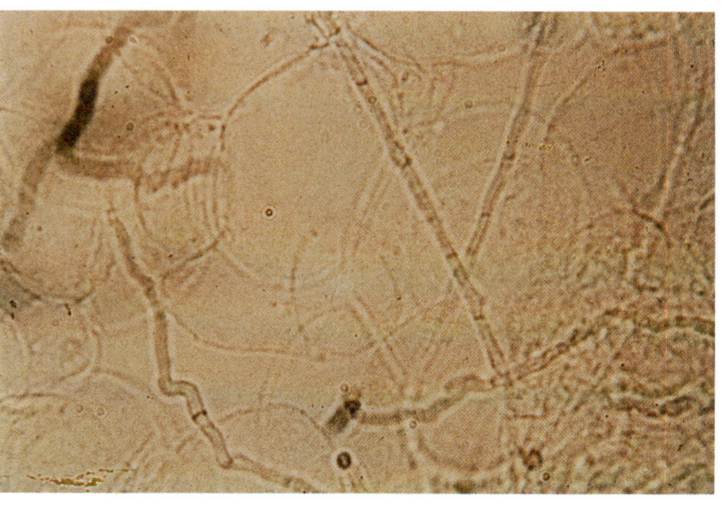

Figure 224 Microscopic demonstration of fungi in a scraping from a scaling lesion after preparation with 10% KOH solution for 30 minutes (dimmed bright-field).

Fungal Diseases

A. Diseases due to Dermatophytes

Diseases caused by dermatophytes are among the most common infectious diseases of the skin. For practical purposes, it is expedient to classify diseases caused by dermatophytes according to body regions, since the clinical symptoms are determined more by the affected region of the body and the patient's resistance to infection than by the species of the microorganism (frequently *Trichophyton rubrum* and *Trichophyton mentagrophytes*). The diagnosis should be confirmed by microscopy and by culture (Sabouraud or Kimmig Agar at 25 °C for 3 weeks).

a) Tinea Capitis

Tinea capitis is classified into tinea capitis superficialis and tinea capitis profunda (kerion Celsi). Children are affected more frequently than adults.

Clinical Features

1. Tinea capitis superficialis is characterized by round, nummular patches without hair that occasionally coalesce into larger areas. There is fine, lamellar scaling without significant inflammatory signs. Stubs of broken hair are visible in the lesion.
2. Tinea capitis profunda presents with a marked inflammatory reaction, pustules, crusts and swelling of the regional lymph nodes. The inflammation originates from the hair follicles which are infected with fungi.
3. The scalp is affected; in men the bearded area can have tinea barbae.
4. The superficial form heals without scars; deep inflammations usually lead to scarring and alopecia.

Therapy

Internal

Systemic antimycotics **(R. 55 to 59)**, to be used for 4-6 weeks.

External

Topical antimycotic therapy alone is not successful against tinea capitis. It can be used in addition to systemic treatment to prevent spreading of infectious material.

b) Tinea Corporis

Clinical Features

1. Sharply delineated, scaling, erythematous lesions with scalloped, accentuated margins and formation of pustules, especially along the edges, are characteristic. The lesions expand slowly. They may be aggravated by sunlight.
2. The lesions can develop anywhere on the body. Pets (cats, dogs, guinea pigs) can transmit the infection to exposed areas of skin (face, arms), especially in children. Lesions can also be found in the gluteal and inguinal regions (tinea cruris).
3. The infection causes moderate to severe itching.

Therapy

Systemic

Systemic antimycotics **(R. 55 to 59)** are very effective against tinea corporis, but external therapy is usually sufficient and is preferable.

External

1. Local antimycotics in a base appropriate for skin type, location, and degree of inflammation – solution **(R. 14b, c)**, lotion or cream **(R. 35a, b)** – for at least 2–3 weeks.
2. Aqueous dye solutions **(R. 14a)** have an antimycotic effect, but since they stain the clothes, they are not readily accepted by outpatients.
3. Corticosteroids are not recommended. They have an anti-inflammatory effect but encourage dissemination of the fungi on the skin.

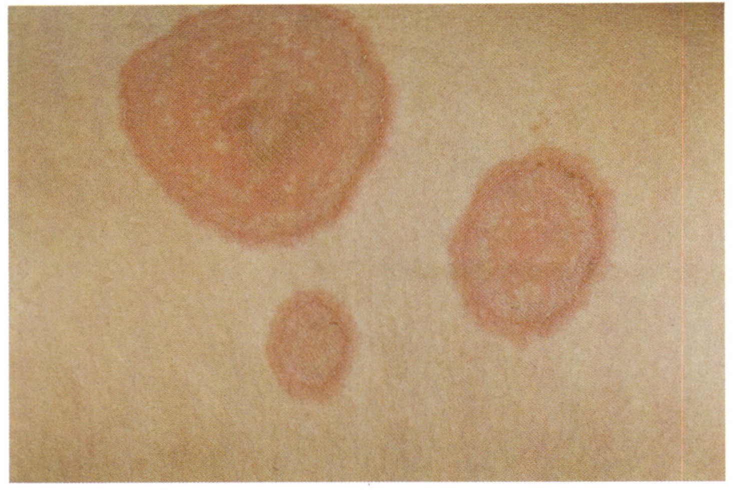

Figure 225 Tinea corporis. Sharply delineated erythematous zones with scaling and pustule formation along the margins.

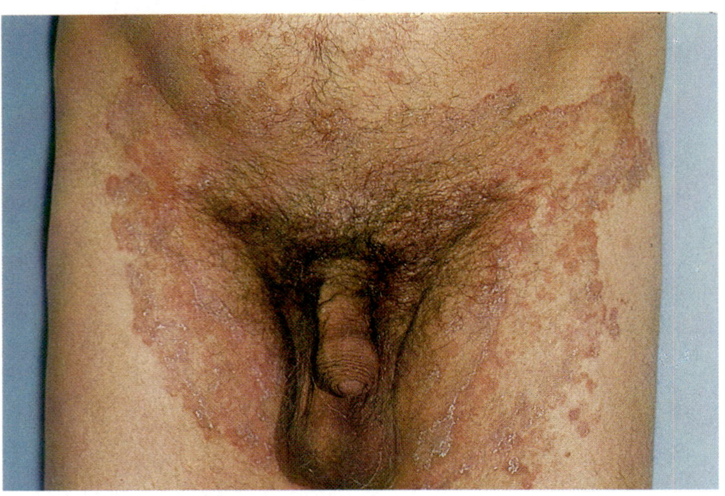

Figure 226 Tinea cruris. Scaly, partially infiltrated erythema with polycyclic borders that expands peripherally. Typical accentuated margin.

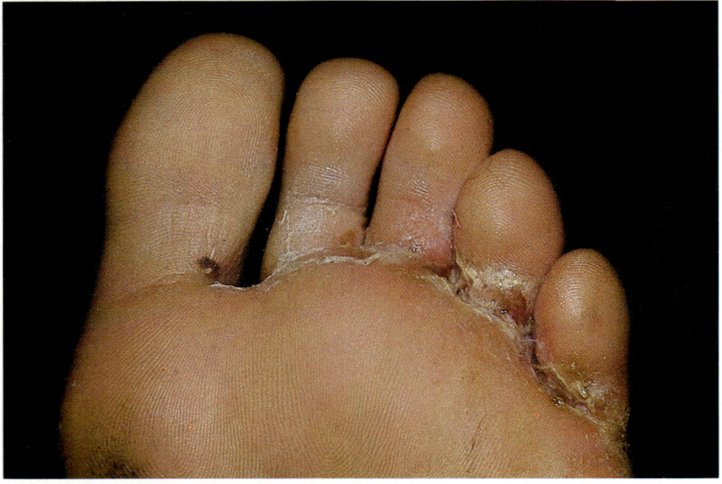

Figure 227 Tinea pedis. Maceration with erosions and scaling originating from the interdigital spaces.

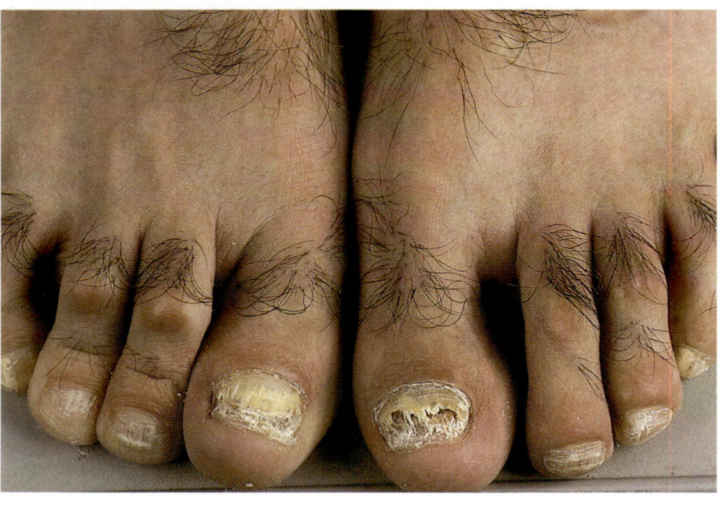

Figure 228 Onychomycosis. Tinea unguium. Thickening, whitish-yellow discoloration and partial destruction of the toenails.

c) Tinea Pedis

Clinical Features

1. Scaling, erythema, maceration, and rhagades are found between the toes.
2. The skin changes are seen most frequently in the fourth interdigital space and they can spread to the dorsum of the toes and particularly the soles of the feet. One or more toenails are often affected.
3. The patient usually complains of itching in the involved area. Prolonged wearing of athletic shoes or rubber boots produces a moist environment, especially in patients with hyperhidrosis, and can lead to acute exacerbation and severe inflammation and vesicular palmoplantar eczema (see page 45). Acute erysipelas (see page 57) can also originate from tinea pedis.

Therapy

1. A moist environment must be avoided; the patient must wear appropriate shoes, not rubber boots or tight shoes, but sandals and cotton socks instead. The interdigital spaces must be kept dry (bland powder).
2. Foot baths with antimycotic additives, e.g., potassium permanganate **(R. 4)**. Dry thoroughly after bathing or even blow dry.
3. Antimycotic powders **(R. 13)** or solutions **(R. 14)** can be used; insert gauze strips between the toes.
4. To avoid reinfection, contaminated socks must be washed in hot water, and disinfection of contaminated footwear is also necessary.

d) Tinea Unguium, Onychomycosis

Constant work in a moist environment damages the nail plate and encourages fungal infection. The patient often has poor peripheral circulation (smoking, acrocyanosis) or occlusive artery disease.

Clinical Features

1. Whitish-yellow discoloration of the nail plate starts at the free end of the nail and advances slowly toward the nail bed. This is followed by thickening and loosening of the nail plate from the nail bed. Finally the nail crumbles.
2. The toenails are affected more frequently than the fingernails.

Therapy

Mycoses of the nail are very resistant to therapy and recur frequently. It is advisable to inform the patient of these problems before treatment is started. If circulation is poor and cannot be improved, antimycotic therapy will not be effective. Before systemic therapy is started, the organisms must be identified microscopically and by culture for the appropriate drug, since onychomycosis can be caused not only by dermatophytes but also by yeasts and saprophyte fungi.

Systemic

1. Terbinafine **(R. 59)** for dermatophyte infection, given for 3 months.
2. Itraconazole **(R. 58)** for 3 to 6 months, depending on the clinical success.
3. Griseofulvin **(R. 55)** is helpful in the treatment of dermatophytes: up to 6 months for fingernails, up to 10 for toenails.

External

1. The thickened nail is softened with 15% urea ointment, followed by application of an antimycotic. Treatment must be maintained regularly until a healthy nail has grown. This therapy is successful only occasionally, even with regular and prolonged application.
2. Extraction of the nail is usually not successful because the fungal infection recurs readily. Damage to the nail matrix from extraction can result in growth of a deformed nail, which is again more susceptible to fungal infection.

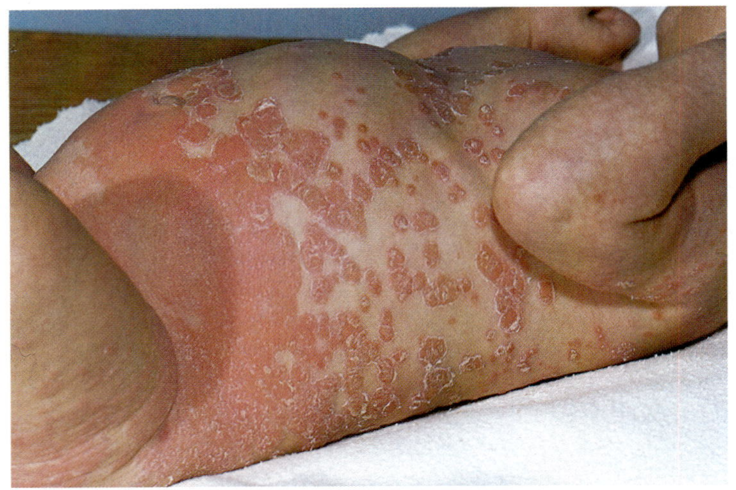

Figure 229 Candidiasis (thrush), originating from a diaper rash. The sharply delineated scaly erythema tapers off into multiple satellite foci. Distinct marginal collarette of scale.

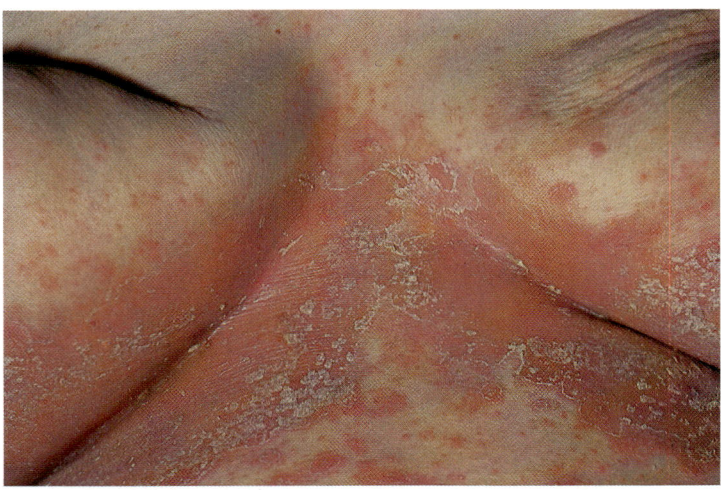

Figure 230 Candidiasis (thrush). Solid red, scaly erythemas with distinct marginal scaling; satellite foci in the periphery.

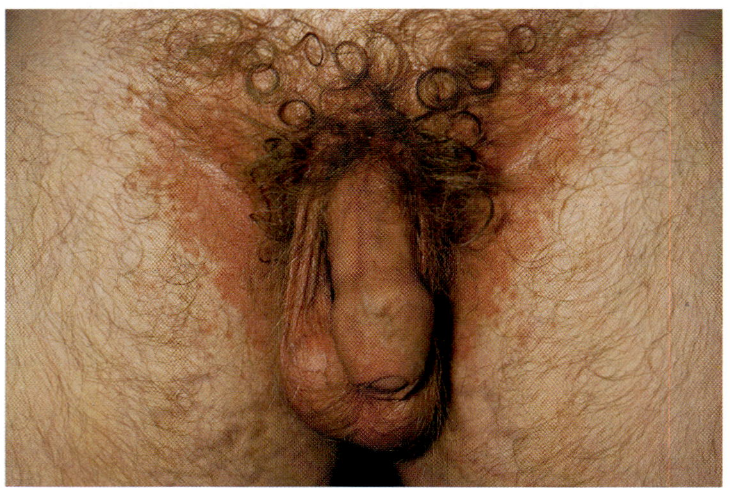

Figure 231 Candidiasis (thrush). Mainly symmetric erythema, tapering off into individual foci, located in the inguinal area and extending to the scrotum.

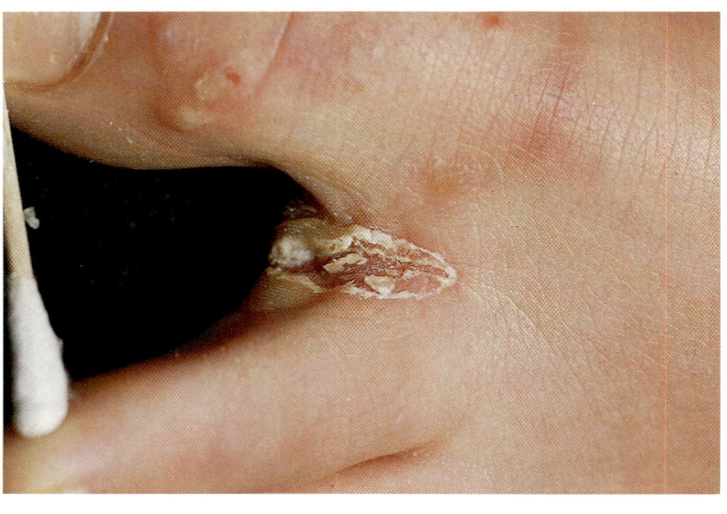

Figure 232 Candidiasis (thrush). Typical morphology in the interdigital space. Rhagade with distinct layer of scales.

B. Skin Diseases Caused by Yeasts (Candidiasis)

Candida albicans is the primary pathogenic yeast. These infections involve the intertriginous areas, the nail wall and occasionally the mucous membranes. Candidiasis can occur as a primary disease but is more often secondary to treatment with broad-spectrum antibiotics or corticosteroids. It also occurs in diabetes mellitus or severe illnesses that impair the immune system (AIDS, malignant lymphoma, systemic lupus erythematosus, pemphigus). These patients may develop life-threatening sepsis following fungal infections of the skin or mucous membranes. Ordinarily, candidal infections are found in infants and small children as well as the elderly. Chronic candidal infections are seen in patients with congenital or acquired defects in cellular immunity.

a) Candidal Infection of the Skin (Thrush)

Clinical Features

1. Bright red, shiny lesions are characteristic; in the intertriginous areas there are often large confluent lesions. In the periphery, small papules with scaling scalloped borders (satellite lesions, typical of thrush) are found.
2. Cutaneous candidiasis occurs predominantly in the intertriginous areas, i.e., in the perianal, inguinal and submammary regions, the axillae and the interdigital spaces of the fingers. In a patient with an impaired immune system, candidal infection can involve the entire skin.
3. The patients often complain of burning and pruritus.

Therapy

Elimination of the predisposing factors is of prime importance, especially increased moisture of the skin which can result from excessive sweating (obesity, fever), incontinence or diabetes mellitus.

Systemic

1. Only for extensive involvement and in patients with increased risk (AIDS, leukemia, cytostatic treatment), systemic use of an antimycotic drug **(R. 56 to 58)** for 1 to 2 weeks.
2. Confirmed intestinal candidiasis is treated with nystatin or amphotericin B orally (these two substances are not absorbed and are locally effective).

Topical

1. The intertriginous areas should be kept dry with powder or zinc lotion and by the insertion of gauze strips.
2. Sitz baths with antimicrobial additives such as potassium permanganate are helpful, followed by blow drying.
3. Pastes containing nystatin **(R. 14a)** are effective. Ointments are not advisable for the intertriginous areas.
4. Dye solutions **(R. 14a)** are acceptable for the perianal region and the vulva and are very effective there.
5. In infants, occlusive, disposable diapers should be avoided in favor of cloth diapers.
6. Reduction of dietary intake of sugar is recommended as an additional measure.

b) Candidiasis of the Mucosa, Candidiasis of the Genital Area

Clinical Features

1. Creamy white, adherent plaques of approximately pinhead to coin size are characteristic. They can coalesce to widespread membranous plaques.
2. The mucous membranes of the mouth and the tongue may be affected. Similar changes occur as candidal vulvovaginitis in women or as candidal balanitis in men. In patients with an impaired immune system, the *Candida* infection can spread from the oral mucosa to the pharynx and esophagus.
3. In candidal balanitis, round or circinate, bright red, smooth lesions on the glans penis and on the foreskin are characteristic.
4. When perianal or perivulvar candidiasis is present, intestinal or vaginal infection must be suspected and appropriate diagnostic examinations performed, and if necessary, appropriate treatment instituted.

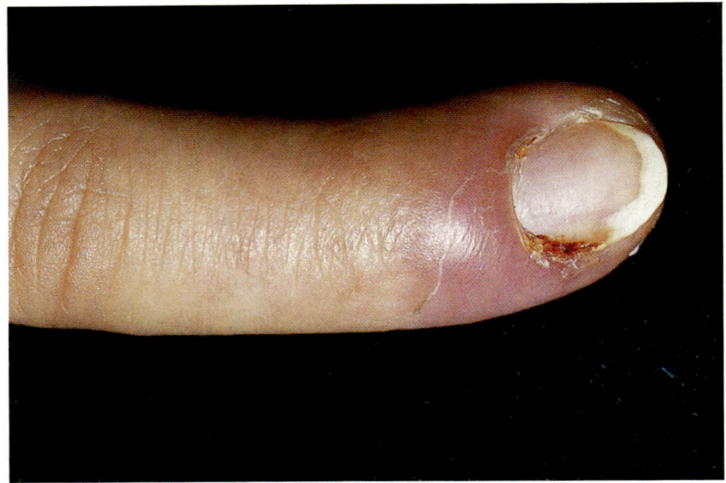

Figure 233 Candidiasis with paronychia. Clinically, this acute periungual inflammation cannot be distinguished from a bacterial infection.

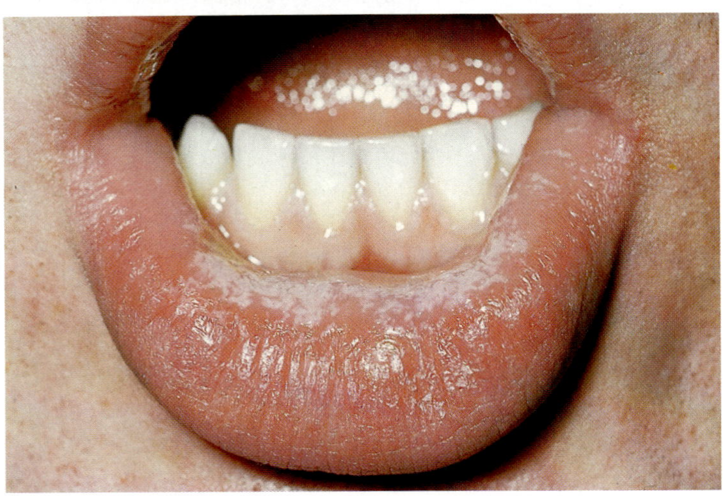

Figure 234 Candidiasis, oral thrush. White plaques with peripheral reticulation. Lesions can be scraped off.

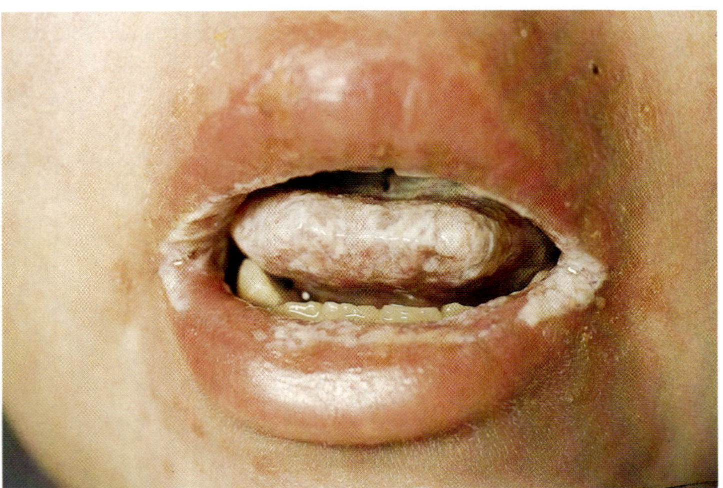

Figure 235 Chronic mucocutaneous candidiasis in a patient with cellular immunodeficiency. Thick white coating on the tongue, in the corners of the mouth (thrush perlèche) and the red of the lips.

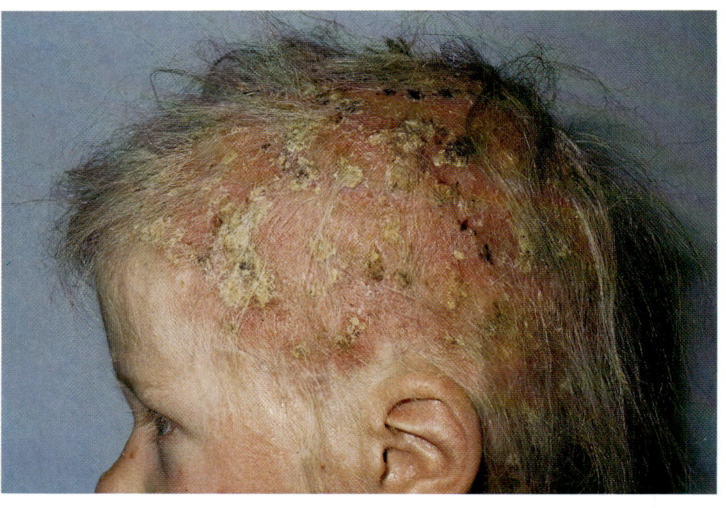

Figure 236 Chronic mucocutaneous candidiasis in a patient with cellular immunodeficiency. Extensive inflammatory infiltration of the scalp, which is covered with crusts.

Therapy

Mucosal Candidiasis

1. Treatment with a suspension of an antimycotic drug (nystatin, amphotericin B, miconazole, etc.) is helpful.
2. In severe cases and in patients at risk (see above), systemic treatment with fluconazole, ketoconazole or itraconazole (**R. 56 to 58**) may be helpful.

Genital Candidiasis

1. Most antimycotic drugs have a similar effect on the treatment of vaginal infection. They are applied as vaginal suppositories or vaginal creams.
2. External application of a cream containing nystatin (**R. 31**) or dabbing with a trimethylan dye solution (**R. 14a**). An alternative is a one-time oral treatment with fluconazole.
3. Sitz baths with potassium permanganate solution soothe the severe pruritus.
4. Concomitant intestinal candidiasis should be treated.
5. In genital candidiasis, treatment of the sexual partner is necessary to avoid "ping-pong infection".

c) Candidal Paronychia

Clinical Features

1. The skin surrounding the fingernail shows marked discoloration and edematous swelling. Pressure on the tissue produces thick purulent material. The cuticle is absent. Chronic infection causes disturbed growth of the nail and occasionally yellow-green discoloration (an indication of secondary infection with *Pyocyaneus*).
2. Since this condition is encouraged by frequent work in a moist medium (dishwashers, cleaning personnel, hair dressers), the fingernails are more frequently involved than the toenails.
3. Chronic paronychia often leads to impaired growth of the nail with transverse ridges.
4. The patient should always be evaluated for diabetes mellitus.

Therapy

1. Elimination of the predisposing factors is of prime importance. Rubber or vinyl gloves worn over cotton gloves will prevent a moist compartment for the hands of persons who work in a wet medium. It is better to avoid this work completely, or at least during the acute phase of the disease. The cuticle should not be manipulated!
2. Antimycotic drugs should be used in solutions or tinctures (**R. 14c**) to transport the effective agent to the site of infection.
3. Hand baths only for short periods of time can be helpful for patients with marked purulent secretion.
4. Consistent adherence to these recommendations usually results in marked improvement, but it may take 2 to 3 months.
5. Short-term systemic treatment with ketoconazole or fluconazole may be indicated should local therapy be unsuccessful. The infectious organisms must be identified before treatment is started.

C. Pityriasis Versicolor

Pityriasis versicolor is a noninflammatory, noncontagious fungal disease caused by the bimorph yeast *Pityrosporum orbiculare (ovale)*. This fungus occurs naturally as a saprophyte in the inguinal area and on the scalp. It produces a substance that interferes with melanin synthesis (azelaic acid). The affected areas are a lighter color and contrast with the surrounding tanned skin. On non-tanned skin, these areas appear light-brown.

Pityriasis versicolor occurs more often during the summer and in hot, humid climates. Patients with seborrhea and hyperhidrosis are affected more frequently. The disease is also found as a concomitant phenomenon during systemic corticosteroid therapy, in patients with immunodeficiencies or during immunosuppressive therapy. Poor body hygiene is not a contributing factor. Patients who are more than 40 years of age are rarely affected.

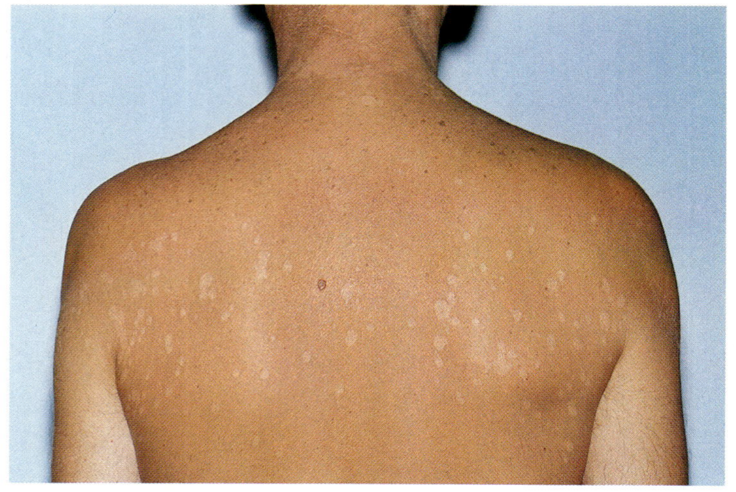

Figure 237 Pityriasis versicolor. Oval-shaped, hypopigmented, minimally scaling lesions.

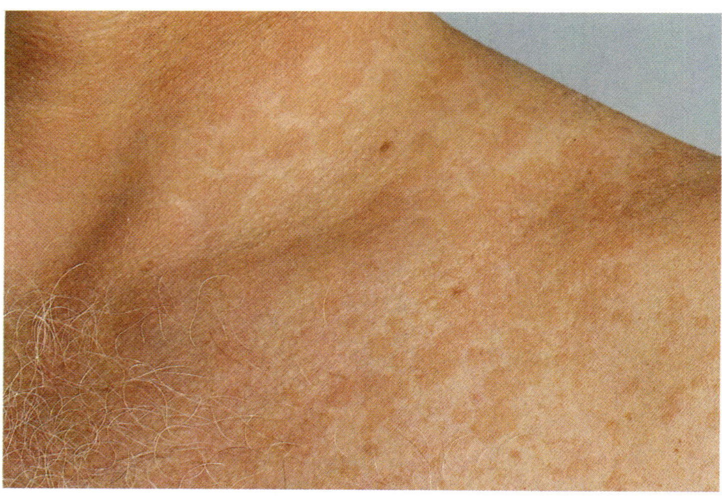

Figure 238 Pityriasis versicolor. The rounded, confluent foci appear brownish on untanned skin.

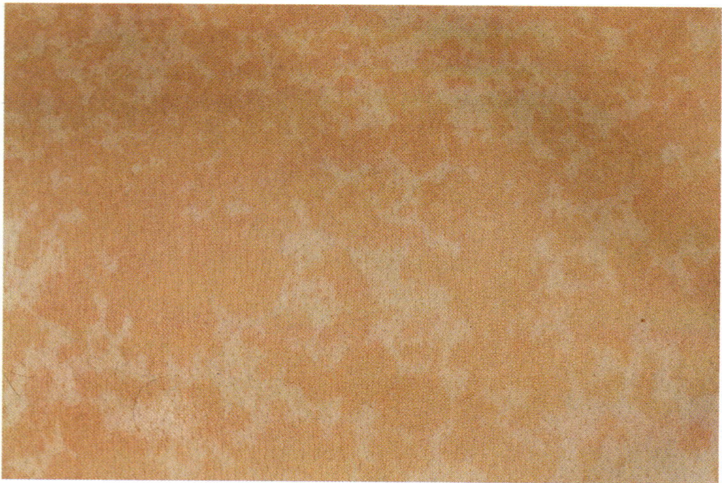

Figure 239 Pityriasis versicolor. Detail.

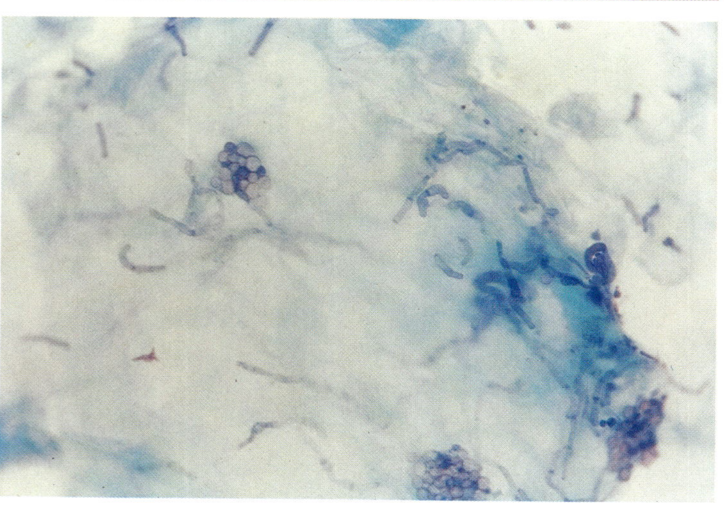

Figure 240 Diagnosis of agent (*Pityrosporum orbiculare*) with azure-stained cellophane tape preparation. Microscopy shows a typical mixture of round yeast cells and hyphae.

Clinical Features

1. Flat, round or oval-shaped lesions that can occasionally coalesce to palm-size lesions are characteristic. Scraping with a wooden spatula produces bran-like scales. The color of these lesions may range from white to red or brown.
2. The lesions are found mainly on the shoulders, chest, back and occasionally the upper arms and thighs.
3. The disorder is mainly a cosmetic problem with occasional mild pruritus. The scales can be removed with cellophane tape and the causative fungi can be easily identified by staining with blue ink, Gram stain or methylene blue solution. The cellophane tape is touched to a scaling lesion once and is then taped to a glass slide with a drop of the staining solution. The specimen can be examined after approximately one minute under 25 X magnification.

Therapy

With all therapeutic measures, it must be kept in mind that the disease recurs readily and is only a cosmetic problem.

1. The most important therapeutic measure is elimination of the underlying hyperhidrosis.
2. Pyrithione zinc cream or ketoconazole should be applied to the entire body, including the scalp (fungus reservoir); the medication should be removed after a few minutes by thorough showering. This treatment is repeated every other day for 14 days.
3. Topical broad-spectrum antimycotics **(R. 35a)** are also effective but must be applied 1–2 times daily for at least 3 to 4 weeks; this can be expensive.
4. Systemic imidazole derivatives are effective **(R. 56 to 58)** but not indicated for this harmless disorder.
5. It is important to inform the patient that it will take 2 to 3 months or renewed suntanning before the depigmented lesions regain the same color as the surrounding skin.

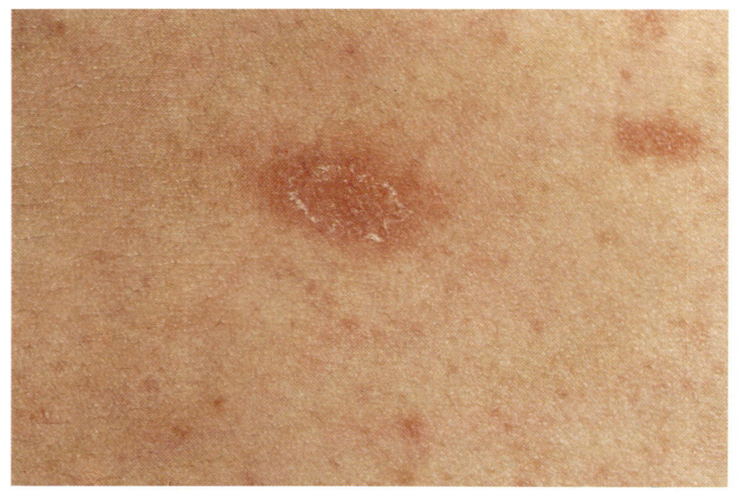

Figure 241 Pityriasis rosea. Fairly large initial lesion with scaly margin (so-called "herald patch").

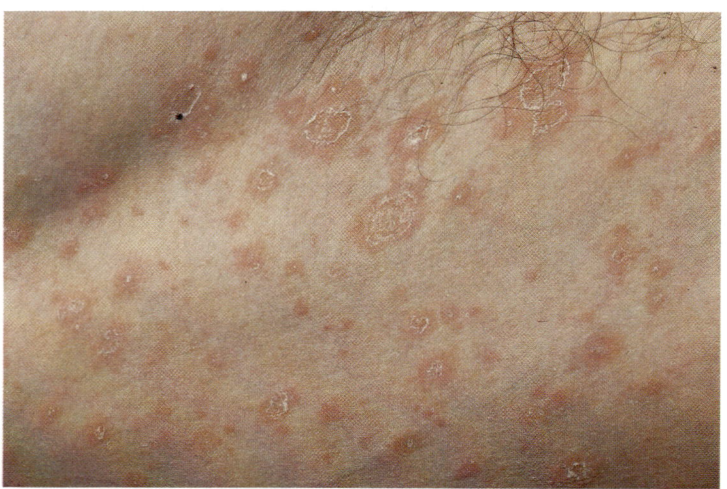

Figure 242 Pityriasis rosea. Rash-like dissemination of round and oval erythemas of various sizes with characteristic collarette of scale.

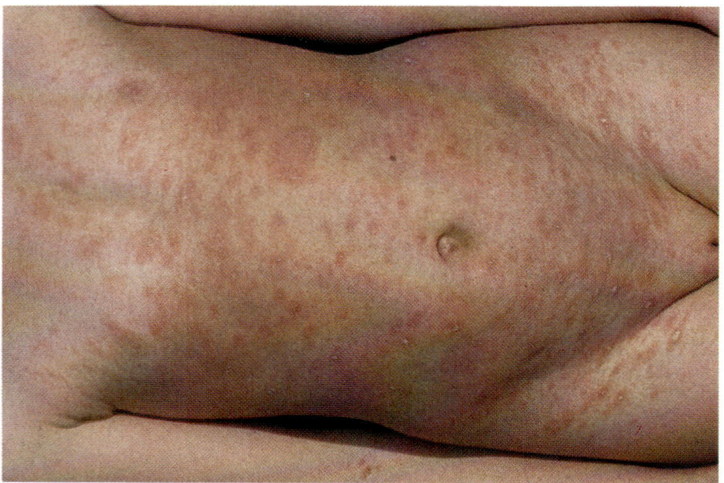

Figure 243 Pityriasis rosea. Maximal development of the disease with herald patch and lesions oriented in the direction of the lines of cleavage in the skin. Typical limitation to the trunk and the proximal parts of the extremities.

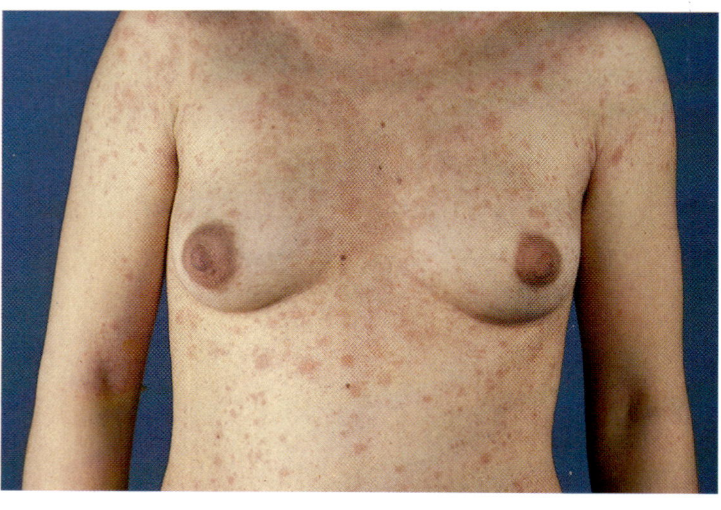

Figure 244 Pityriasis rosea. Exanthema involving mainly the trunk. The usual distinct collarette of scale is absent here.

Pityriasis Rosea

The cause of this common, non-recurrent disease is unknown. A virus etiology is suspected because the disease usually occurs during the spring. The skin changes have a characteristic appearance and a typical location that is important for the diagnosis. Pityriasis rosea develops slowly to the full-blown picture over a period of 5 to 10 days and lasts approximately 3 to 6 weeks. Young adults, adolescents and children are affected most frequently. Pityriasis rosea-like eruptions are known to occur after treatment with certain drugs such as captopril, clonidine and gold.

Clinical Features

1. The first symptom usually is a 2 to 5 cm, round or oval-shaped, reddened, scaling lesion with accentuated border, the so-called "herald patch", which is generally found on the trunk.
2. Several days to 3 weeks later, symmetric eruptions of similar, but smaller, pale-red to pinkish-brown lesions with silvery scales appear.
3. The lesions are located on the lateral and anterior parts of the trunk, especially on the mid-chest. With more extensive involvement, they can also be found on the proximal parts of the extremities. The foci are often oblong with the long axis running parallel to the lines of cleavage in the skin, especially on the sides of the trunk. A collarette of scale is usually found between the center and the margin of the individual focus. Pale red patches without collarette often appear simultaneously.
4. The face and the distal parts of the extremities are rarely involved.
5. Pruritus is minimal and is present only intermittently.
6. Secondary eczema is often found in the affected region, because the skin of these areas can be irritated easily, e.g., by cortisone ointments.

Therapy

1. The disease usually disappears spontaneously after 3 to 6 weeks, even without treatment. Therapy is not required in most patients, but mild topical therapy with an aqueous zinc lotion **(R. 20a)** may be helpful.
2. For inflammation, a corticosteroid shake mixture **(R. 22)** has been found useful.
3. Other measures, such as corticosteroid ointments, hot baths and frequent washing with soap, as well as wool clothing should be avoided because they irritate the lesions and delay healing.

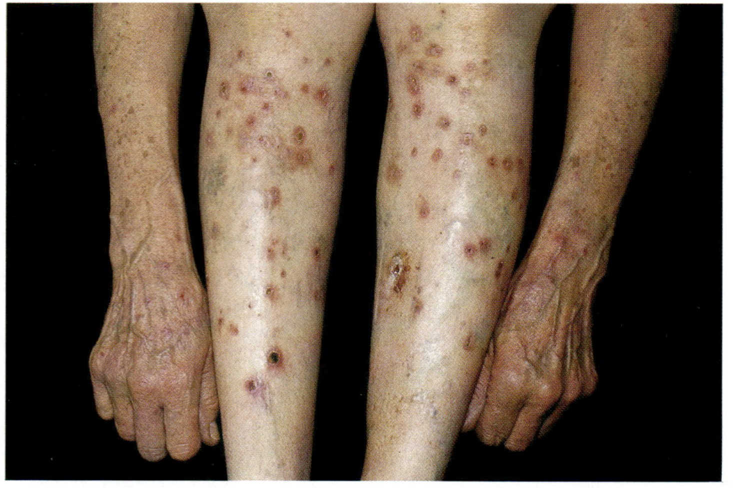

Figure 245 Prurigo. Nodules with circumferential inflammatory reaction on the extensor aspects of the extremities, which have been scratched open due to intense itching.

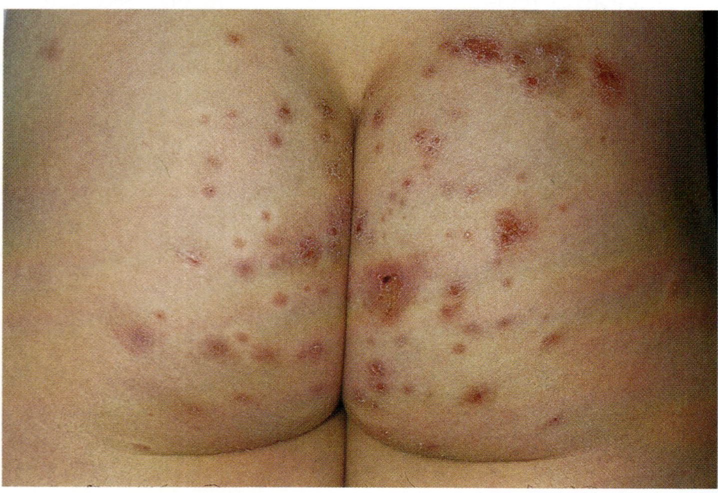

Figure 246 Prurigo. Acutely inflamed, mostly excoriated nodules in the gluteal region.

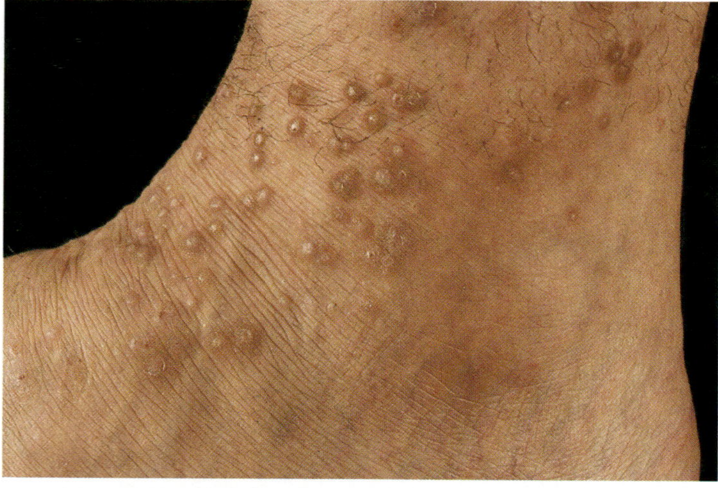

Figure 247 Prurigo. Firm, distinctly pigmented and intensely itching nodules of long duration.

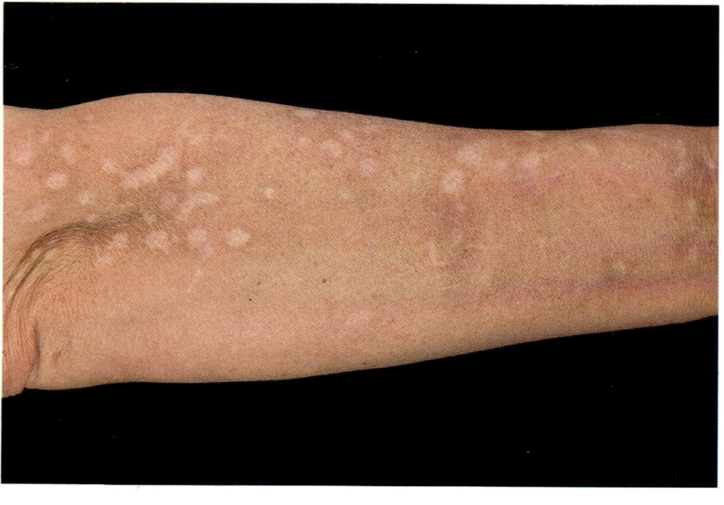

Figure 248 Prurigo. Residual scarring. Round, depigmented lesions with hyperpigmented margins.

Prurigo, Prurigo Nodularis

These conditions are special forms of skin reactions characterized by severely itching papular eruptions. There is no recognizable local cause. In some cases, the development of skin changes is followed by marked itching, in other cases, the lesions are produced by constant scratching. Evaluation must include a thorough work-up to exclude possible systemic diseases such as diabetes mellitus, impaired kidney function, liver diseases, hematologic disorders, drug abuse and helminthic infection of the intestines. A skin disease caused by parasites (scabies, lice) must also be ruled out. Finally, one must remember that prurigo can be a late manifestation of atopic dermatitis in adolescents and adults (see page 41). In many patients, the cause of prurigo cannot be found, despite exhaustive examination. The disease can run a short and acute course, particularly in childhood, but it can also have a prolonged, chronic course over many years.

Clinical Features

1. The prime lesion in prurigo is a firm seropapule (a wheal-like reaction topped by a small vesicle). The vesicle is usually destroyed by scratching and is thus rarely observed. More often, one finds lentil-sized, centrally excoriated papules. Later, one may occasionally see deep, punched-out excoriations.
2. Prurigo occurs mainly on the extensor sides of the extremities, less often on the trunk and rarely on the face, contrary to acne excoriée, which is caused in a similar manner (see page 3). The palms, the soles of the feet and the mucous membranes are never involved.
3. The lesions heal, often with long-lasting hyper- or depigmentation. Deep excoriations result in permanent scars. Prurigo papules on the lower legs are especially tenacious.
4. The excoriations are restricted to the prurigo papules, which is typical for this condition. Linear excoriations are rare. Characteristically, the patients report that the extreme pruritus of the individual lesions is reduced significantly immediately after they are scratched open ("as soon as it bleeds").

Therapy

1. Clarification of the etiology is of prime importance. In those cases in which the cause can be found, the underlying disease must be treated. If a psychiatric problem is suspected (delusions of parasitosis), evaluation and treatment by a psychiatrist are indicated.
2. Antihistamines are useful, especially those with a sedative component **(R. 62)**. For severe cases, neuroleptic drugs in low doses may be indicated (e.g., Haldol, 5 drops 3 times a day.).
3. A topical anesthetic in a medium appropriate for the condition of the skin may be helpful (lotion for acutely irritated skin, pastes and especially ointments for long-standing lesions without irritation of the surrounding skin), occasionally with the addition of a tar preparation (e.g., liquor carbonis detergens 5% or tumenol 5%).
4. Corticosteroid ointments **(R. 38a, b)** should be used only for severe inflammatory, eczematous reactions.
5. Intralesional injections of corticosteroids **(R. 46)** can be helpful for persistent, circumscribed lesions.

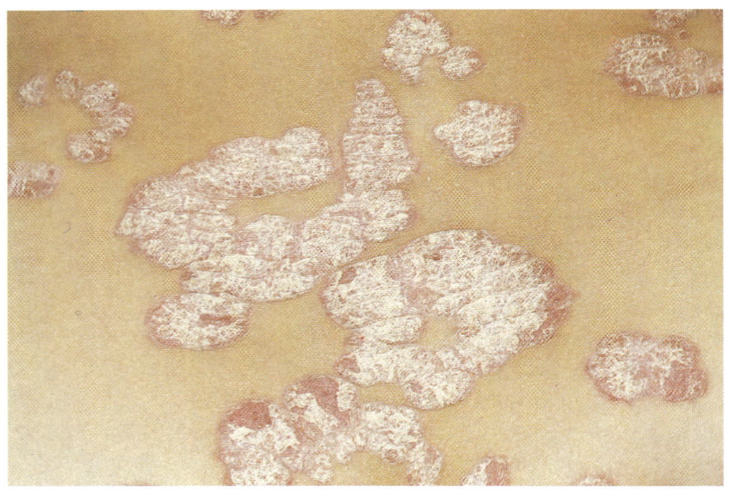

Figure 249 Psoriasis vulgaris. Sharply demarcated, scaling, reddened, individual guttate plaques.

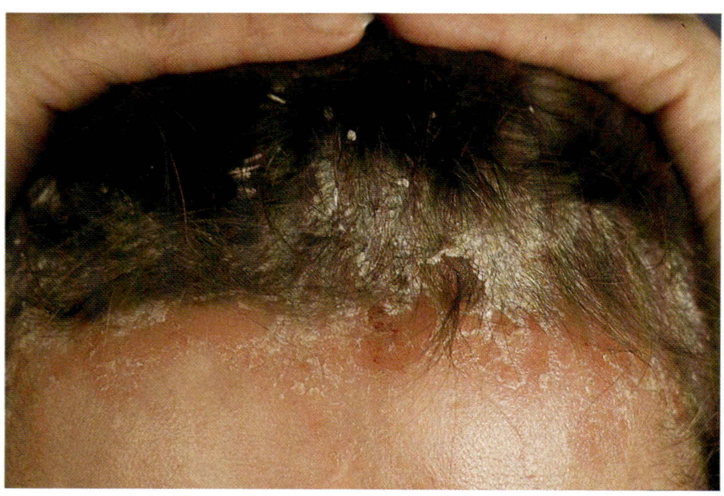

Figure 250 Psoriasis vulgaris. The lesion involves the scalp with typical ribbon of extension to the forehead.

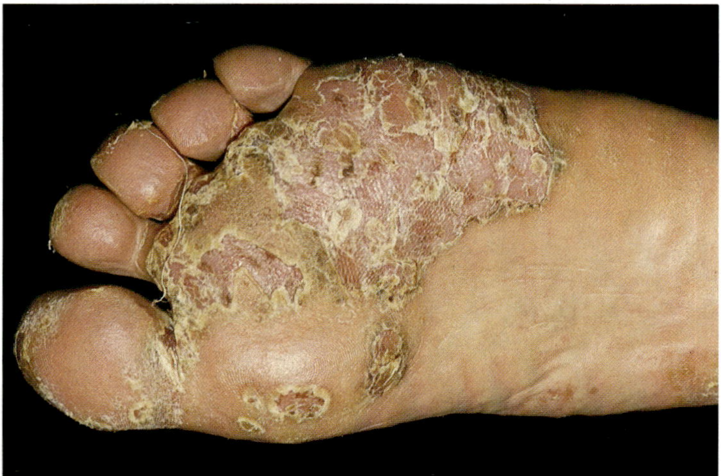

Figure 251 Pustular psoriasis. Involvement of the sole of the foot with development of pustules which are characteristic for this location.

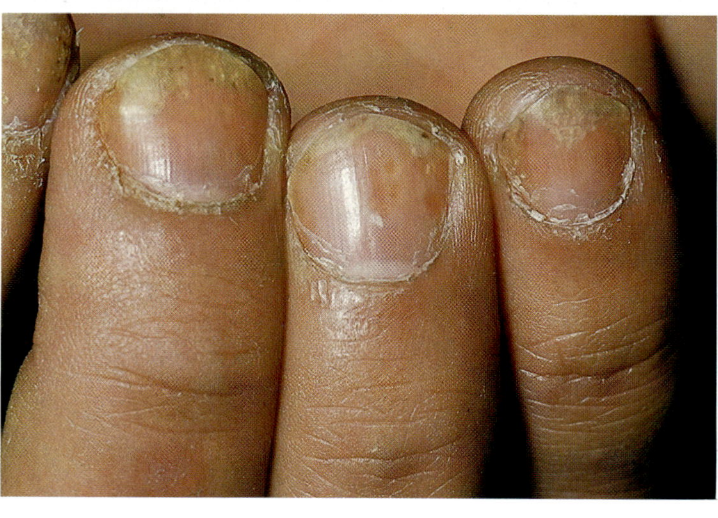

Figure 252 Psoriasis vulgaris. Involvement of the nails with oil stain-like discolorations that can involve a large part of the nail.

Psoriasis

Psoriasis is one of the most frequent skin diseases in the United States, with an estimated prevalence of 1 to 2 percent of the population. The tendency to develop psoriasis is inherited; the cause of the disease is unknown. Onset can be at any age, most often in young adults, rarely, however, in children and the elderly. The course of the disease varies considerably from individual to individual. It usually runs an extremely chronic course, with phases of remission and exacerbation. Certain factors are necessary for the manifestation of psoriasis, and they vary considerably for individual patients. They include external factors such as irritation of the skin by pressure, injuries and sunburn. Psoriasis can also develop in pre-existing skin diseases, such as drug eruptions, other eczematous diseases or allergic contact dermatitis. This characteristic tendency of the skin of psoriatic patients to react to external stimuli with the development of psoriatic lesions is known as isomorphic response or Koebner's phenomenon. Endogenous factors may also provoke development of psoriasis. These include chronic alcohol abuse, emotional stress, certain drugs, especially beta-blockers as well as lithium, chronic infectious diseases (so-called focal inflammations) and obesity. Patients with psoriasis are usually in good health unless they develop an acute exacerbation (e. g., pustular psoriasis, psoriatic erythroderma or psoriatic arthritis). The cosmetic disfiguration, however, often reduces the quality of life significantly and may even lead to latent danger of suicide.

Clinical Features

a) Psoriasis Vulgaris

1. One sees erythematous patches of varying size (lentil- to palm-size lesions), sharply delineated from the surrounding skin with a round or polycyclic border. Particularly characteristic are the thick, imbricated and adherent whitish scales that cover the lesions and that can be removed with the fingernail as small chips.
2. Psoriasis has a predilection for the elbows, knees, scalp, and sacral region.
3. The fingernails are frequently involved and show pitting, with the appearance of "oil droplets" when subungual keratoses are present. In advanced cases, the nail separates from the bed, becomes brittle and crumbles, and the paronychium is then involved.
4. Subjective symptoms are usually absent. Occasionally, the lesions become irritated and itch, especially on the scalp and in intertriginous areas.

b) Pustular Psoriasis

The spectrum of this type of psoriasis extends from chronic pustular involvement of palms and soles (psoriasis pustulosa, type Königsbeck-Barber) to generalized development of pustules on the entire skin with a severe, occasionally life-threatening course (psoriasis pustulosa, type Zumbusch). Pustular psoriasis can develop from psoriasis vulgaris, or it can develop suddenly without any prior psoriasis.

c) Psoriatic Arthritis

This is a chronic, destructive arthritis in patients with psoriasis and involves mainly the interphalangeal joints, the spine and the large joints. Rheumatoid factors are negative. Skin lesions or at least changes in the nails are usually present. Prolonged involvement can lead to severe deformities.

d) Erythrodermic Psoriasis

Psoriasis can develop secondarily into erythroderma, in which the entire skin is erythematous and shows massive scaling. A prolonged course of this disease can lead to significant fluid and protein losses, and the patient is severely ill. This form is sometimes caused by irritating topical treatment, especially excessive UV-radiation.

Therapy

At the present, there is no cure for psoriasis. Therapeutic measures can only produce a remission of symptoms. At best, the disease can be converted from an active to a latent state; or at least, scaling and itching can be reduced and thus substantially improve the cosmetic appearance. The

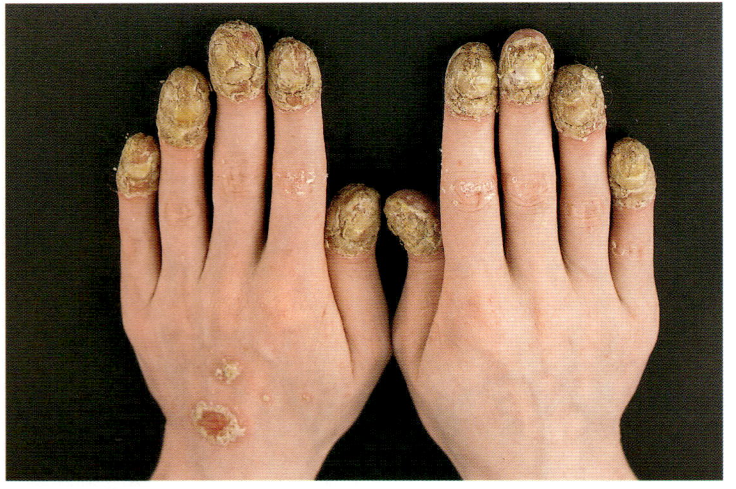

Figure 253 Psoriasis vulgaris. Affected nails with thickening and crumbly decomposition and concomitant involvement of the paronychium.

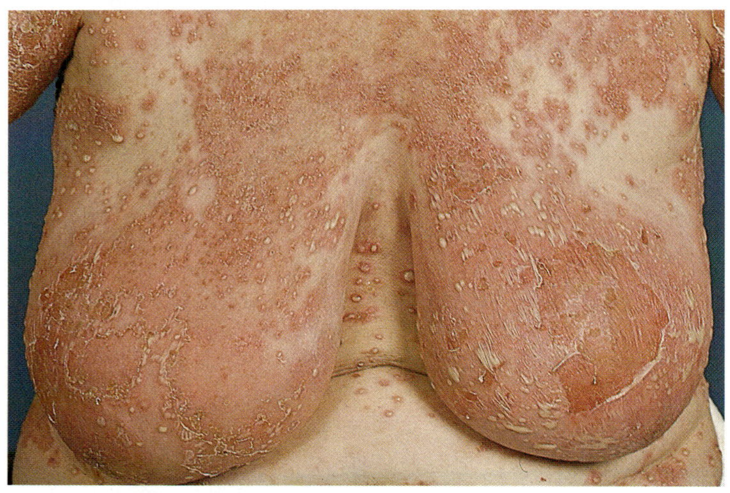

Figure 254 Pustular psoriasis. Acute stage with crops of pustules on an extensive circinate erythema. Area of desquamation of the upper layers of the epidermis on the left breast.

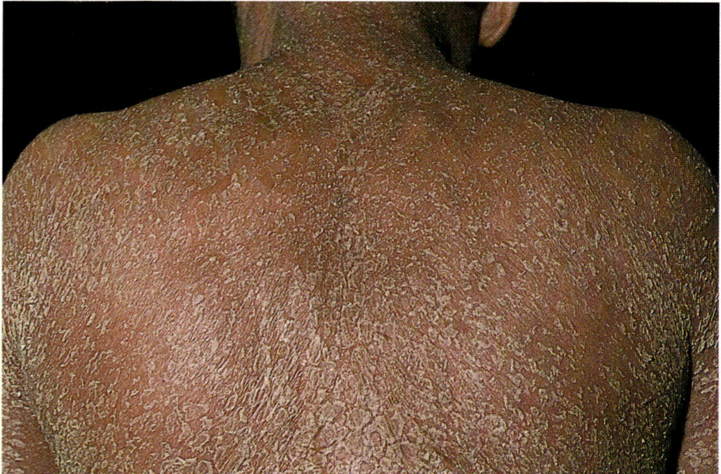

Figure 255 Psoriatic erythroderma. Universal involvement of the skin with erythema, scaling and thickening.

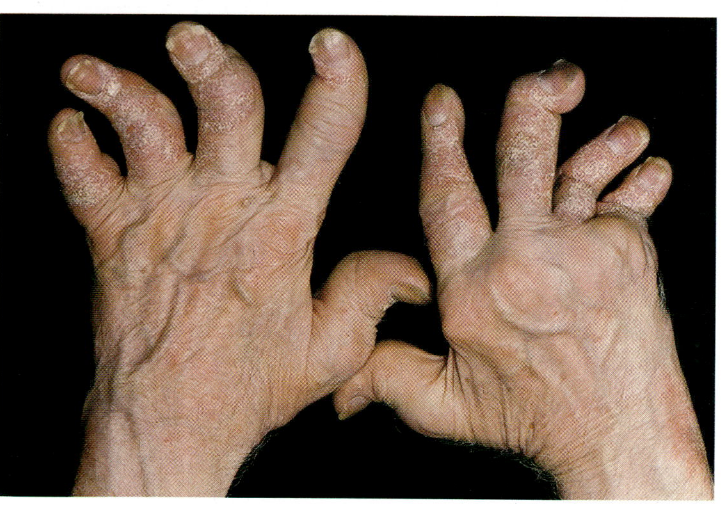

Figure 256 Psoriatic arthritis. Marked deformity of the fingers with significant limitation of movement. Skin and nails show typical psoriatic alterations.

unpredictable course of psoriasis produces phases in which intensive therapy is necessary; at other times, the patient is practically free of symptoms, and no treatment is required. The patient needs psychologic guidance during the long course of the disease. It is especially important that he or she learns to distrust so-called "miracle cures".

Systemic

Systemic therapy should be limited to patients with severe disease whose symptoms cannot be controlled by other measures.

1. Retinoids, especially acitretin **(R. 64)**, have a very good antipsoriatic effect, especially against pustular psoriasis, psoriatic erythroderma and psoriatic arthritis.
2. Topical and systemic corticosteroids produce good results. However, there is usually an exacerbation of symptoms, occasionally to a more severe form (pustular psoriasis), when treatment is discontinued. Therefore, systemic corticosteroids should be used only in exceptional cases.
3. Immunosuppressive substances, such as cyclosporine A and methotrexate, have a good antipsoriatic effect, even in low doses. The risks of this therapy must be kept in mind, especially with long-term therapy.

Topical

1. It is very important to remove the thick layer of scales with salicylic Vaseline (3–5%) and with baths to which soft soap has been added.
2. Anthralin, 1/64–2% **(R. 37)** is still the best topical antipsoriatic drug. Since high concentrations lead to rapid irritation and dermatitis of the healthy surrounding skin, the optimal dose must be found by starting with a low dose and carefully increasing the concentration. The substance has the added disadvantage that its oxidation products cause lasting stains on underwear and sanitary facilities. Attempts have been made to modify anthralin therapy (short contact anthralin therapy [SCAT]) in order to reduce these undesirable side effects. Anthralin therapy requires great therapeutic experience, especially when dealing with extensive psoriasis. These patients should always be referred to a dermatologist who has adequate experience with this therapy.
3. Coal tar products have a distinct antiproliferative effect. The disadvantages are unpleasant odor, and they cause staining of skin and clothing. Bituminous coal tar also causes increased photosensitivity.
4. In general, corticosteroids cannot be recommended as the primary topical therapy for psoriasis. It is true that they produce a rapid remission of psoriatic lesions, but the lesions recur as soon as treatment is discontinued. The chronic character of psoriasis requires long-term therapy, which may lead to undesirable corticosteroid side effects. With topical treatment of extensive lesions, systemic effects can occur from resorption of the drug through the skin. However, local treatment with corticosteroids is indicated for certain sites: corticosteroid tinctures **(R. 18)** for the scalp and the auditory canal, corticosteroid creams **(R. 38a, b; R. 39b)** for the face and in skin folds.
5. UV-therapy: The effectiveness of ultraviolet light on psoriatic lesions has been known for a long time. UV-therapy is carried out as selective ultraviolet therapy (SUP) with long-wave UV-B light, or as photochemotherapy, with a combination of a photosensitizing drug such as 8-methoxypsoralen (methoxsalen) and UV-A light (PUVA; PUVA bath). Because of the possible risks involved with photochemotherapy, this method should only be used by a dermatologist who has experience with this treatment and the necessary equipment. The advantages of a UV-therapy are that it requires relatively little time and that topical treatment is not necessary with its use, except for moisturization of the skin and removal of scales before UV-treatment is started. The disadvantage is that since treatment is usually necessary for a long time, the risk of cutaneous carcinoma from the cumulative dose of artificial UV-radiation is increased significantly.
6. As a rule, psoriasis in the stage of eruption should be treated with relatively mild procedures (no anthralin, no photochemotherapy, no fatty ointments).
7. Psoriasis of the scalp is treated like seborrheic dermatitis (see page 49). Additionally, a shower cap over an occlusive foil may be used at night to enhance penetration of the active scale-removing medication.

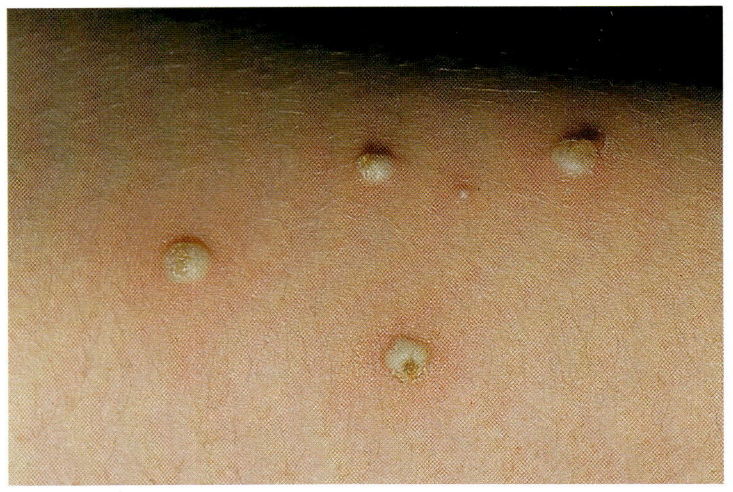

Figure 257 Follicular pustules. Purulent inflammation of the hair follicle. Pustules with surrounding erythema.

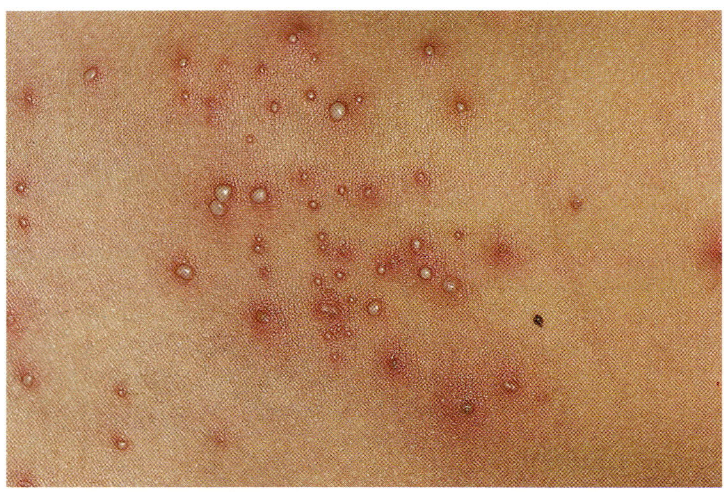

Figure 258 Follicular pustules. Extensive dissemination of pustules surrounded by inflammatory reaction.

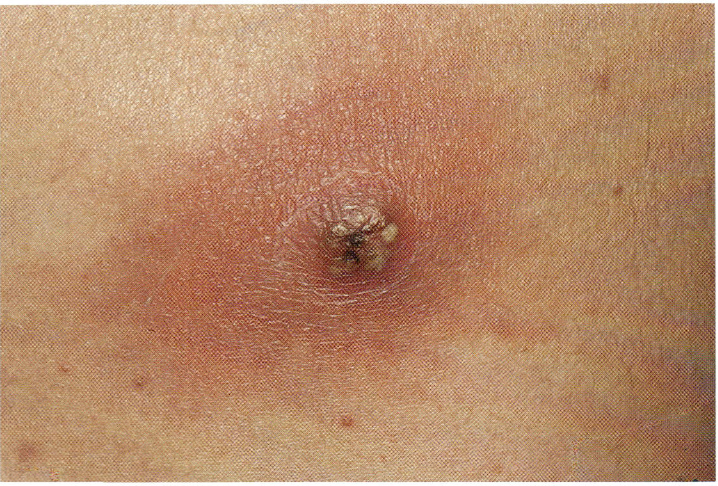

Figure 259 Furuncle. Acute inflammatory tumor with central purulent core.

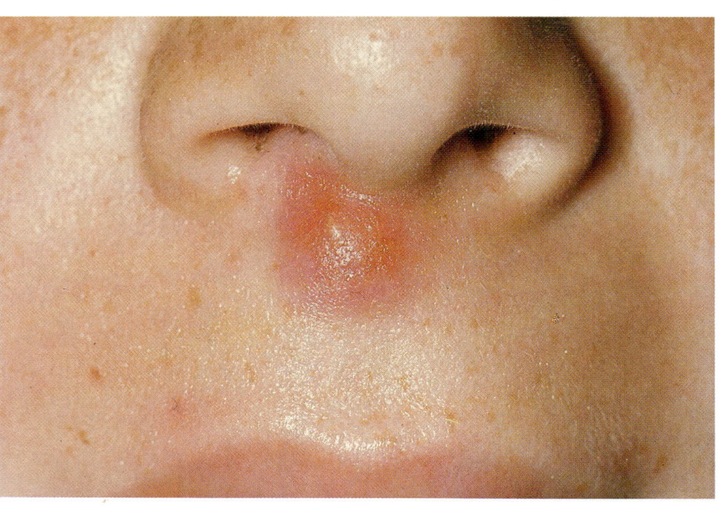

Figure 260 Furuncle at the entrance to the nose.

Pyodermas

A. Folliculitis, Follicular Pustules

Follicular pustules are infections usually caused by *Staphylococcus aureus*. Single or multiple follicular pustules (infections of the pilosebaceous apparatus) can be caused by a variety of factors: Local or systemic impairment of the immune system and an increase or alteration of the bacterial flora entering the follicles, e.g., from influenza or fever of other origin, chronic diseases with immunosuppression (AIDS, diabetes mellitus, etc.), immunosuppression caused by drugs, oily skin due to constant contact with oil or prolonged application of fatty ointments, as well as in patients with atopic dermatitis. Follicular pustules can develop into furuncles.

Clinical Features

1. Follicular pustules are often pierced by a hair and often surrounded by an erythematous zone.
2. The pustules occur only in those areas of the skin that have hair follicles; they do not develop in the palms and on the soles. Pustules occur most frequently on the face and neck (folliculitis barbae), the chest, the back and the extremities.

Therapy

Before treatment is started, it is important to evaluate the patient for systemic or local causes, underlying diseases, occupational exposure to oil, etc.

1. The pustules are evacuated and dabbed with a disinfectant solution **(R. 17)**, or dried out with aqueous zinc lotion. Erythromycin acne preparations are also helpful, as well as benzoyl peroxide.
2. The bacterial flora of the skin can be reduced by frequent washing with detergents **(R. 5)**.
3. Systemic treatment with antibiotics is not necessary.

B. Furuncle and Furunculosis

This is a deep-seated, infectious folliculitis and perifolliculitis with a core of pus. Furuncles develop in patients with transient or permanent local or systemic impairment of the immune system. They often occur as single lesions. Other patients may develop recurrent furuncles over a prolonged period of time (recurrent furuncles, furunculosis). This disease affects mainly young men who are otherwise healthy. The patients must be examined for a variety of etiologies, such as alcoholism, drug abuse, diabetes mellitus, leukemia and other malignant diseases, AIDS and chronic diseases of the liver.

Clinical Features

1. The slightly raised inflammatory erythema with a central core undergoes central necrosis and pus formation within a few days. The core can rupture and drain, or the furuncle can also be resorbed and regress.
2. Trunk and extremities are affected most frequently; the face is involved occasionally.
3. There is lymphangitis and enlargement of the regional lymph nodes. In rare cases, sepsis can complicate the course.

Therapy

Local therapy is sufficient in most cases. In furuncles of the nose and upper lip, the infection can spread through the angular vein and cause thrombosis of the cavernous sinus or meningitis. These cases require special therapeutic care.

General

Patients with systemic symptoms or an impaired immune reaction, and especially those with furuncles of the face should have bed rest. Patients with furuncles of the nose or upper lip should not speak or chew.

Systemic

1. Furuncles of the face must be treated with systemic antibiotics. Furuncles at other sites require antibiotics only when generalized symptoms or impairment of the immune system is present. In those cases, penicillinase-resistant antibiotics **(R. 47)** are preferable. Determination of the organisms and their antibiotic sensitivity must always precede!

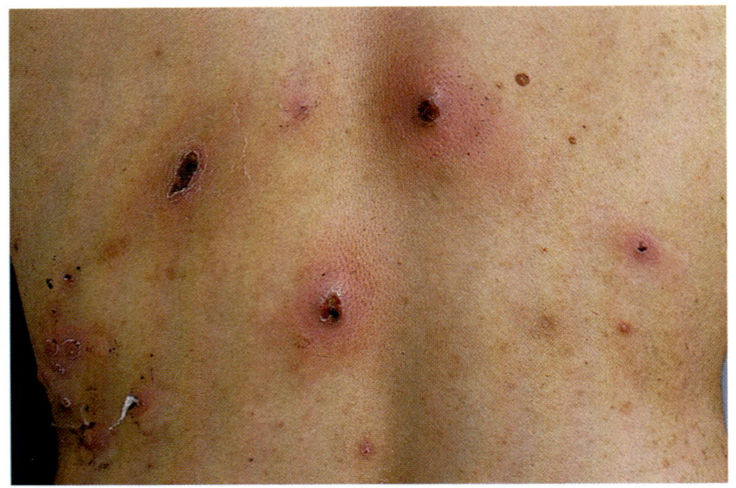

Figure 261 Furunculosis. Multiple furuncles in a patient with diabetes mellitus.

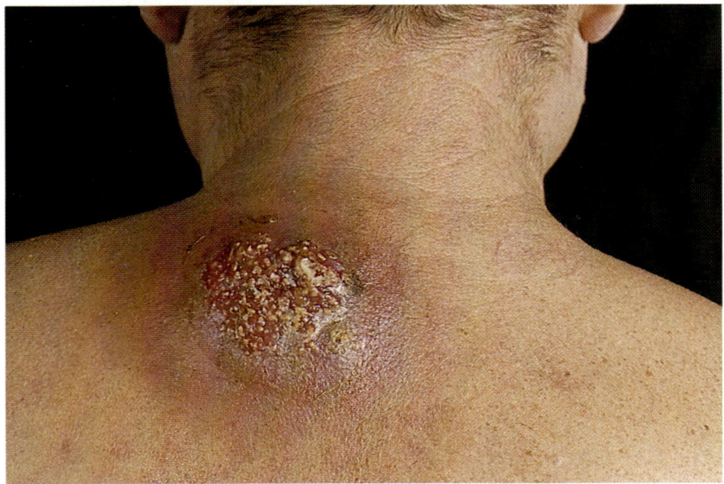

Figure 262 Carbuncle of the neck. Severe involvement with extensive, acutely inflamed swelling and multiple small purulent foci.

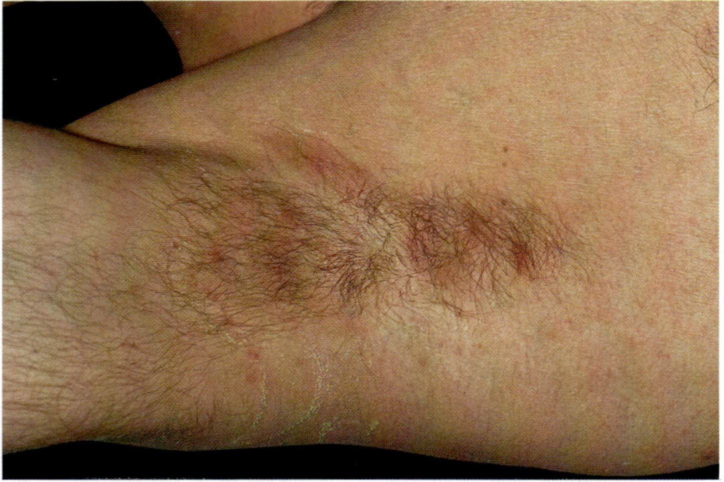

Figure 263 Abscesses of the sweat glands. Painful nodular inflammation in the right axilla.

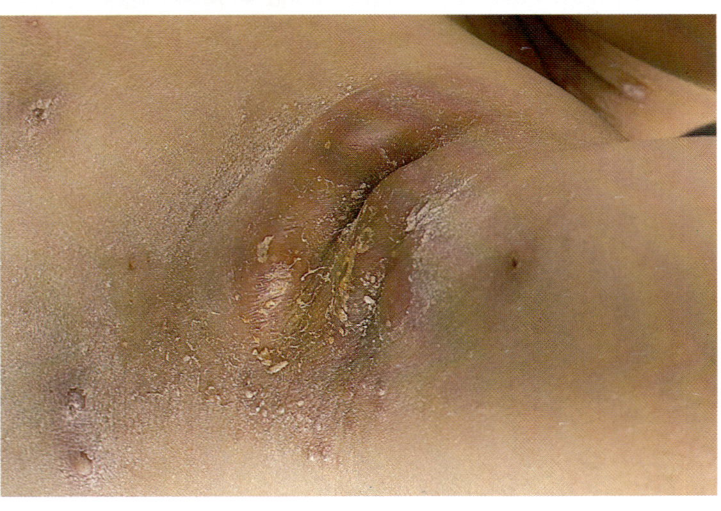

Figure 264 Abscesses of the sweat glands. Painful nodular and abscess-forming inflammation in the left axilla surrounded by individual pustules.

2. For recurrent furuncles, treatment with an immunostimulating substance or autovaccine therapy can be tried.
3. Substitution of immunoglobulins is indicated only in patients with antibody deficiency.

External

1. Ichthyol ointment (**R. 41b**), covered with a dressing is helpful.
2. Cold packs (ice cubes) enhance resorption in the early stages.
3. Local heat application (infrared light) induces hyperemia and expedites suppuration.
4. When an abscess has formed, it should be drained with a stab incision.

C. Carbuncle

Clinical Features

The special anatomy of the back of the neck favors the formation of painful inflammatory conglomerate tumors, which are actually aggregated furuncles.

Therapy

In addition to the therapeutic measures described for furuncles, generous incision under general anesthesia is necessary at an early stage to drain the pus.

D. Sweat Gland Abscesses

These abscesses are found mainly in the apocrine glands of the axillary, inguinal and perigenital regions. Multiple recurrent sweat gland abscesses (so-called suppurative hidradenitis) are usually a symptom of acne conglobata and frequently occur in such patients, in addition to the other symptoms of that condition (see page 5).

Clinical Features

1. Nodular swellings with and without pus are seen. In severe cases, inflammatory erythema occurs later with formation of fistulae and irregular rope-like scarring.
2. Areas of predilection are the axillae, inguinal, perianal and perigenital areas.
3. In advanced cases, the abscesses can be very painful.

Therapy

Treatment is often difficult. The abscesses tend to recur over a prolonged period. Minor surgical procedures (incision of abscesses, excision of small nodules) are often performed but should be avoided if at all possible. They do not prevent a recurrence and often cause the formation of fistulae which makes the condition worse. Patients with extensive involvement may require major surgery with excision of the entire involved area, followed by plastic closure of the defect (e.g., latissimus dorsi plasty). These are major, technically difficult operations and should be performed by a surgeon with experience in these procedures.

Systemic

1. Isotretinoin (**R. 65**) is the most effective treatment in advanced cases.
2. In comparison, treatment with systemic antibiotics is generally not very effective.
3. Immunostimulating substances have been tried with little or no success.

Topical

Topical therapy contributes little because the pathologic changes are located deep in the dermis. Washing with disinfectant soaps reduces the bacterial flora of the skin.

E. Impetigo Contagiosa

Impetigo contagiosa is the most frequent bacterial skin disease in children. The diagnosis is usually easy to make, and therapy is rapidly successful in most cases. This superficial skin disease is caused by streptococci, or less frequently, by staphylococci. The infection is transmitted by direct skin contact and develops rapidly. Several children in one family are often involved (contact infection). The children should be kept out of school or kindergarten for a few days to avoid spreading the disease. Impetigo occurs more frequently in poor socioeconomic conditions, but this does not necessarily imply that the disease is generally due to lack of cleanliness. Children with atopic dermatitis are particularly prone to developing impetigo Furthermore,

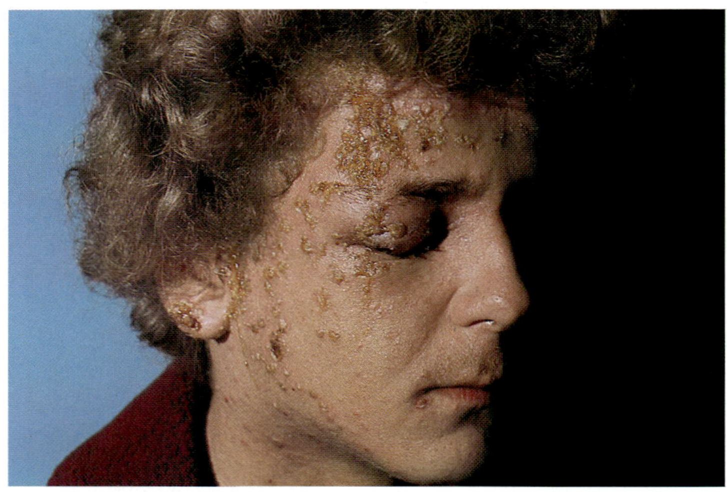

Figure 265 Impetigo contagiosa. Yellow crusts and pustules in a planar or circinoid distribution. The skin is otherwise unchanged.

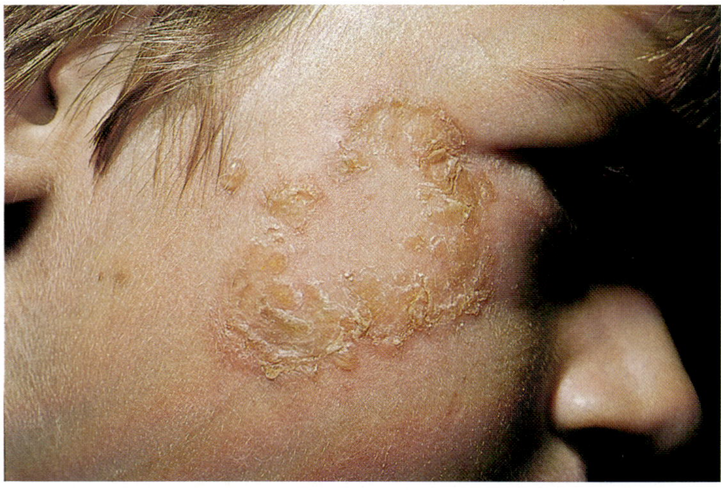

Figure 266 Impetigo contagiosa. Annular lesion with layered, yellow, crusty coating.

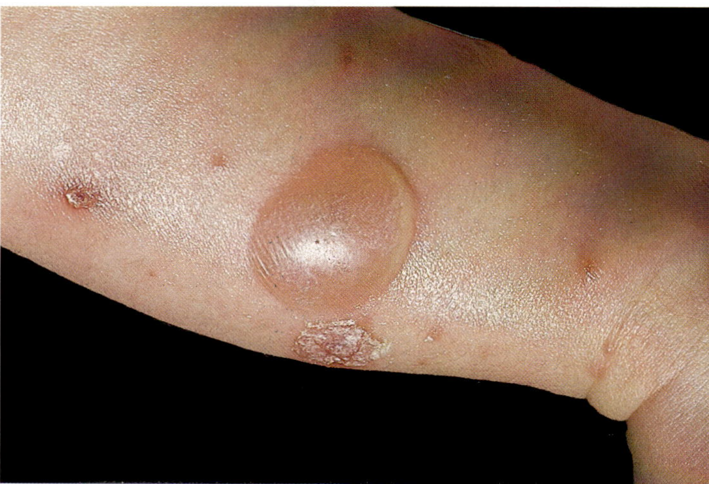

Figure 267 Impetigo contagiosa. Bullous form of the disease, often seen in children.

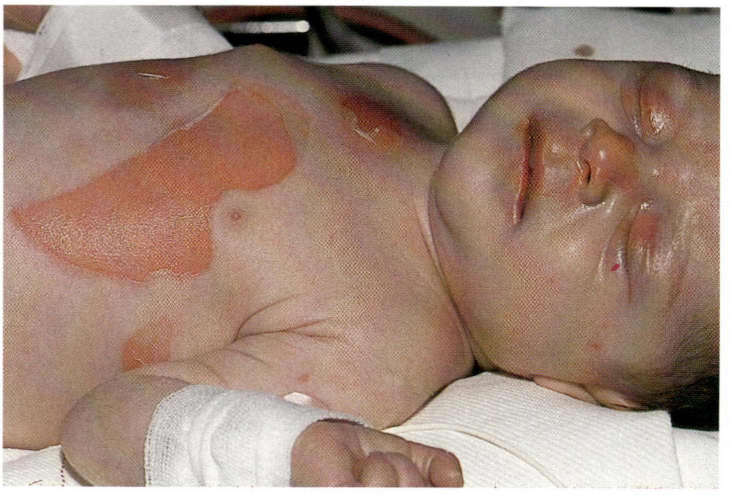

Figure 268 Staphylococcal scalded skin syndrome (Ritter's disease). Bullous infantile impetigo in its maximal form. Bullae or remnants of bullae with extensive desquamation of the upper epidermis.

impetigo occurs more frequently in hot and moist climates. Complications of impetigo, such as glomerulonephritis or sepsis, are rare today. Impetigo should not be confused with secondary bacterial infection (impetiginization) of pre-existing skin diseases, such as scabies, eczema or insect bites.

Clinical Features

1. Honey-colored to dark yellow, layered crusts form round, centrifugally expanding lesions. These lesions often have a distinct margin or the crust is only on the margin, so that the lesions are irregular with circinate borders. Sometimes there is a slightly erythematous base.
2. Occasionally, vesicles and erosions predominate instead of crusts.
3. Areas of predilection are the face and occasionally the intertriginous areas (axillae, inguinal region), but the disease can affect any part of the body.
4. Moderate pruritus is present. There are no systemic symptoms.

Therapy

Topical therapy is promptly effective in most cases and usually sufficient.

1. A topical ointment or cream (such as Aureomycin ointment or Polysporin ointment), or simply soft zinc paste 2 times daily.
2. A disinfectant full bath **(R. 4)** also helps to loosen the crusts.
3. Systemic antibiotic therapy **(R. 47, 51)** is only necessary for widespread vesicular impetigo or when septic complications are present.

F. Staphylococcal Scalded Skin Syndrome

This maximum form of vesicular staphylococcal impetigo (formerly known as dermatitis exfoliativa neonatorum [Ritter von Rittershain]) is known today as SSSS – staphylococcal scalded skin syndrome. It can develop very rapidly in small children and usually occurs as a secondary disease after a bacterial infection such as otitis media or infection of the umbilicus. In most cases, it is caused by *Staphylococcus aureus* of group II, phage type 71.

Clinical Features

1. The disease is characterized by large bullae, ruptured bullae and erythema.
2. The entire skin can be involved. The bullae are found predominantly in areas exposed to mechanical forces.
3. The mucous membranes are practically never involved, contrary to toxic epidermal necrolysis.
4. This is a severe generalized disease with high fever and malaise. The patients often have difficulty drinking. Immediate hospitalization and antibiotic treatment are necessary (penicillinase-resistant penicillin).

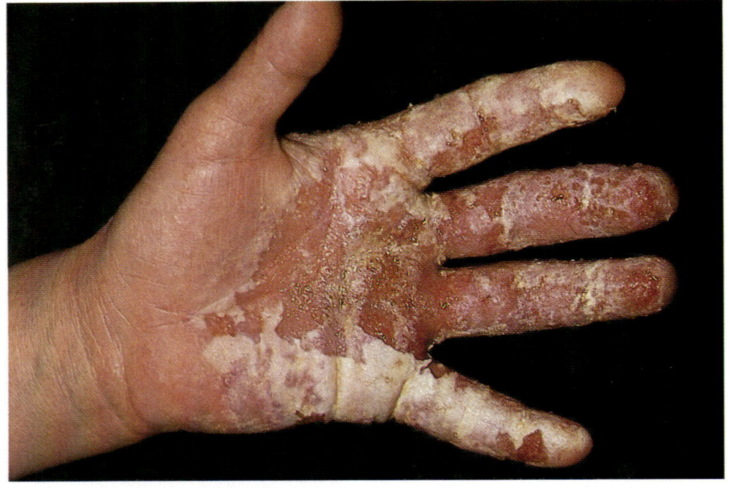

Figure 269 Acute radiation dermatitis. Acute erosive-ulcerative inflammatory radiation reaction after radiation accident.

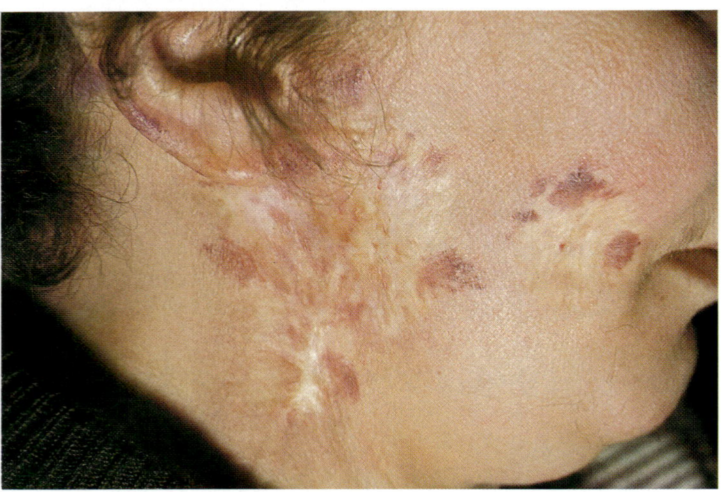

Figure 270 Radiation dermatitis. Figurated scar corresponding to the irradiated field. Adjacent to it are remnants of the irradiated nevus flammeus.

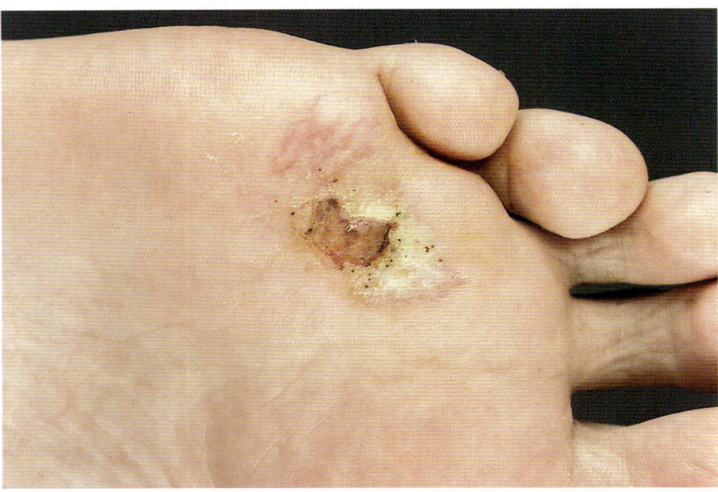

Figure 271 Radiation dermatitis. Sequel of radiation treatment of plantar warts.

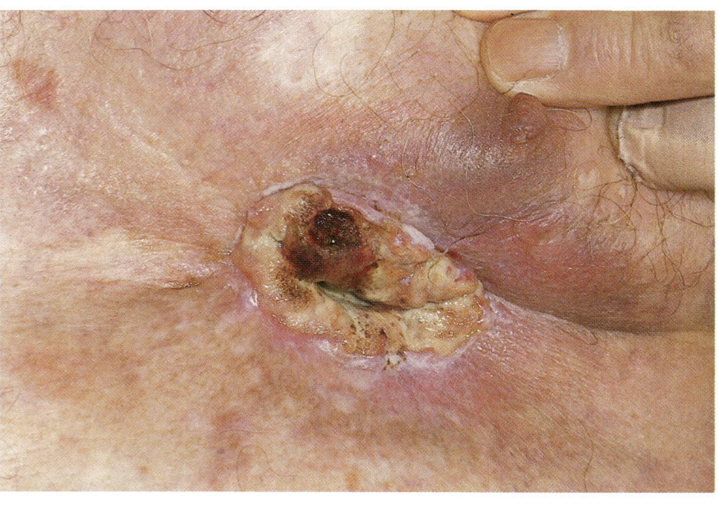

Figure 272 Squamous cell carcinoma secondary to radiation dermatitis.

Radiation Damage to the Skin

Irradiation of the skin with ionizing radiation (x-rays, grenz rays, beta rays, gamma rays) causes dose-dependent damage to the skin. Acute radiation dermatitis consists of an inflammatory reaction due to direct injury to the cell. Chronic radiation damage to the skin occurs as a summation effect after multiple exposures to low-level radiation. These changes can be due to local radiation to the skin or to deep irradiation of internal organs. Similar alterations are also seen following accidents in nuclear installations, as the accident at Chernobyl has shown. Radiation damage to the skin is seen less frequently today, because radiation for benign and inflammatory disorders of the skin is not used very often anymore, and better methods for irradiation of internal organs (rotational irradiation, fast electrons) have been developed.

A. Acute Radiation Dermatitis

Clinical Features

This acute reaction of the skin to ionizing radiation is classified into 3 stages according to the degree of severity. The mildest form (first-degree acute radiation reaction) consists of erythema, which appears after about a week, followed by hyperpigmentation, which lasts for a long time. Higher doses produce a more intensive inflammatory reaction, with edema, blistering and long-lasting erosions (second-degree acute radiation reaction), which is always followed by a chronic radiation dermatitis (see below). The most severe form of acute radiation injury to the skin is characterized by complete tissue destruction and deep necroses. After demarcation, an ulcer develops which is very resistant to treatment (third-degree acute radiation reaction). This type of radiation reaction is always the result of an overdose of radiation.

Therapy

An adverse, acute radiation reaction can be treated with topical corticosteroids to combat inflammation. Systemically, pain medications with anti-inflammatory action, such as aspirin or other nonsteroidal anti-inflammatory drugs are given.

B. Chronic Radiation Dermatitis

Clinical Features

This stage develops following second- or third-degree acute radiation reaction, and also as a result of a high total radiation dose that was given in fractionated, low-level individual doses. After a latency period of 2–10 years, the skin becomes thin and vulnerable, with telangiectasias, spotty hyper- and depigmentation and thickened connective tissue (radiation fibrosis). Deep, poorly healing ulcers develop in the center of these areas even after mild trauma (radiation ulcer). In addition, one sees keratotic changes (radiation keratosis). Radiation ulcers and radiation keratoses can eventually lead to radiation carcinoma, the most severe and dreaded complication of radiation injury. Suspicious lesions should always be evaluated by tissue biopsy.

Therapy

1. Topical therapy of radiation dermatitis consists of frequent moisturization of the skin with a mild ointment **(R. 33b, c)** and protection from any great mechanical stress to prevent the development of ulcers.
2. Long-standing radiation ulcers that fail to heal, especially those with malignant changes, must be treated surgically by excision followed by skin graft coverage. These procedures are technically difficult and not without risk, especially when the radiation fibrosis extends to the bone.
3. Topical corticosteroids should be avoided here because the skin is already thin and vulnerable.

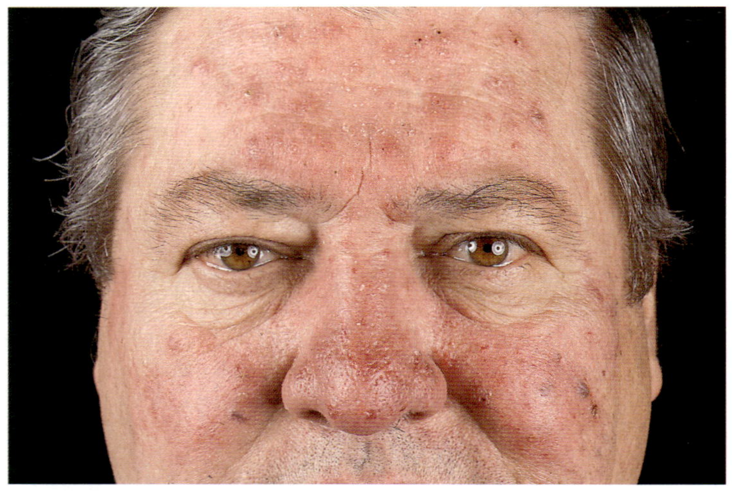

Figure 273 Rosacea. Erythema and papules on nose, cheeks and forehead. Distinct involvement of the conjunctiva.

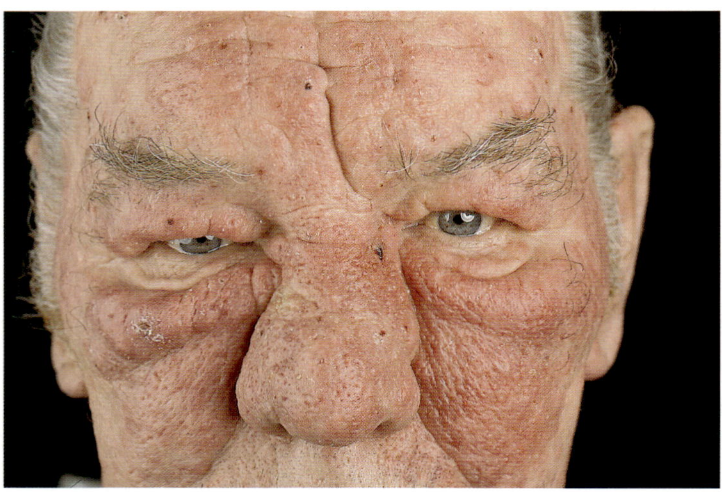

Figure 274 Rosacea. Planar, papular infiltrates in typical location (nose, cheeks, forehead) with marked hyperplasia of the sebaceous glands (rhinophyma).

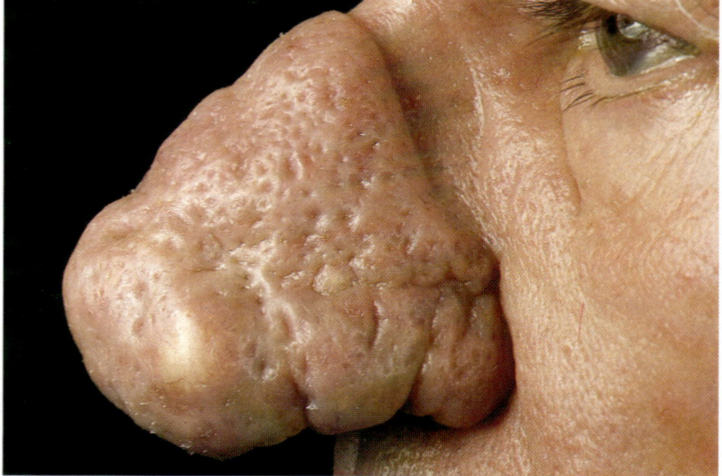

Figure 275 Rhinophyma. Distinctly sharp demarcation from pressure from the frame of the patient's glasses. Other symptoms of a facial rosacea are absent.

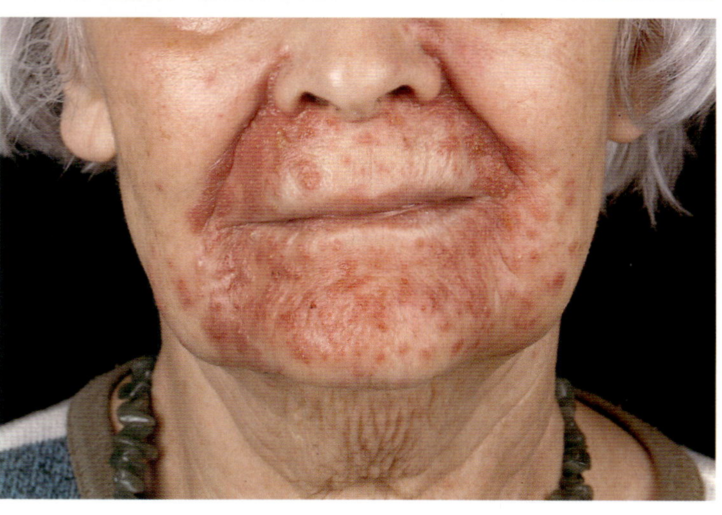

Figure 276 Perioral rosacea-like dermatitis (steroid rosacea) following long-term topical corticosteroid application.

Rosacea and Rosacea-Like Dermatitis

A. Rosacea

Rosacea is a common chronic skin disease affecting mainly the face. It manifests itself in middle-aged persons and involves both sexes with the same frequency. The most disfiguring type, rhinophyma, occurs almost exclusively in men. The cause is unknown. Alcohol abuse, poorly balanced diet, or hyperseborrhea are associated with rosacea only in isolated cases.

Clinical Features

1. Persistent erythema, papules, and pustules, as well as large inflammatory nodules and plaques can be present, depending on the severity of the disease. In contrast to acne, there are no comedones, even though the patient may have oily skin.
2. Areas of predilection are the cheeks, nose, forehead and occasionally the chin. Involvement often takes the shape of a "butterfly".
3. Involvement of the eyes with blepharitis, conjunctivitis, keratitis, and iridocyclitis can occur as complications of rosacea.

Therapy
Systemic

1. Systemic antibiotic therapy with tetracyclines can be tried in cases of rosacea (e.g., minocycline) when topical therapy is unsuccessful. Treatment is started with normal doses and is later reduced to a low maintenance.
Additional systemic therapy is necessary only in severe cases of rosacea.
2. Isotretinoin **(R. 65)** in doses of 0.2 to 1 mg per kilogram of body weight is given for 10–16 weeks.
3. Metronidazole, 250 mg per day for 10 days to a maximum of 20 days is helpful. Long-term treatment with metronidazole is contraindicated because of the risk of polyneuropathy and possible carcinogenic effects.

Topical

The skin of rosacea patients becomes irritated very easily. Irritating substances or bases (salicylic acid, sulfur, fatty ointments) should be avoided.

1. The skin should be washed with detergents that have strong or weak defatting effects, depending on the type of skin.
2. Anti-inflammatory and antibacterial medications in a non-irritating base or benzoyl peroxide in a gel form 3–5% **(R. 25a)**.
3. Metronidazole is also effective when applied topically (1-2%).
4. Topical corticosteroids have no place in the treatment of rosacea. They can be effective for a short period of time, but the disease recurs after treatment is discontinued. Long-term therapy can result in "steroid damage" to the skin, which is very unpleasant in the face (erythema, telangiectasias, exacerbation of the rosacea, hypertrichosis).
5. Hot drinks, exposure to steam and alcohol consumption increase the symptoms and should be avoided. Dietetic measures have no effect on rosacea.

B. Perioral Rosacea-Like Dermatitis (Steroid Rosacea)

This disease occurs almost exclusively in women. Long-term use of fluorinated or strong corticosteroids, as well as the use of excessively oily cosmetics have been identified as causative agents.

Clinical Features

Pinhead-sized inflammatory papules appear on an erythematous base in the perioral region with a narrow, unaffected area surrounding the lips. The disease involves the surrounding skin only in severe cases.

Therapy

If the patient has been on corticosteroid therapy, it must be discontinued. This can be the most difficult step, because the skin changes are usually exacerbated at first. The treatment should be supplemented with moist dressings **(R. 1)** or lotions **(R. 20a)**. Ointments and creams with a strong lubricating effect should be avoided. If the condition is resistant to therapy, systemic tetracyclines (doxycycline or minocycline) at a normal dose should be given, which can later be reduced to the lowest possible maintenance dose.

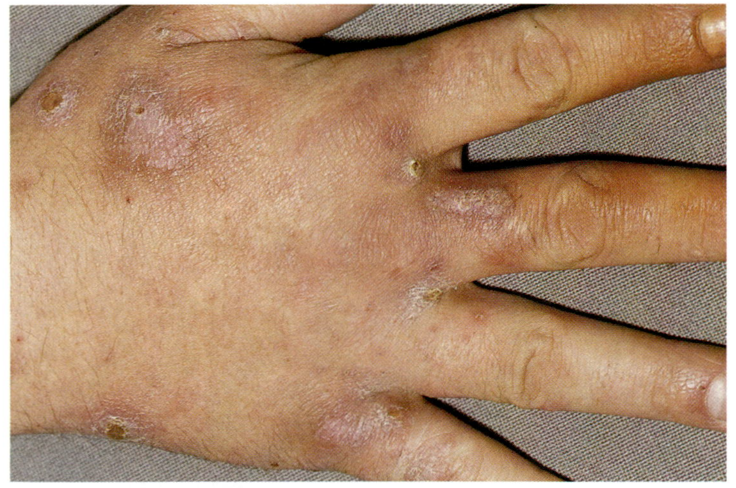

Figure 277 Scabies. Eczematous papules and burrows mainly in the interdigital areas.

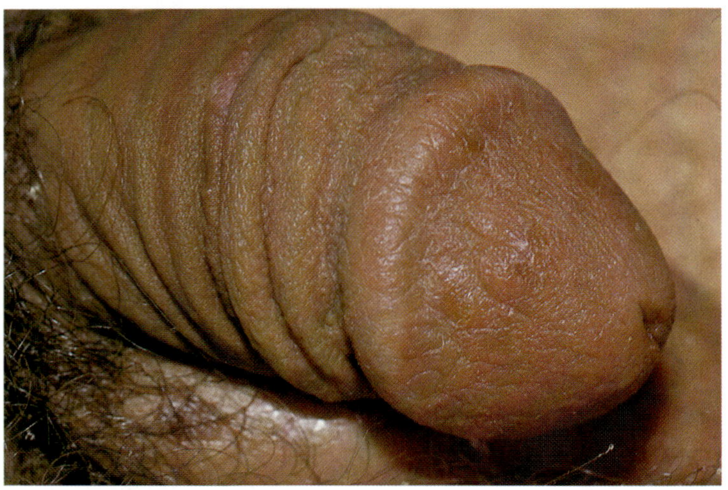

Figure 278 Scabies. Typical location of the papules in a man: Body and glans of the penis.

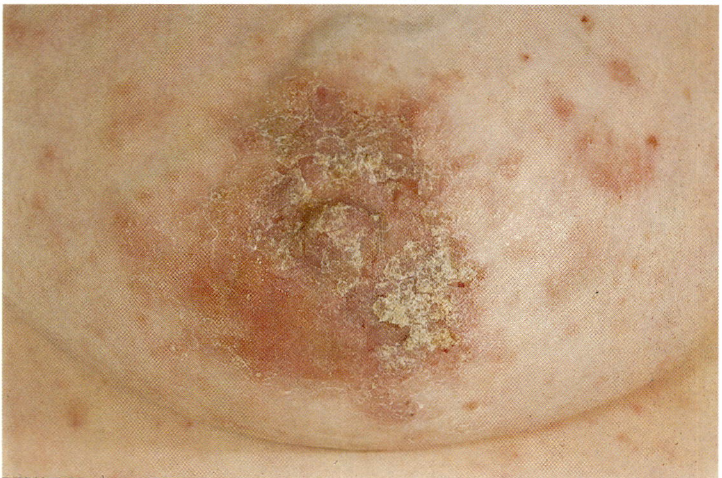

Figure 279 Scabies. Nonspecific eczematization. Typical location in a female patient: Region of the mamilla.

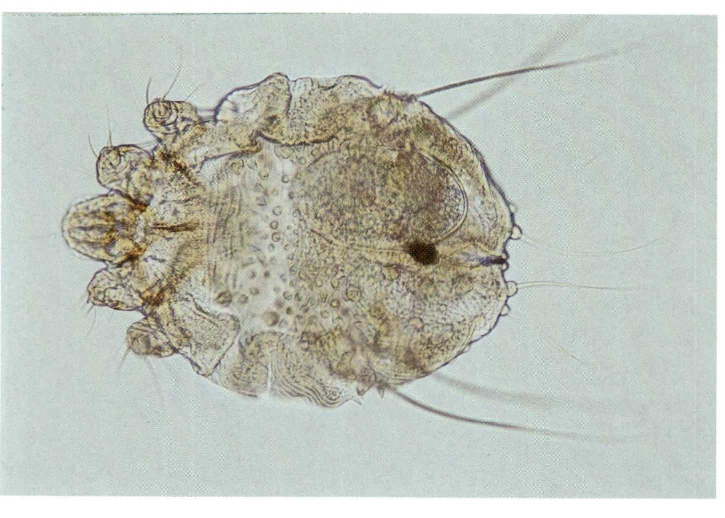

Figure 280 Scabies mite. Magnification 120x.

Scabies

The causative organism is the almost invisible itch mite, Sarcoptes scabiei. Scabies occurs epidemically through close physical contact in families, nursing homes, orphanages, etc. It is an infectious disease that affects all social levels and is not associated with poor bodily hygiene. It can also be transmitted by sexual intercourse, and in these cases, the diagnostic work-up should include other sexually transmitted diseases.

The disease is recognizable by the burrows and papules the female mite makes to deposit her eggs. These are always found in typical locations and are characterized by inflammatory reactions, formation of yellow crusts, weeping, pain and marked pruritus. Diagnosis is confirmed by demonstration of the causative organisms. The mites are removed from the burrows with a thin injection needle or the papules can be excised with a curette. Although this procedure can be difficult, it is desirable to establish the diagnosis. The incubation period is approximately 3 weeks. It is important to identify the source and treat all contact persons.

Clinical Features

1. Skin-colored or reddened, pinhead-sized papules or raised burrows, several millimeters to 1 cm long, are often but not always visible. Eczematous eruptions with punctate erosions, crusts, and scales predominate, as well as secondary scratch marks.
2. These frequently uncharacteristic changes are located chiefly in the finger clefts and in the perimamillary and genital regions. The axillary folds, umbilical area and buttocks are often involved.
3. Of diagnostic significance are pinhead to pea-sized nodules on the shaft of the penis in men and in the mamillary region in women. In adults, the face and scalp, as well as palms and soles are practically never involved. In children, vesicular eruptions are frequently seen on palms and soles.
4. Intensive itching which is worse at night, as well as other infected persons in the environment are additional important diagnostic clues.
5. Infection with Norwegian scabies, or crusted scabies, is characterized by the formation of heavy crusts on erythematous skin. It occurs mainly in persons with impaired immunity. In contrast to common scabies, these crusts are heavily infested with mites and are very contagious. They are often the source of scabies epidemics in hospitals and nursing homes.

Therapy

1. An antiparasitic drug (lindane, benzoyl benzoate or crotamiton, **R. 40**) should be rubbed into the skin from neck to toes for 3 days. The medication is applied at bedtime and should be washed off in the morning. Bed sheets and clothing are then also changed. Since the drug is absorbed more readily in children (toxicity), their treatment should be limited to one side or one quadrant for only a few hours at a time. Crotamiton should be used during pregnancy.
2. Bed sheets and clothing used during the 2 days before treatment should be boiled or aired for 5 to 7 days to avoid reinfestation with mites that develop from the eggs. The mite can survive only 12–24 hours away from the human skin.
3. Pruritus, as well as eczematous lesions and post-scabious papules can persist for several days or weeks after the mites have been killed. Application of corticosteroid creams **(R. 38a, b)** for 1–2 weeks is helpful.
4. Antihistamines **(R. 61, 62)** may be indicated for severe pruritus.
5. All infected persons must be treated to avoid re-infections (ping-pong infections).

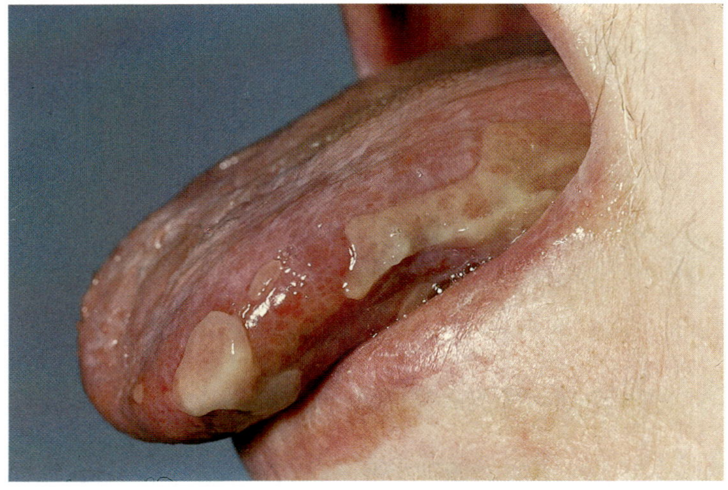

Figure 281 Drug-induced erosive-ulcerative stomatitis. The tongue is involved with fibrin-covered erosions.

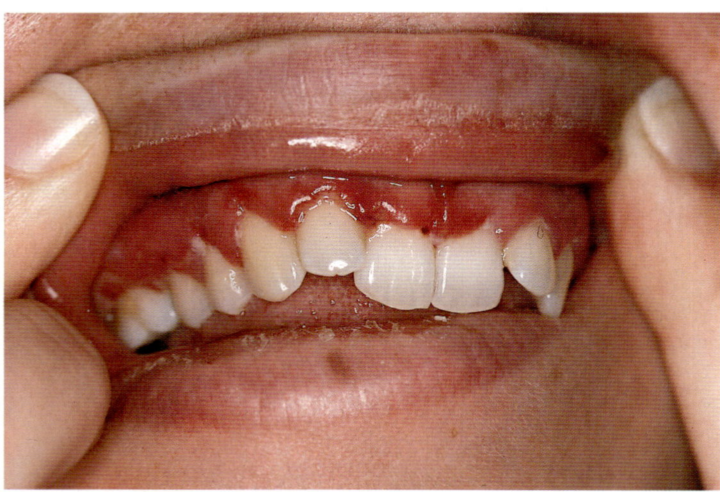

Figure 282 Acute gingivitis. Part of a herpetic gingivostomatitis.

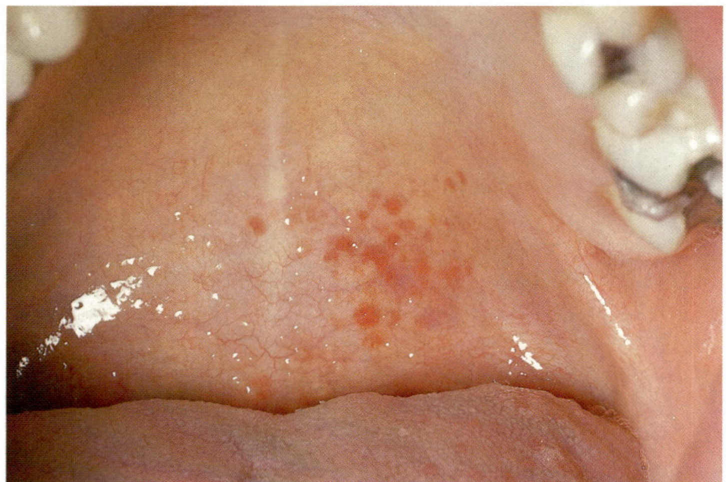

Figure 283 Herpangina Zahorsky. Vesicles on the hard and soft palate are arranged unilaterally and in groups. The vesicles in this case have become hemorrhagic.

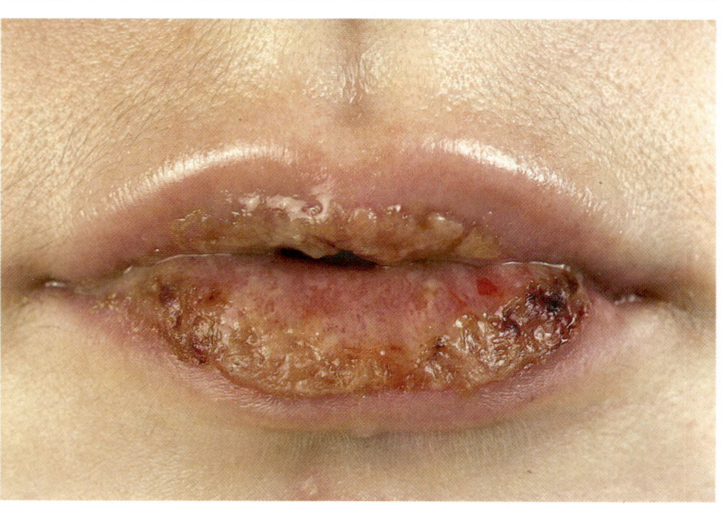

Figure 284 Stomatitis as part of an erythema multiforme. Typical crust formation on both lips.

Stomatitis, Inflammation of the Oral Mucosa

Stomatitis is an inflammation of the total oral mucosa or major parts of it. It is merely a symptom and requires further diagnostic clarification. Recurrent aphthae (see page 11) are not associated with stomatitis. As a rule, stomatitis is a self-limited disease that develops its maximum form within 1 week and then subsides within 2–3 weeks. Stomatitis can appear as part of a viral infection, an undesired drug reaction, or an erythema multiforme. It can also be caused by bacterial infections (pyogenic gingivostomatitis), or it may be due to other permanent or transient immunosuppressive disorders such as xerostomia, leukemia and debilitating systemic diseases.

Clinical Features

1. Erosions, fibrinous coatings, ulcers, and foul-smelling detritus are present in the anterior part or the entire oral mucosa. Ulcers of the oral mucosa nearly always heal without scars, in contrast to the skin.
2. The gingiva is often involved in the form of gingivitis or gingivostomatitis.
3. The lesions are painful at rest as well as from chewing or speaking. Not infrequently, the patients also complain of an unpleasant, often metallic taste (parageusia).
4. With severe stomatitis, there are blood clots in the mouth and hemorrhagic crusts on the lips, especially when stomatitis is part of an erythema multiforme.
5. Generalized symptoms such as weakness and malaise can be attributed to the underlying disease and not to the stomatitis.

Therapy

It is very important to clarify the cause of the stomatitis, so that specific therapy can be directed to the underlying disease. Symptomatic treatment consists of the following measures:

1. Rinse frequently with lukewarm water or a mild astringent (**R. 16b**).
2. The diet should be liquid, later soft.
3. Bed rest is the most important general measure for severe stomatitis.
4. Systemic corticosteroids are indicated only for severe stomatitis, but not for infectious stomatitis, such as herpetic gingivostomatitis.

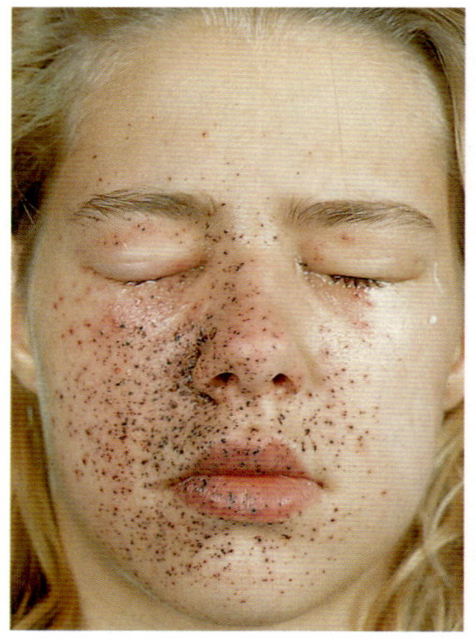

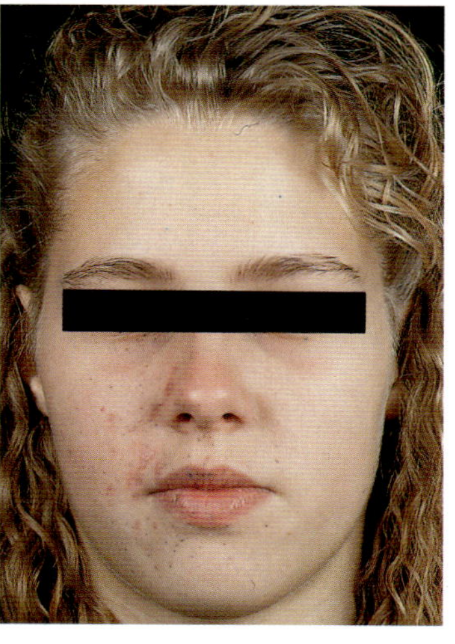

Figure 285 Left: Powder injected by a shot from a gun filled with blanks. Right: Appearance following mechanical cleaning under general anesthesia.

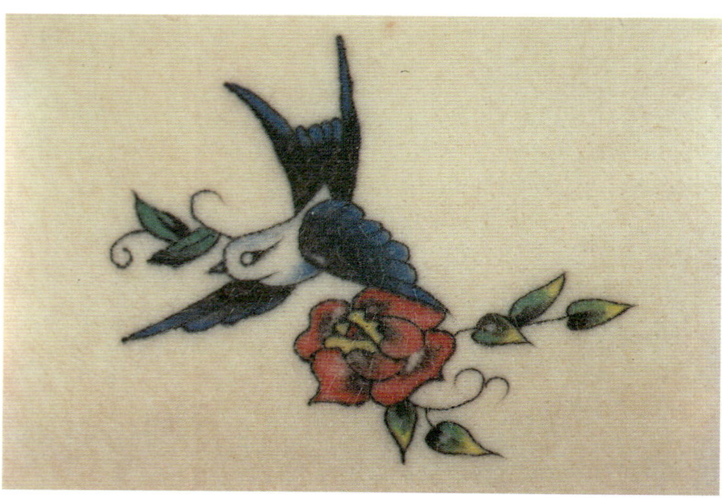

Figure 286 Decorative tattoo.

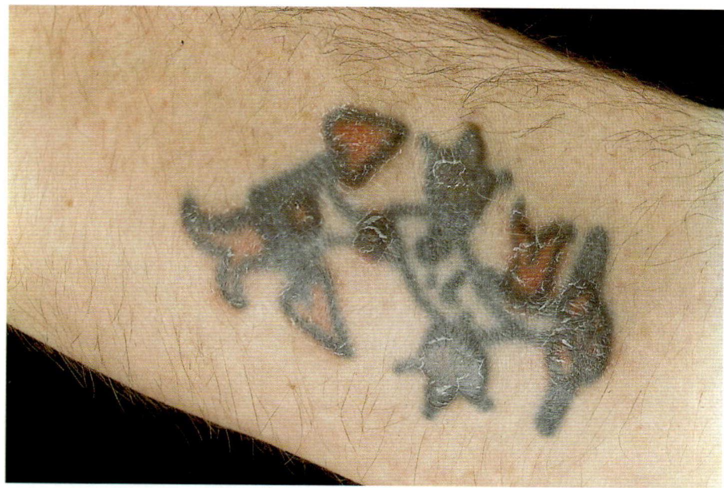

Figure 287 Decorative tattoo with formation of a granuloma where HgS was introduced. Sensitivity to mercury was demonstrated by epicutaneous testing.

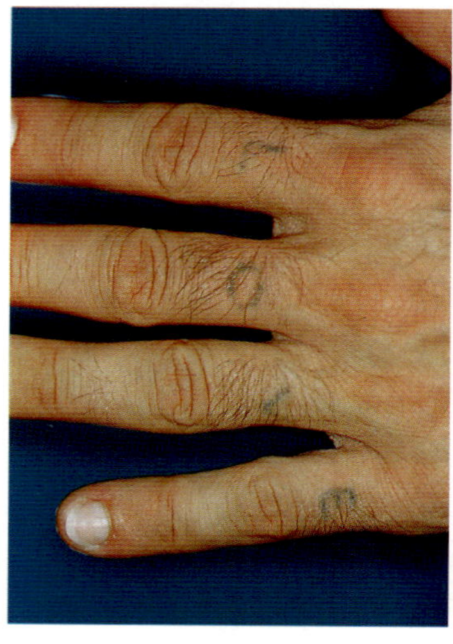

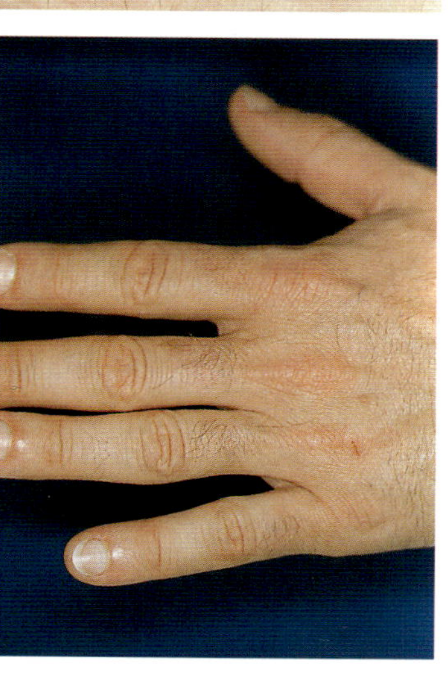

Figure 288 Left: decorative tattoo on the fingers. Right: Appearance following removal with a ruby laser.

Tattoos

Tattoos are deposits of foreign material in the skin. This can occur accidentally with stone dust, coal dust, gunpowder, or metal dust such as iron, copper, silver or similar exogenous materials. It can also be a decorative tattoo. Decorative tattoos are classified as so-called lay tattoos, in which the pigment is usually ink or india ink that is injected at irregular depth into the skin, or as so-called professional tattoos, which are often extensive, multicolored ornamental tattoos which are uniformly superficial so that the colors are more vibrant. Lay tattoos are usually made by adolescents to show that they belong to a certain group, or they are often found in drug addicts and prisoners. They are also seen in military personnel, especially seamen who originally learned about tattoos in Southeast Asia. Currently, decorative tattoos are frequently seen in the greater population because they have become fashionable.

Tattoos have medical significance when the decorated individuals wish to have them removed. The most common reason is that the ornaments are considered a stigma of an earlier phase in life with which they no longer identify. This occurs much more often with the so-called lay tattoos that are so often found on exposed regions of the body such as the dorsum of the hand and fingers and rarely in the face.

Clinical Features

1. The motives depicted in the tattoos vary significantly. They can be tattoos of a blood type (e.g., members of the SS had these tattoos on the inside of the left upper arm), the number on the inside of the forearm of concentration camp inmates, as well as group designations for prisoners (e.g., 3 dots on the back of the hand) or large ornamental designs. Occasionally, tattoos are performed for cosmetic or esthetic reasons, to change the shape of the eyebrows, the contours of the lips, as so-called permanent make-up, but also after operative procedures, such as a tattoo of the areola mammae after surgery of the breast.
2. Intolerance to the pigments in the tattoo is seen occasionally (most frequently to the heavy metals chromium and mercury). Transmission of infections (hepatitis, syphilis, HIV) is possible with contaminated instruments but can be avoided with the necessary precautions.

Therapy

1. At present, the best method for removing tattoos is photothermolysis with a laser. Different types of equipment are used, depending on the color of the pigment used for the tattoo. Black, blue and green tattoos can be removed successfully with a calibrated ruby laser. For red and yellow colors, an alexandrite laser, which uses a higher wave length, or a Nd-YAG laser are better.
2. Smaller, linear tattoos can usually be excised with good cosmetic results.
3. The use of high frequency milling tools to remove large tattoos cannot be recommended as treatment of choice because the therapeutic result depends largely on the depth of the pigment. Especially in lay tattoos, some of the pigment is often deep in the subcutis and cannot be removed completely, or a conspicuous scar can result.
4. Primary treatment of large tattoos caused by foreign material (accidents, deposits of gunpowder, etc.) should be early mechanical removal with a sterile brush. This treatment is painful and usually requires general anesthesia.

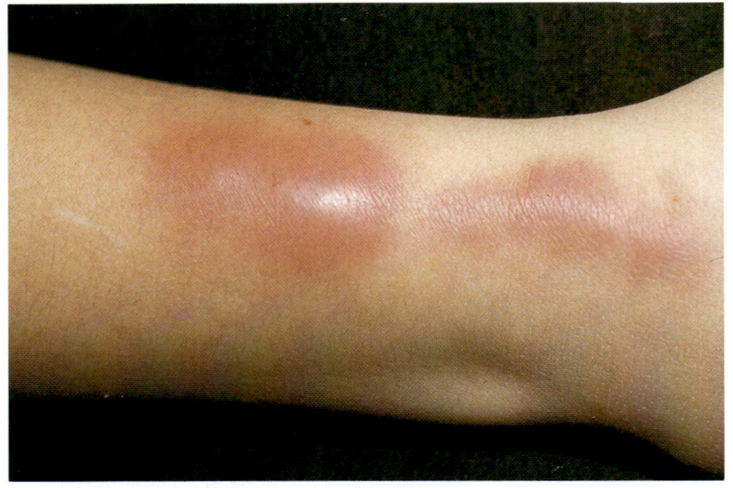

Figure 289 Acute thrombophlebitis. Rope-like, acute inflammatory infiltration along the course of a superficial vein.

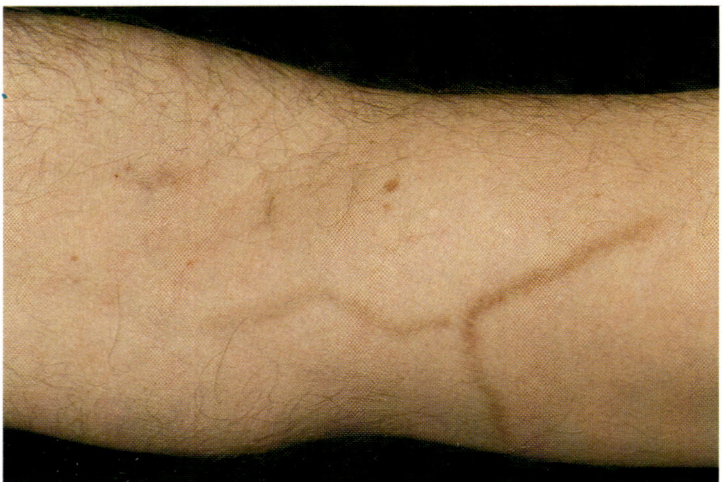

Figure 290 Pigmentation along the veins as sequel of a medication-induced thrombophlebitis.

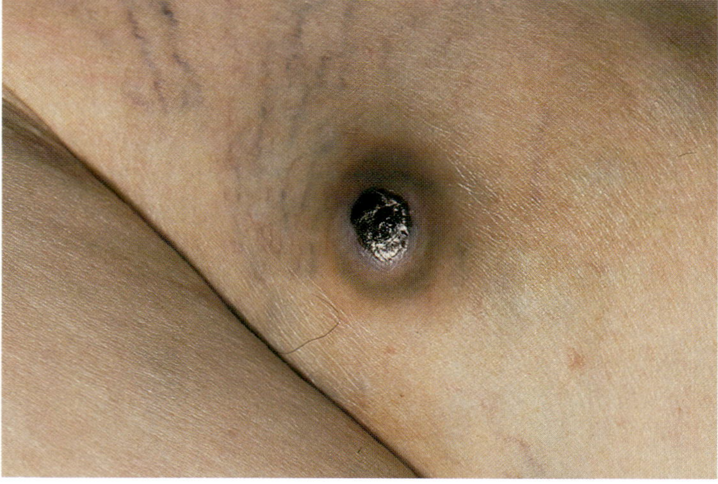

Figure 291 Ulcerated varix.

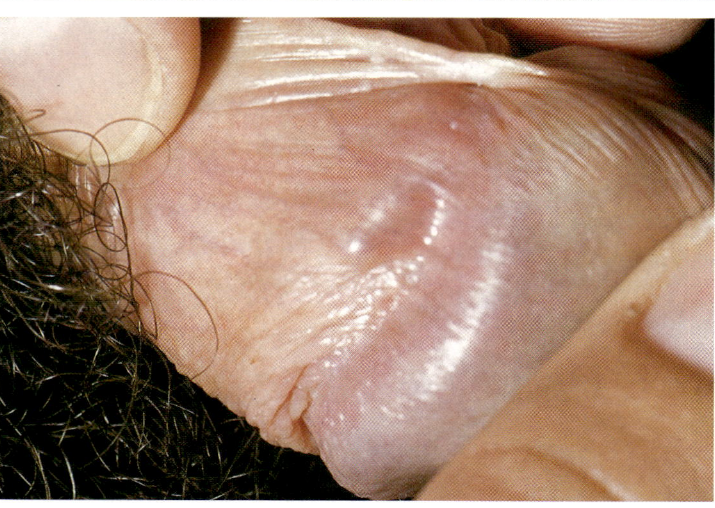

Figure 292 Phlebitis of the sulcus coronarius. Rope-like, occasionally painful induration of a vein in the sulcus coronarius.

Thrombophlebitis

Thrombophlebitis is a primary inflammation of the superficial veins with secondary formation of a thrombus. Injury to the vein wall can be caused by injection of medications that irritate the vein, an indwelling venous catheter, or blunt trauma. Thrombophlebitis is also seen in patients with varicose veins and with certain generalized disorders such as Behçet's disease, typhus and neoplastic disease. Since the thrombus generally adheres firmly to the vessel wall, embolization is extremely rare in thrombophlebitis.

Clinical Features

1. A rope-like, firm, very painful inflammatory infiltrate can be felt in the area of the affected vein with marked erythema of the overlying skin.
2. Iatrogenic thrombophlebitis is naturally found almost exclusively in the arms. Otherwise, thrombophlebitis occurs much more frequently in the legs, in women more than in men.
3. A systemic reaction with fever, elevation of the sedimentation rate, leukocytosis and malaise is evident in many cases.
4. When massive inflammation is present, circumscribed necrosis can occur with subsequent development of a postphlebitic ulcer.

Therapy
Systemic

1. Drugs that suppress prostaglandin synthesis, such as aspirin 1–3 g per day or indomethacin 50 to 100 mg per day, are helpful. These medications have anti-inflammatory and analgesic effects.
2. Anticoagulant therapy (heparin 3 x 5000 IE s.c.) is necessary only for bedridden patients.

Topical

1. Cooling with alcohol dressings (**R. 1**) is helpful.
2. Topically applied diclofenac has a local antiphlogistic effect.
3. The effectiveness of external heparinoid therapy is still questionable. Nevertheless, most patients feel relief from these topical medications.
4. The patient should be made ambulatory with compression bandages.
5. When nodular necrosis is present, the clot should be removed through a stab incision (Protect the eyes from spurting blood!). This is then followed by a compression dressing.

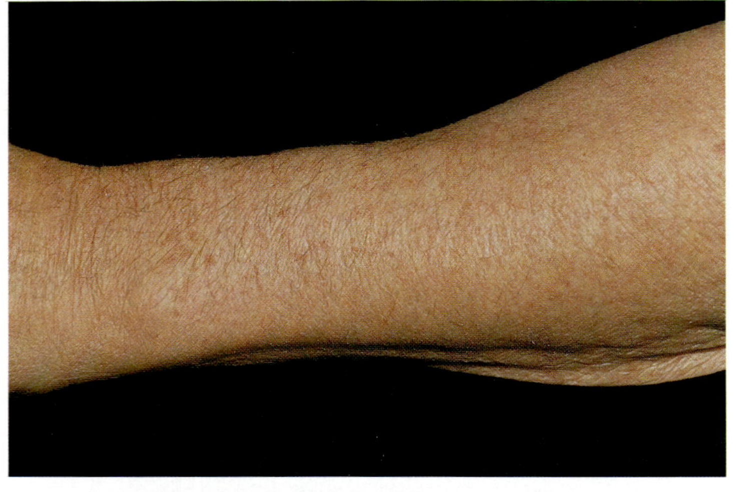

Figure 293 Dryness of the skin. Fine scaling in a patient with decreased turgor of the skin.

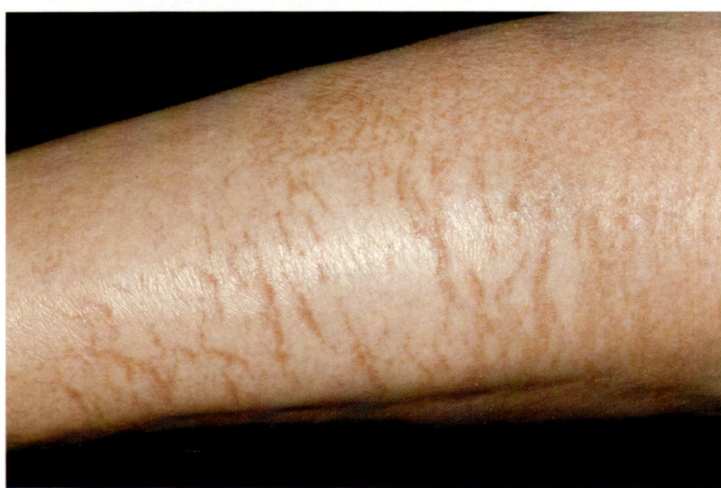

Figure 294 Dry skin with eczematization. Scaling with fissures and subsequent eczematization.

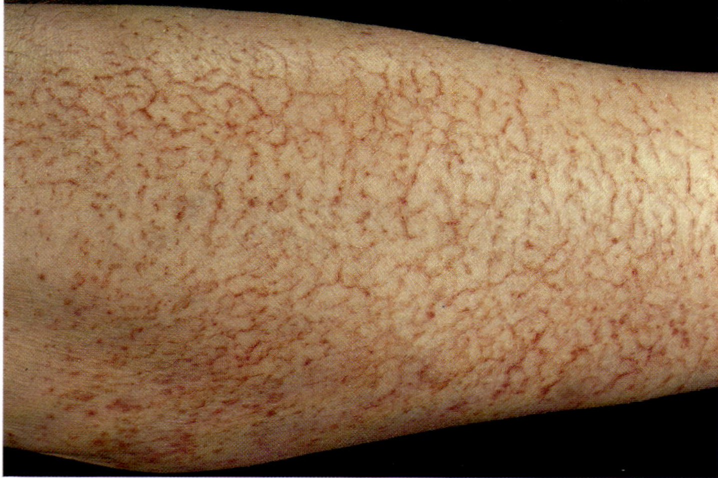

Figure 295 Eczema due to desiccation. Distinct hemorrhagic reticular eczema in fissures caused by the desiccation.

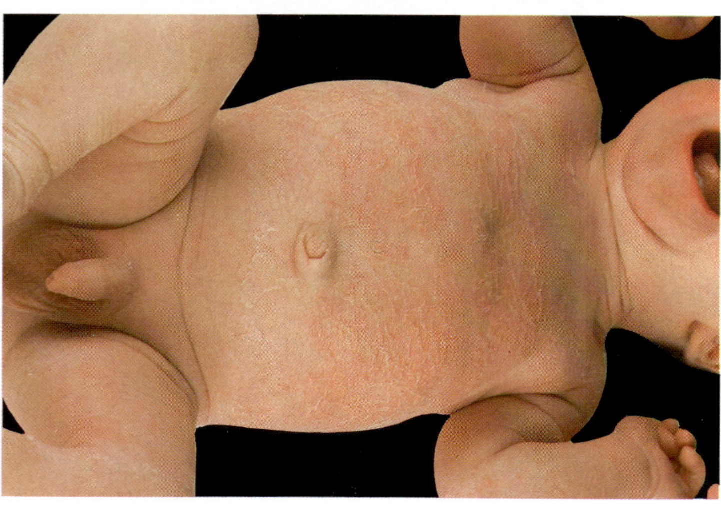

Figure 296 Ichthyosis vulgaris, so-called "fish skin disease". Marked scaling on trunk and extremities.

Dry Skin, Ichthyosis

A. Dry Skin

Unpleasant dryness of the skin (xerosis) is a frequent symptom with many causes. It is found especially in older persons with otherwise healthy skin at times of low humidity (winter, central heating), from too frequent washing and bathing, in patients with atopic dermatitis (see pages 41–45) and in patients with congenital ichthyosis. It can also occur as an adverse effect of some medications, such as spasmolytics with atropine-like effect, synthetic retinoids (acitretin, isotretinoin), beta receptor blockers, H_2 receptor blockers (cimetidine, ranitidine) and tamoxifen.

Clinical Features

1. Unpleasant dryness of the skin is often only a subjective symptom without visible skin changes. Sometimes fine scaling of the skin and pruritus develop later.
2. In the elderly, dry skin is accompanied by loss of turgor in all the skin. It can be pinched into folds which disappear much more slowly than normal.
3. Scaling, superficial fissures and pruritus develop as a result of the dryness, which may later lead to secondary eczematization or eczematization in the fissues of the dry skin (eccema craquelé). This is found especially on the lower legs, less often on the arms and trunks of older people.

Therapy

1. Dry skin can be effectively improved by repeated topical application of fatty creams or ointments which contain water, with or without the addition of urea **(R. 33b, 42b)**. In patients with atopic dermatitis, this should be repeated several times daily. Oil baths can also help.
2. To improve the indoor climate, the room temperature must be lowered and the air humidified.

B. Ichthyosis, Fish Skin

This is a group of several inherited disorders of keratinization that can vary considerably in severity and are characterized by coarse, dry, scaly skin.

Clinical Features

1. The skin is abnormally dry, with scaling that can be fine like bran, or with larger plaques, or with rhomboid-shaped markings like reptile skin.
2. In the most common form, ichthyosis vulgaris, the flexor surfaces of the joints are spared, yet they are affected in the more severe types of ichthyosis.
3. The functions of the sebaceous and sweat glands are usually impaired. This can lead to thermoregulatory disturbances in hot weather and with intense physical activity.

Therapy

Causal therapy is not possible, but topical treatment can improve appearance and symptoms. Many patients find long-term treatment too troublesome and apply the medication only sporadically or discontinue it altogether.

1. Ointments containing urea **(R. 42b)** are helpful for keratolysis and improve the water-retaining capacity of the skin.
2. Topical treatment can be supplemented by oil baths to lubricate the skin. A lubricating ointment should be applied immediately after bathing **(R. 33b)** to avoid excessive dehydration of the skin.
3. Severe cases may benefit from acitretin **(R. 64)**.
4. Occupations that cause degreasing of the skin (long-term contact with soaps, detergents, organic solvents, cement) should be avoided.

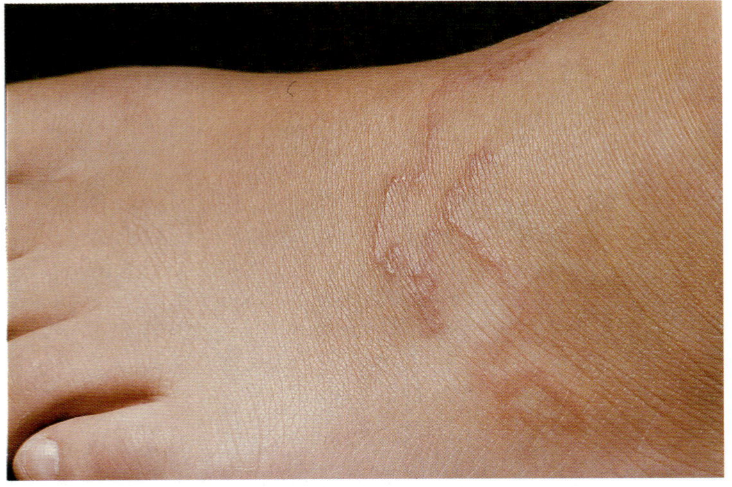

Figure 297 Creeping eruption. Winding burrows of a larva migrating in the skin (larva migrans).

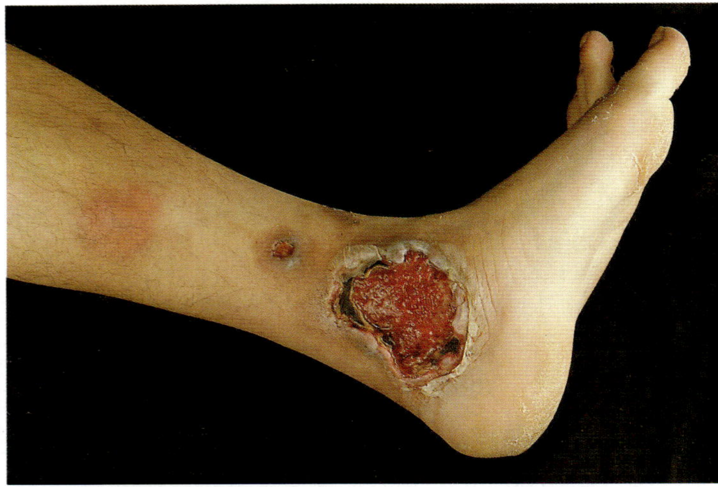

Figure 298 Bacterial ulcers following a hike in a tropical grassy landscape.

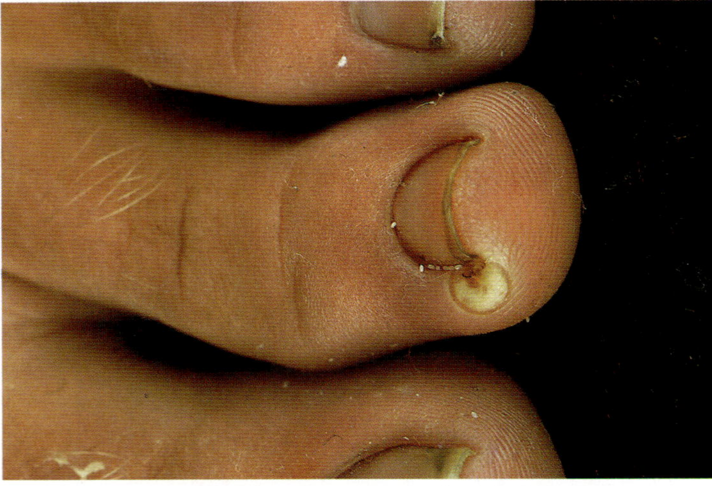

Figure 299 Sand flea infestation. Typical location.

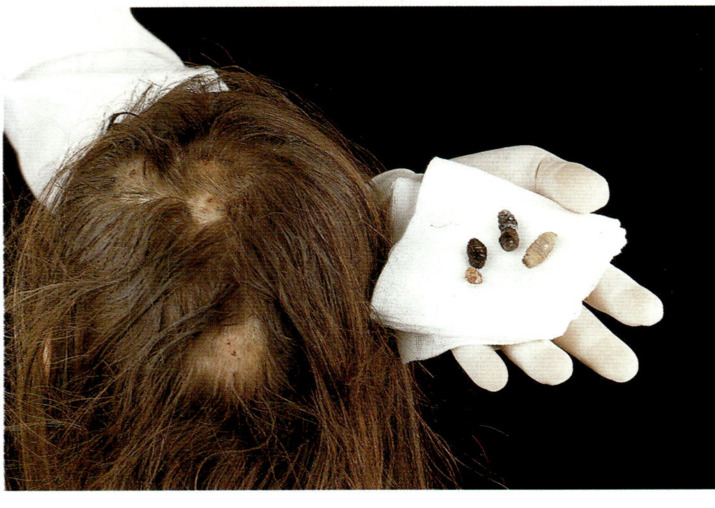

Figure 300 Larvae developing in the skin after a bite by a botfly, *Dermatobia hominis*, in South America. Small abscesses, each containing a larva.

Vacation Dermatoses

A. Creeping Eruption

Creeping eruption (larva migrans) is caused by larvae of different worms (predominantly *Ankylostoma brasiliense*) which burrow into the superficial layers of the skin. Clinically, one sees a wandering, thin, erythematous, serpentine, raised, tunnel-like lesion, occasionally with vesicle formation. The larvae migrate a few millimeters to several centimeters a day. They are located a few millimeters in front of the winding linear burrows. Spontaneous healing usually occurs within a few weeks. Systemic symptoms (fever, pulmonary infiltrates) may require treatment with an anthelmintic (albendazole).

B. Bacterial Ulcers

Bacterial ulcers on the legs and feet are some of the most frequent skin diseases acquired during vacations in tropical countries. They are caused by bacteria that enter the skin through contact with plants or insects during hikes in grasslands or underbrush. Several ulcers with inflammatory erythema and surrounding edema in the ankle region and proximal to it are typical. They develop slowly and are often very resistant to treatment. Systemic antibiotic therapy with a broad-spectrum antibiotic is often necessary, especially when the patient has general symptoms. The antibiotics should be given for 8 to 10 days. Moist dressings with or without disinfectant additives are useful as topical therapy, as well as topical antibiotics **(R. 34)**.

C. Sand Flea Bites

Sand flea disease, tungiasis, is found in Central and South America and in West Africa. A small, hyperkeratotic swelling with a central opening develops a few days after the sand flea bite. The terminal segments of the flea are occasionally visible in this opening. Sand flea bites in humans are found under the toenails, between the toes and on the heels, rarely on the calf or knee. The infections are rarely seen on the upper half of the body, because the sand flea can only jump approximately one meter. Development of pustules and ulcers is possible. Treatment of uncomplicated cases consists of enlarging the opening with a needle and removing the sand flea. This is then followed by topical disinfection. If extraction is not possible, the sand flea can be killed by closing the opening with any ointment or turpentine, because the flea breathes through it.

D. Furunculoid Myiasis Caused by Human Botflies

Furunculoid myiasis can be caused by one of two species of flies, the tumbu fly in Africa (*Cordylobia anthropophaga*) and the botfly (*Dermatobia hominis*) in Central and South America. Clinical symptoms usually begin in the first larval stage, approximately one week after implantation of the eggs. Itching, especially at night, and burning pain are frequent symptoms. Beginning in the second week, a serous fluid exudes from the central opening of a small, ball-shaped prominence, followed by increasing furunculoid swelling which can cause exquisite pain from the fourth week on. Many times there is impetiginization with lymphangitis. The swelling increases to the size of a pigeon's egg shortly before the larva emerges, which causes no pain. A small stab incision is often necessary to remove the larva. The larva can be brought to emerge spontaneously within 48 hours by closing the air hole with vaseline or other ointments.

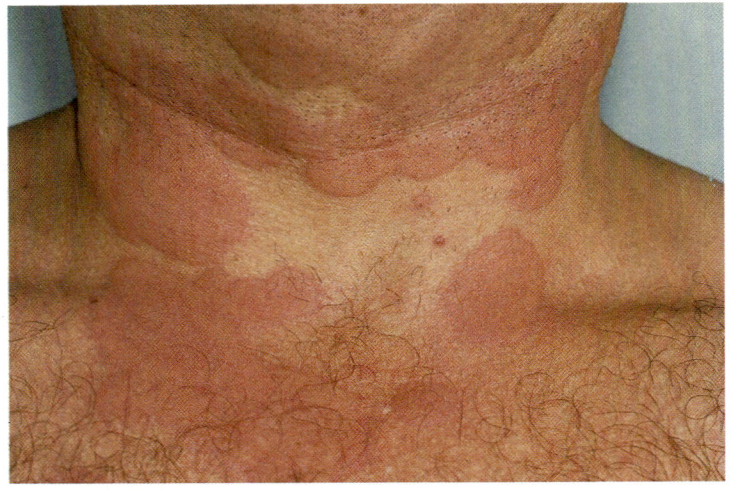

Figure 301 Urticaria. Transient wheals on neck and chest.

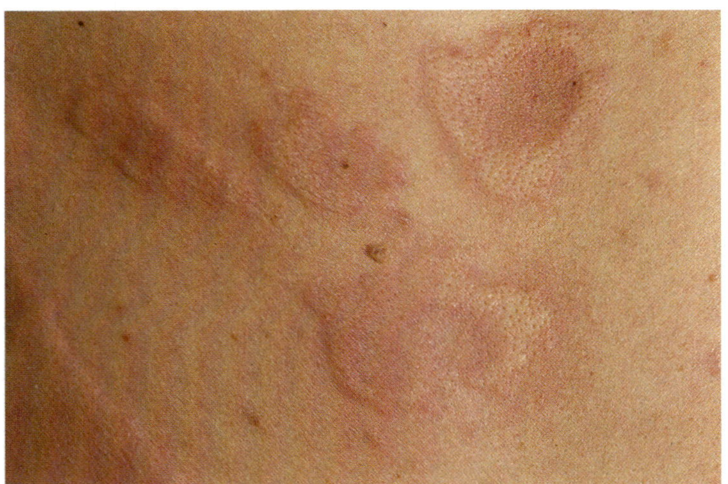

Figure 302 Urticaria. Wheals with raised margins. Pressure from the edema causes pallor of the raised margin.

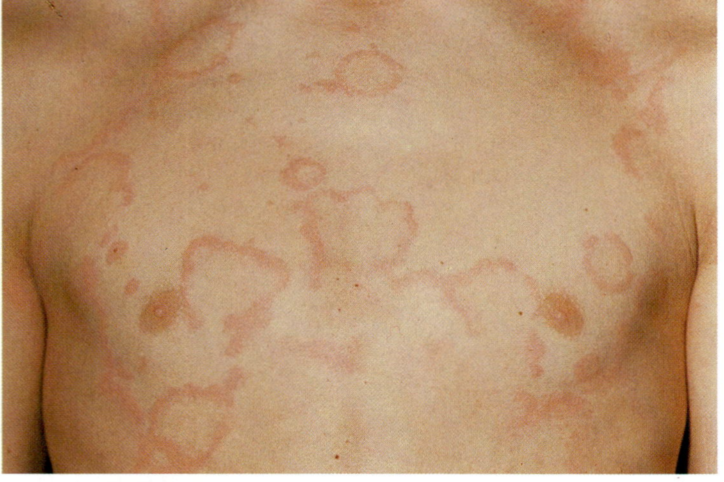

Figure 303 Urticaria. Wheals with raised margins. Coalescence of individual foci produces gyrate lesions.

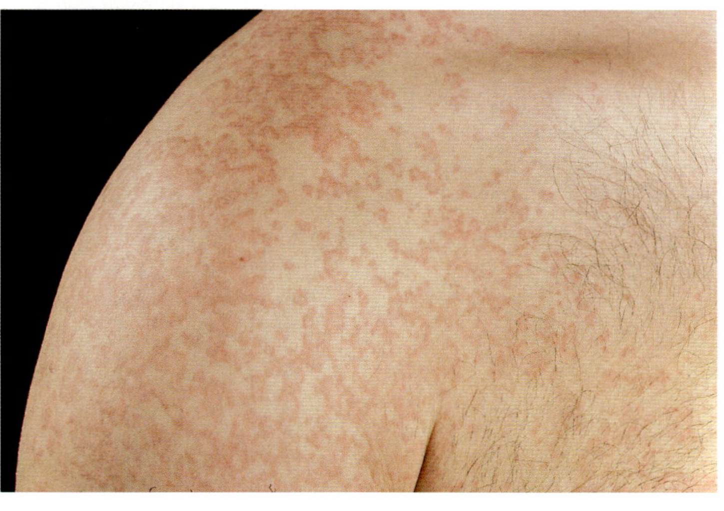

Figure 304 Cholinergic urticaria. Typical urticaria with papules and small spots.

Urticaria and Angioedema (Quincke's Edema)

Urticaria is characterized by transient edemas (wheals) in the upper and middle layers of the skin, while angioedema is an edema of the deep layers of the skin (subcutis). The causes of these polyetiologic symptoms are more or less identical. The factors that lead to urticaria can also result in the much rarer angioedema. Nonallergic causes are much more frequent than allergic ones. Urticaria or angioedema are sometimes accompanied by symptoms of shock: drop in blood pressure, flushing, profuse sweating, dyspnea, sensations of constriction, tachycardia and other shock symptoms. Angioedemas due to hereditary or acquired deficiency of C1-inhibitor differ completely from the above-mentioned types of angioedemas with respect to clinical features and treatment (see below).

A. Urticaria

A non-recurring urticaria, i.e., one which lasts not more than 4 to 6 weeks, is called acute urticaria. Urticaria that lasts longer than 6 weeks or has recurrent attacks is termed chronic urticaria. Causative factors of acute urticaria can be medications (almost all drugs, especially antibiotics, in particular penicillins and cephalosporins, as well as analgesics and x-ray contrast media), infections (virus infections such as hepatitis A, bacterial infections such as tonsillitis), the toxins of bee and wasp stings, food, preservatives in drugs and food, and fruit acids. Such factors are found in approximately 50% of all patients with urticaria.

The causes of chronic urticaria can be identified very rarely (in less than 5%), despite the most thorough work-up. Acetylsalicylic acid (aspirin) often causes a new outbreak of the condition in many of these patients. Traces of preservatives or food dyes can also be causative factors.

More easily identified are urticarial reactions which can be prompted by physical irritation (cold, heat, pressure or sunlight) and that are sporadic or have a familial tendency. Factitious urticaria (red urticarial dermographism) and finally cholinergic urticaria (minute urticarial foci, developing after physical or emotional stress) are other frequent types of urticaria.

Clinical Features

1. Transient, slightly elevated, round wheals without involvement of the epidermis are characteristic. The individual eruption usually persists for 24 hours or less.
2. Marked edema makes the wheals appear whitish. They can have a raised margin and can coalesce into circinate lesions.
3. Pruritus is almost always present and usually severe.
4. All areas of the body can be involved, most frequently the trunk and the extremities.
5. The special anatomy of the penis, vulva and oral mucosa results in edema formation instead of wheals.

Therapy

Determination and elimination of the cause is the most important measure. A thorough history often clarifies the diagnosis in acute urticaria. Patients with chronic urticaria must be informed that it may not be possible to find the causes to avoid disappointment.

Systemic

As long as no shock symptoms are present in patients with acute urticaria, oral antihistamines, preferrably without a sedative component **(R. 61, 62)** are sufficient, e.g., loratadine (Claritin) or cetirizine (Zyrtec). For chronic urticaria, cyproheptadine (Periactin) or hydroxyzine (Atarax, Vistaril) can also be tried. Calcium has practically no therapeutic value. Severe cases of acute urticaria should be treated with the measures described for angioedema (see below). Shock symptoms must receive appropriate treatment, depending on their severity (see page 79).

Topical

Topical treatment is rarely necessary because the symptoms are transient. Local antihistamines are not very effective; they can even cause an allergic or photoallergic contact dermatitis.

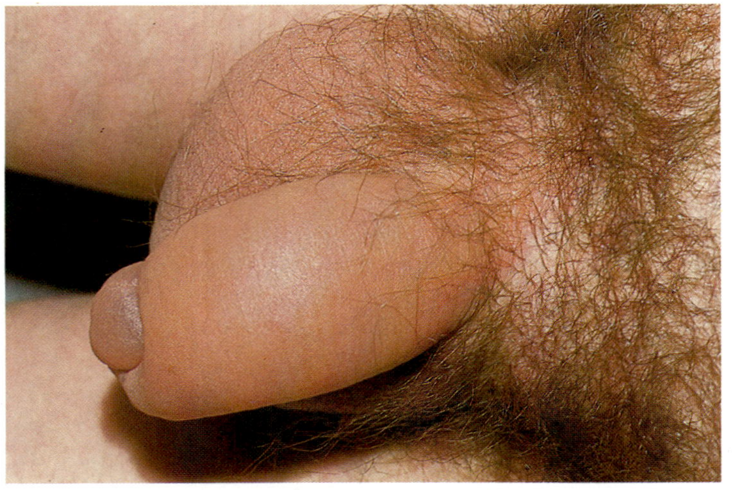

Figure 305 Urticaria. Diffuse edema of the penis. Wheals do not form at this site due to the special texture of the connective tissue.

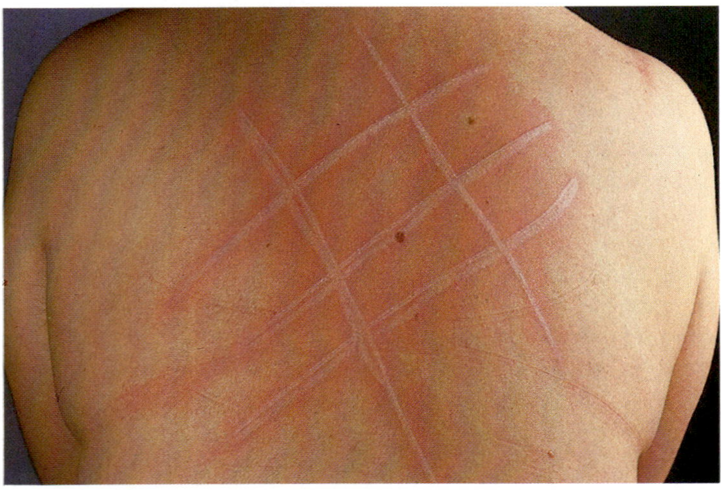

Figure 306 Urticarial dermographism. Wheal formation following linear pressure to the skin.

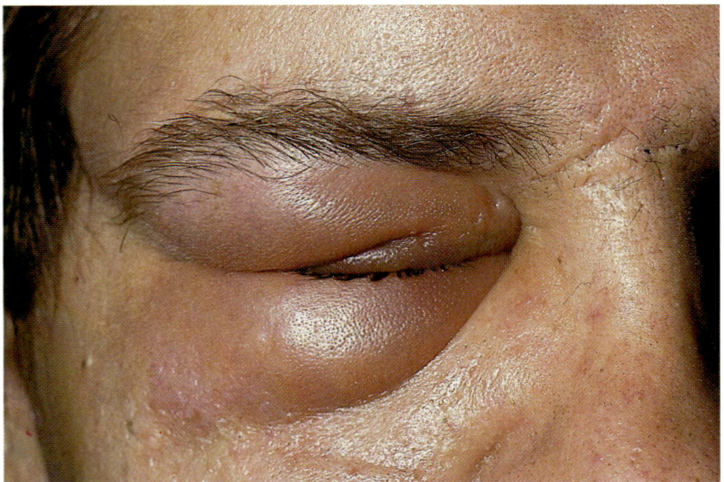

Figure 307 Angioedema. Unilateral massive transient edema, which in this patient is typically located in the lid area.

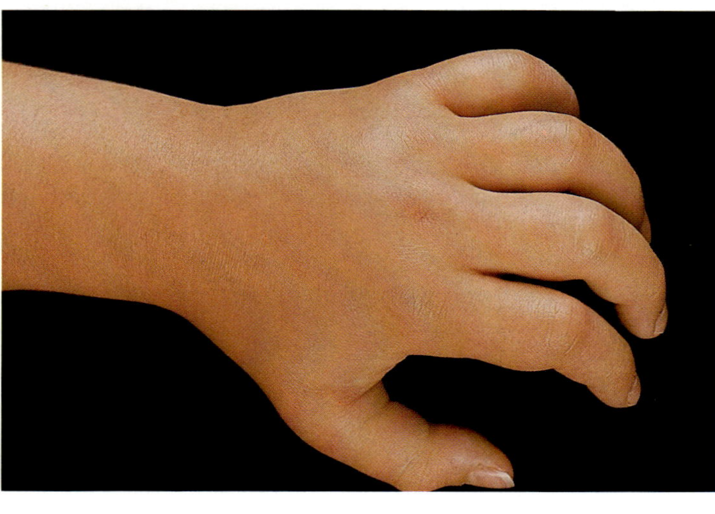

Figure 308 Hereditary angioedema with massive swelling of the hand.

Prophylaxis Many patients with chronic urticaria react to acetylsalicylic acid and other non-steroidal analgesics or antirheumatic drugs with a new attack, occasionally with the symptoms of anaphylactic shock. For this reason, analgesics should be used very selectively with these patients.

B. Angioedema (Histamine-Mediated)

Angioedema can occur as an acute one-time event or as a chronic recurrent problem, simultaneously or alternating with urticaria. Chronic recurrent angioedema can also occur without urticaria. The possible causes of angioedema are just as manifold as those of urticaria and are more or less identical with these (see page 153). Just as with chronic urticaria, there are recurrent angioedemas for which the cause cannot be found even after thorough evaluation ("idiopathic angioedema").

Clinical Features

1. Skin-colored, mostly unilateral swelling which persists for 2 to 5 days.
2. The periorbital region and the lips are usually involved, but the swelling can occur on any part of the skin.
3. Subjectively, there is a feeling of tension and occasionally moderate pruritus and tension pain.
4. Swelling of the oral mucosa or swelling of other internal organs can occur simultaneously or as an isolated finding.

Therapy It is important to exclude hereditary angioedema because this disorder requires an entirely different approach (see below). For the usual forms of angioedema, determination of the cause is the most important goal.

1. Angioedema can only be managed with systemic treatment; intravenous antihistamines (e.g., 1–2 ampullae of clemastine) or intravenous corticosteroids, if necessary, are the drugs of choice.
2. If laryngeal edema is developing, the posterior wall of the pharynx must be sprayed with epinephrine, combined with systemic application of antihistamines, corticosteroids or, if necessary, epinephrine i.v. (0.5 ml 1:1000 solution in 20 ml 0.9% saline solution, given very slowly intravenously!). In extreme cases, intubation or tracheostomy may be necessary.

C. Hereditary and Acquired Angioedemas Caused by C1-Inhibitor Deficiency

This very rare disease differs completely from the histamine-mediated angioedema, which is part of or equivalent to an urticaria. It is characterized by familial occurrence of angioedemas in the skin, by attacks of pain in the gastrointestinal tract, or edema attacks in other internal organs. The disease is caused by an inherited deficiency of C1-inhibitor. Urticaria is never present in this disorder. In very rare cases, lack of C1-inhibitor and its clinical symptoms can be acquired.

The clinical appearance is characterized by recurrent angioedemas of the skin, painful convulsive attacks in the gastrointestinal tract, and occasionally even glottis edema with danger of suffocation.

In emergency cases with impending edema of the glottis, treatment consists of substitution of the C1-inhibitor (Berinert HS). Fresh frozen plasma, intravenous epinephrine, intubation or tracheostomy may be necessary, depending on the symptomatology. Corticosteroids alone are not effective enough or not at all. For long-term prophylaxis, danazol (Danocrine) in a dose of 50 to 200 mg per day is given. These patients are best referred to a center with specific experience in the treatment of this rare disorder.

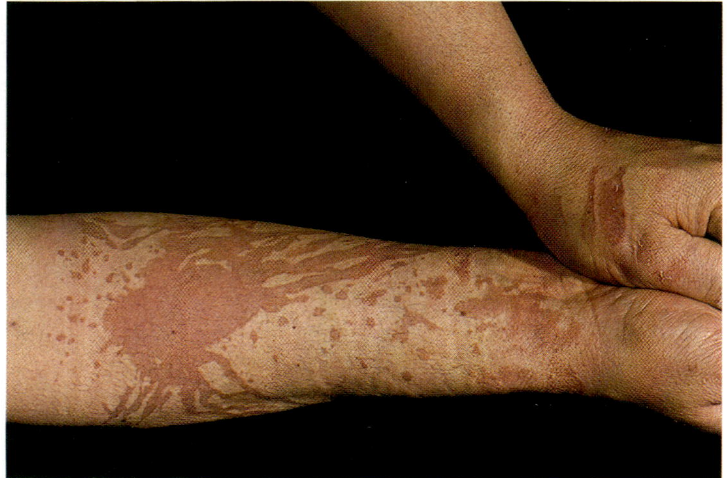

Figure 309 Hydrofluoric acid burn. Sharply demarcated erythema limited to the contact area.

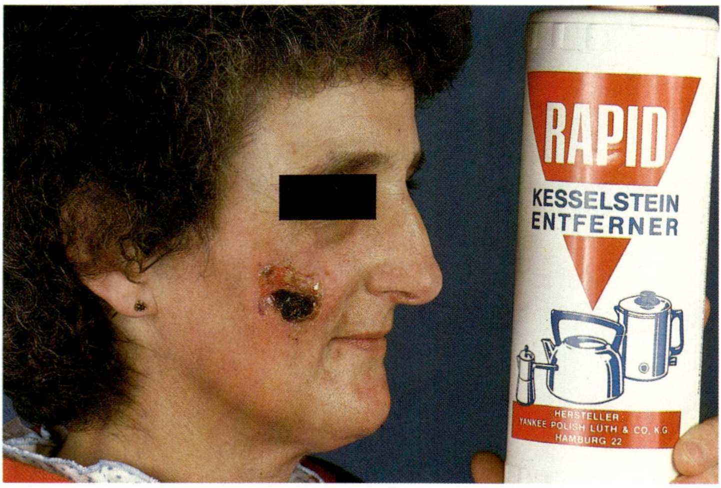

Figure 310 Acid burn caused by boiler scale remover containing amidosulfuric acid. Partially demarcated necrotic tissue on the right cheek.

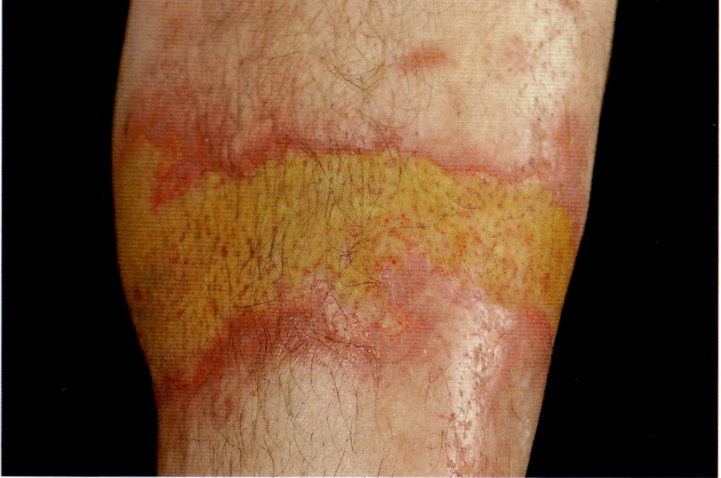

Figure 311 Chemical burn caused by cement. Typical, sharply demarcated necrosis at the zone of contact with the shaft of the boot.

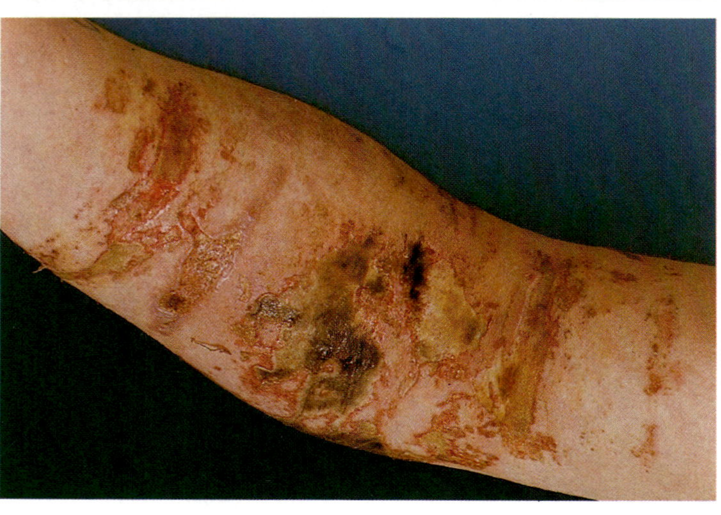

Figure 312 Chemical burn caused by a solution used for pretzel making. Partly demarcated necroses and shallow ulcerations with beginning re-epithelialization.

Chemical Burns

A large number of industrial substances, as well as some household cleaners, can lead to skin injuries of varying degrees. The severity of the injury depends on how aggressive the substance is and how long it acts on the skin. Self-inflicted chemical burns (artifacts, see page 13) and chemical burns in the context of a suicide attempt are relatively rare. Since many chemical reactions on the skin can produce the symptoms of a chemical burn, these reactions have a wide spectrum. The causative chemicals can act as oxidizing or reducing agents, as alkalis, as dehydrating substances, or as cell toxins. Colliquation necroses caused by lyes can spread and are often more extensive than those caused by acids.

Clinical Features

1. The injury is limited to the contact site, usually to an uncovered area of the body. Clinical signs can range from erythema, edema, or blister formation to the formation of white to black necroses, depending on the severity of the injury.
2. The extent of the injury cannot be estimated before demarcation of the necroses occurs.
3. The amount of pain varies. In the acute stage, chemical burns are usually pain free. Pain starts with the perifocal inflammatory reaction. Deep necroses can be less painful than superficial necroses, since sensory nerve fibers are also damaged.

Therapy

1. The causative substance must be washed off immediately with copious amounts of fluid, preferrably water (not less than 20 minutes!). This is more important than wasting valuable time searching for a specific antidote.
2. Subsequent care does not differ significantly from that described for burns (see page 159): Especially for deep necroses, removal of necrotic tissue by surgical debridement, followed by coverage of the defect with skin grafts where necessary. This produces a much better functional and esthetic end result than spontaneous healing with scar formation.
3. Following emergency care of a chemical burn, one should always consult a poison control center regarding possible systemic effects of the causative substance, or refer the patient to such a center for evaluation and treatment.
4. Tetanus prophylaxis is recommended.

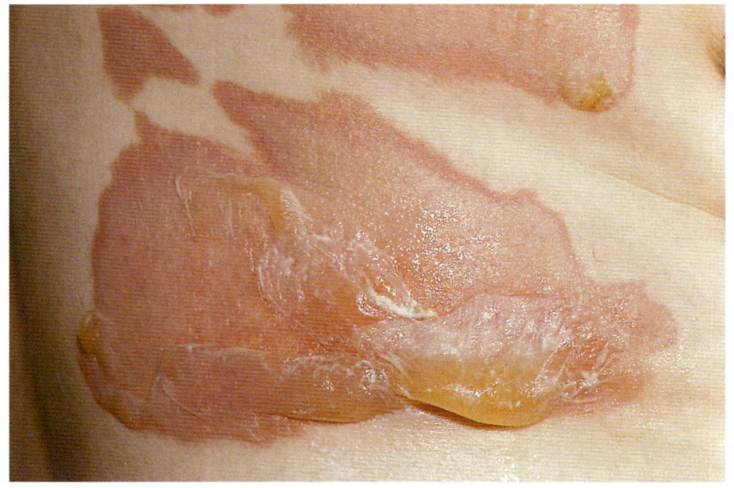

Figure 313 Second-degree burn with erythema and blister formation. Weeping erosions following exposure to hot steam.

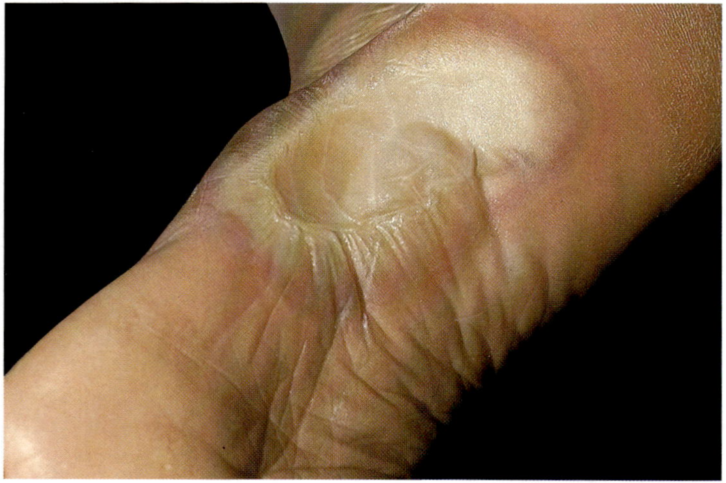

Figure 314 Third-degree burn. Whitish areas of necroses with blister formation and marginal erythema caused by a hot water bottle in a patient with loss of sensation. The patient complained about "cold feet" while under spinal anesthesia.

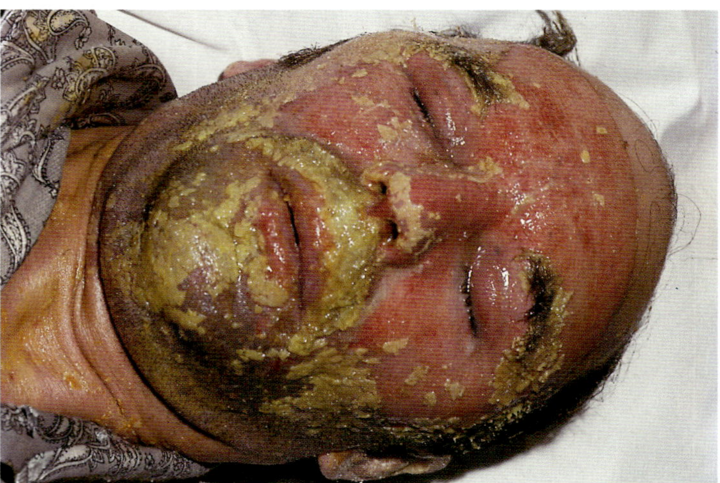

Figure 315 Extensive second-degree burn caused by liquid plastic.

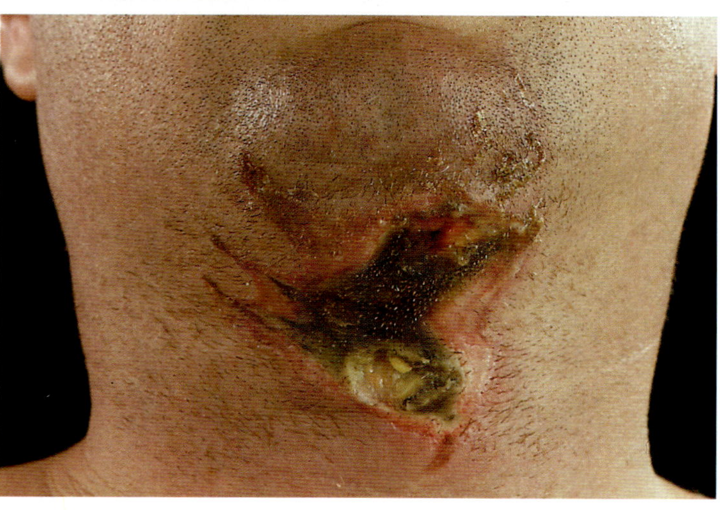

Figure 316 Burn caused by high voltage current in the larynx area. Necrosis at the entrance site of the light arc.

Burns, Scalding

Burns are caused by industrial or household injuries, traffic accidents or during catastrophic events. They are classified according to the extent of tissue damage. Systemic effects of burns, especially shock symptoms immediately after the injury, as well as protracted toxic shock from absorption of toxins 3 to 5 days later, must always be kept in mind. Burns are initially sterile, but bacterial contamination occurs rapidly, and infections, usually mixed infections, occur frequently. Infections in the hospital are caused chiefly by Staphylococcus, Streptococcus and Pyocyaneus.

Systemic effects are due not only to the depth of the burn but also to its surface area (rule of nines). Burns of more than 9% of the body surface always cause cardiovascular symptoms (shock symptoms), which often predominate initially. Other possible systemic complications during the first few weeks include sepsis, anemia, transcutaneous loss of protein and a derangement of carbohydrate metabolism.

Clinical Features

First-degree burn

Only the epidermis is involved. Clinically, there is painful erythema and edema (see sunburn).

Second-degree burn /IIa

Damage to the epidermis and the upper layer of the corium with blister formation. The injury heals in approximately 2 weeks without scar formation.

Second-degree burn/IIb

Only the keratinocytes in the deeper parts of the hair follicles are vital. Therefore, the injury heals slowly and with scar formation.

Third-degree burn

This causes complete destruction of epidermis and corium and the adjacent subcutis. Fourth-degree burn (provided this term is used) includes damage to muscles, tendons and even bones.

Therapy

All third-degree burns and extensive second-degree burns (IIa and IIb) must be treated in the hospital. Patients with severe burns should be referred to a burn center. The exact extent of a burn can often be determined only after surgical excision of the necroses. Before transporting the patient to the hospital or burn center, shock prevention must be initiated (intravenous line, infusion of an electrolyte solution, pain management), even if shock has not yet occurred.

Systemic

Minor first- and second-degree (IIa) burns:

1. Pain management, if necessary.
2. Tetanus prophylaxis is recommended.
3. When signs of wound infection occur, sensitivity of the organism must be determined, followed by appropriate systemic antibiotic therapy.

Local

1. Cooling with cold water and wet dressings with disinfectant additives **(R. 2)**.
2. Treatment of clean, superficial erosions by applying a corticosteroid cream for 2 to 3 days usually results in rapid improvement and pain relief.
3. Immediate removal of blisters and epidermal remnants permits accurate evaluation of the tissue damage. It also reduces the nutrients for possible infecting organisms. This is followed by application of a hydrocolloid dressing or a sterile fatty gauze (e.g., vaseline gauze).
4. Local application of antibiotics or sulfonamides is not recommended because of possible contact allergy and because they promote resistance of the organisms.

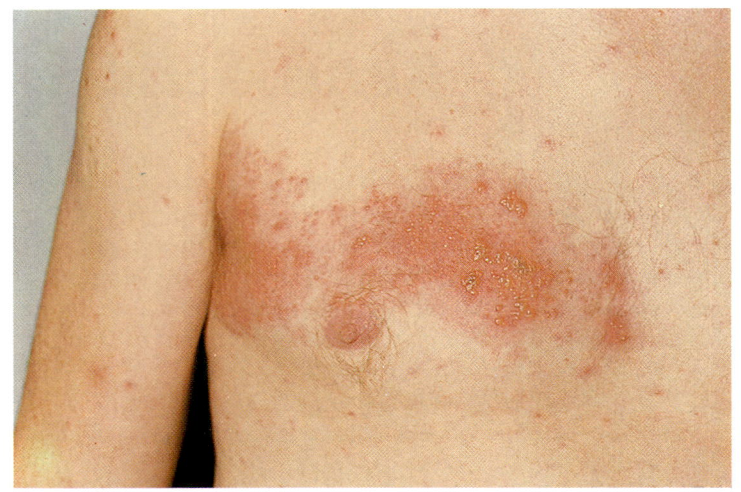

Figure 317 Herpes zoster. Segmental erythema with grouped blisters. Note the isolated blisters outside the segment (aberrant blisters).

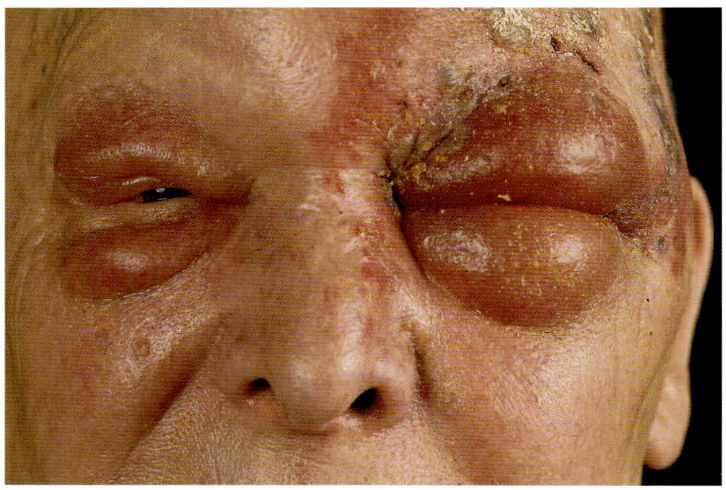

Figure 318 Herpes zoster in the region supplied by the trigeminal nerve (first division; ophthalmic zoster). Marked swelling of the eyelid, secondary also on the contralateral side.

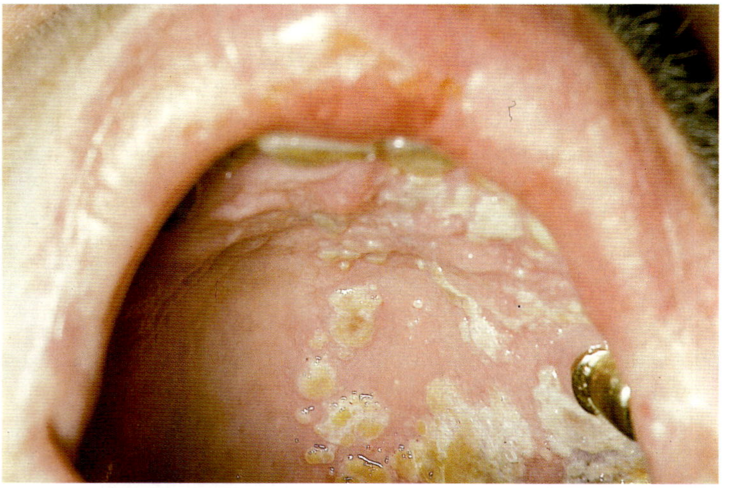

Figure 319 Herpes zoster in the area supplied by the second division of the trigeminal nerve. Typical intra-oral involvement with unilateral blister formation.

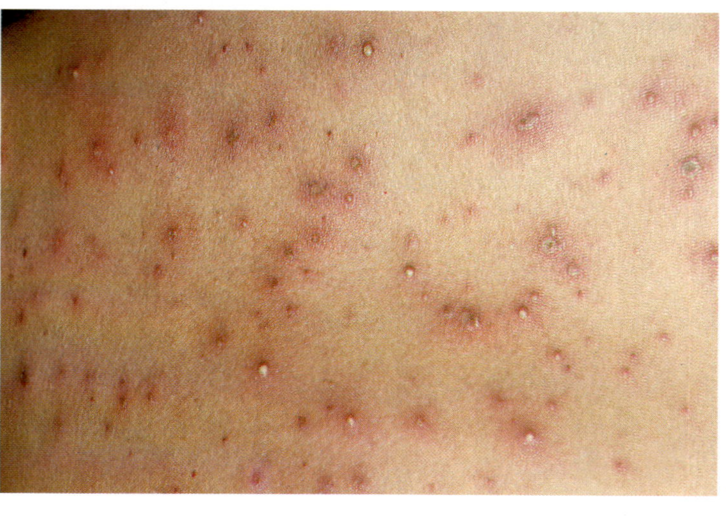

Figure 320 Disseminated herpes zoster. Dissemination of individual blisters over the entire skin, distinguishable from chickenpox only by concomitant involvement of a segment.

Herpes Zoster, Shingles

Herpes zoster is the secondary manifestation of an infection with the varicella zoster virus. It can occur at any age but is much more common in older people. In the elderly, the course of the disease is more severe and the eruptions are frequently followed by prolonged and severe neuralgia. When herpes zoster occurs with Hodgkin's disease, HIV-infection or other immunosuppressive diseases, the illness can run a life-threatening course (meningitis, encephalitis, sepsis).
A patient who has severe involvement with blister formation on the entire skin (generalized herpes zoster) should always be evaluated for a malignant disease. A syntropy between the involved dermatoma and diseases of the internal organs associated with the affected neural segment has often been postulated but never confirmed.

Clinical Features

1. The disease is characterized by groups of vesicles that appear in batches on an erythematous base and then develop into pustules. In more severe cases, the vesicles can become hemorrhagic or necrotic (hemorrhagic zoster, gangrenous zoster). The vesicles develop in one neural segment with occasional dissemination of individual vesicles over the entire skin (generalized or varicellous zoster).
2. The zoster eruption is practically always unilateral and is limited to one or rarely several adjacent, unilateral neural segments. The first division of the trigeminal nerve and the thoracic region are affected most frequently. Lesions of the eye (conjunctivitis, keratitis, iritis) entail the risk of permanent visual damage and require ophthalmologic care. Vesicles on the bridge and tip of the nose are indicative of eye involvement.
3. The skin eruptions are preceded and accompanied by pain in the segmental dermatoma. In older patients, this pain can persist as a very troublesome neuralgia. In children, herpes zoster is often painless. Motor nerves can also be involved and result in pareses (disturbance of oculomotor function and visual accommodation, facial nerve paresis). The regional lymph nodes are usually enlarged and tender.
4. Infection occurs only by direct skin contact. Patients with impaired immunity against varicella are also at risk.

Therapy
Systemic

Acyclovir **(R. 60)** has a virostatic effect. In mild cases, it is given orally (800 mg, 5 times per day), in more severe cases intravenously (5-10 mg per kg body weight 3 times daily). Valacyclovir (Valtrex tablets, 1000 mg, 3 times per day) is also effective. Another oral virostatic drug with systemic effects is famciclovir **(R. 60)**. In immunocompromised patients, the course of the disease can be mitigated by varicella hyperimmune globulin, given in the early phase of the disease (very expensive). In young patients and in cases with a mild course, no systemic therapy is necessary.
Systemic symptomatic therapy is aimed at pain relief. It must be kept in mind that a constant level of the analgesic must be maintained for adequate relief of pain, which means that the drug must be given at regular intervals determined by its half-life. With this method, even severe pain can often be treated with relatively mild to moderate analgesics such as paracetamol (acetaminophen), acetylsalicylic acid, and indomethacin, especially when they are combined with drugs that raise the pain threshold such as thioridazine (Mellaril) or carbamazepine (Tegretol). Severe pain that cannot be relieved by these methods may occasionally require the use of strong analgesics (tramadol or other opiate agonists). "Neurotropic vitamins" (B_1, B_6, B_{12}) have often been recommended for this disease, but their therapeutic effectiveness has never been proved. Systemic corticosteroids can be used as prophylaxis for post-herpetic neuralgia; their possible side effects must be taken into account.

Topical

Wet compresses or painting with a zinc shake mixture can be helpful in the early stage of vesicular eruption. Crusts and dried-up vesicles are best removed with an indifferent ointment. Capsaicin (0.025% in an ointment base), applied 3 to 4 times daily, often provides significant pain relief in post-herpetic neuralgia. Nerve blocks may be indicated for severe post-herpetic neuralgia that cannot be otherwise relieved.

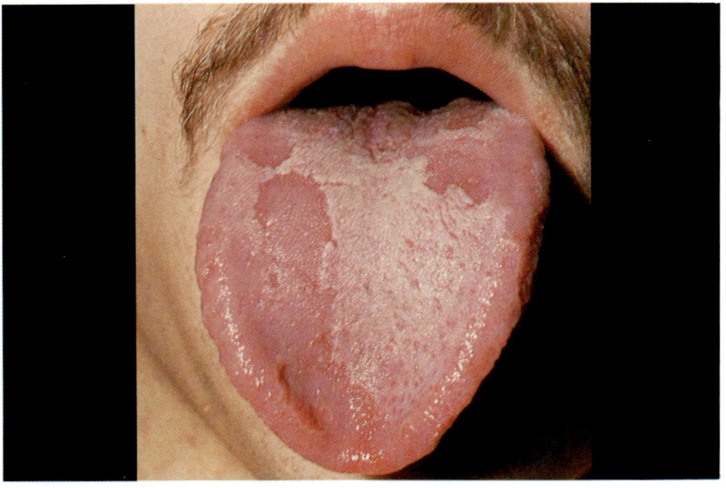

Figure 321 Geographic tongue. Decreased keratinization of the filiform papillae of the tongue in round confluent areas. This is a rapidly changing harmless condition.

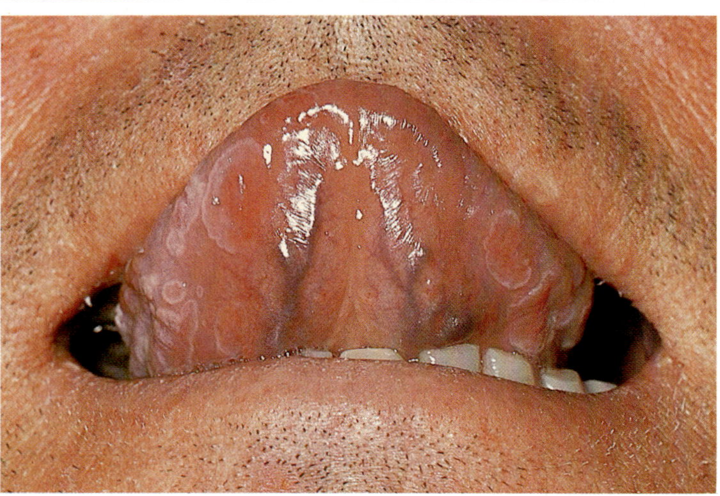

Figure 322 Geographic tongue. Lesions with raised margins on the underside of the tongue.

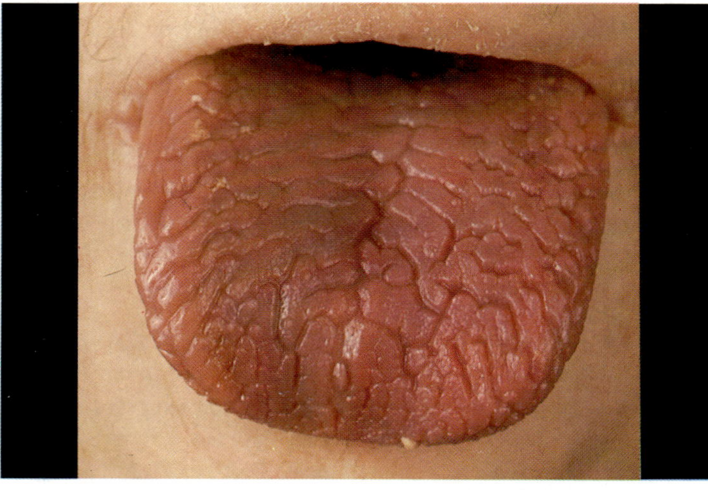

Figure 323 Fissured tongue.

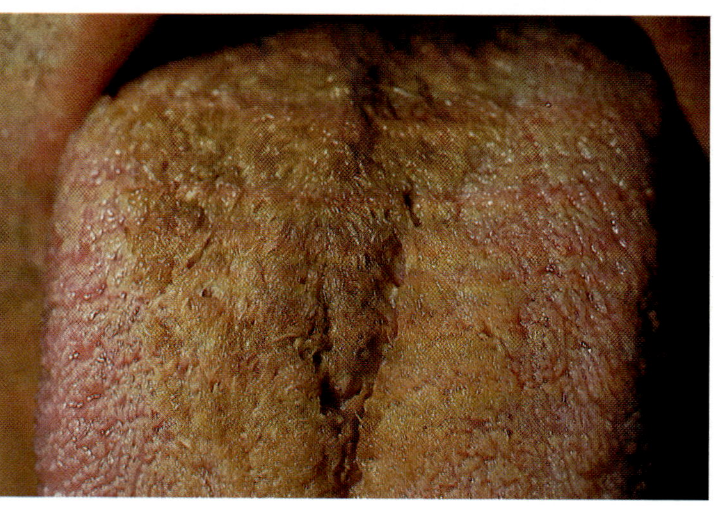

Figure 324 Black hairy tongue. Elongation and brownish discoloration of the filiform papillae of the tongue extending anteriorly and laterally.

Alterations of the Tongue

The tongue is affected in the course of many generalized diseases, especially as part of aphthous or erosive ulcerative stomatitis (see page 143), many viral infections or as adverse drug effects. There are other alterations of the tongue which are harmless but often disquiet patients who are affected with them.

A. Geographic Tongue, Exfoliatio Areata Linguae

These are transitory migrant plaques of unknown etiology, the appearance of which changes rapidly. They represent focal hyperkeratinization of the filiform papillae.

Clinical Features

1. The disorder is characterized by one or several round patches that are darker than the normal surface of the tongue and have a whitish or yellowish margin.
2. The patches develop and grow rapidly within a few days to form gyrate lesions.
3. Usually only the dorsal surface of the tongue, especially its edges, and rarely the oral mucosa, are affected.
4. Subjective symptoms are minimal; there may be mild tenderness, aggravated by sour foods.

Therapy

The patient should be informed that the condition is harmless. No effective treatment is available.

B. Fissured Tongue, Lingua Plicata

The physiologic grooves of the tongue are enlarged. This is usually a harmless congenital condition. In rare instances, it can be associated with chronic swelling of the lips and facial nerve paresis (Melkersson-Rosenthal syndrome).

Clinical Features

1. There are deep grooves on the dorsal surface of the tongue that are often shaped like the veins of a leaf. Sometimes erosions develop at the bottom of the grooves from the lack of the saliva's rinsing and cleansing action.
2. The condition is rarely painful, except when spicy or sour food is eaten.

Therapy

Treatment is necessary only for deep erosions, for which disinfectant mouthwashes (e.g., hexetidine) are useful.

C. Black Hairy Tongue, Lingua Villosa Nigra

The condition is due to increased keratinization of the filiform papillae. In addition, the dark color is enhanced by embedded food remnants and chromogenic bacteria. Black hairy tongue often occurs without recognizable cause. Occasionally, it can develop after treatment with broad-spectrum antibiotics, or rarely after treatment with corticosteroids or mouth washing with chlorhexidine or hydrogen peroxide.

Clinical Features

1. Black or greenish-brown discoloration of the elongated filiform papillae is characteristic. The changes begin at the base of the tongue and spread anteriorly and laterally, forming a triangular field pointing forward.
2. Usually there are no subjective symptoms.

Therapy

The changes can be removed partially with a toothbrush. Black hairy tongue regresses spontaneously after several weeks or months, or occasionally after several years.

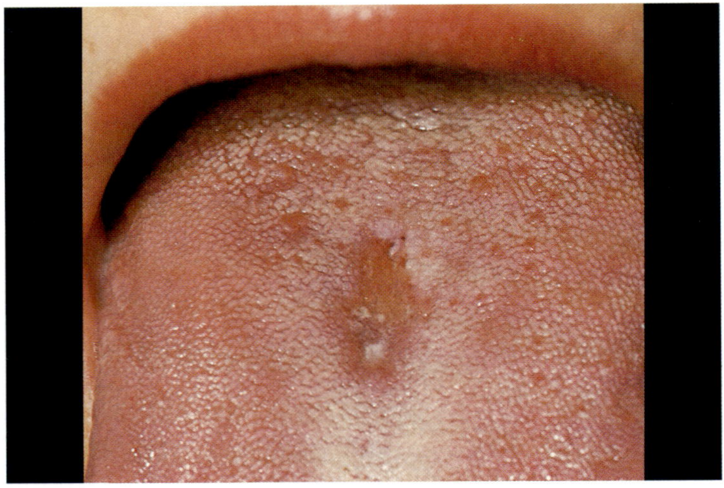

Figure 325 Median rhomboid glossitis (glossitis rhombica mediana). Rhomboid depression of the posterior section of the tongue medially and dorsally.

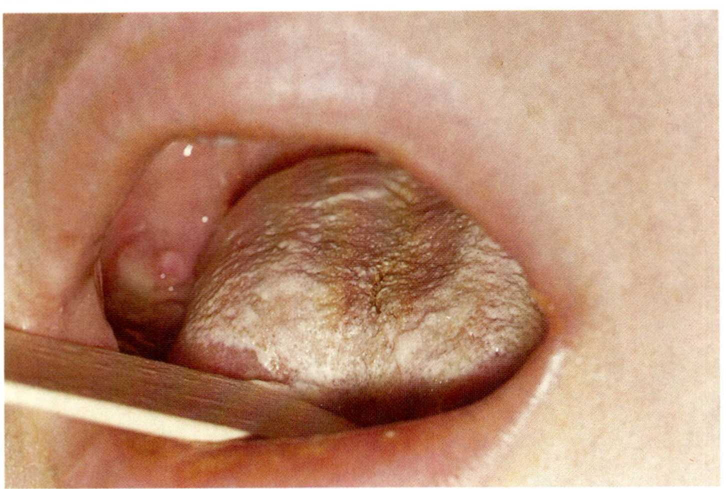

Figure 326 Increased coating of the tongue in a patient with erosive stomatitis and cheilitis.

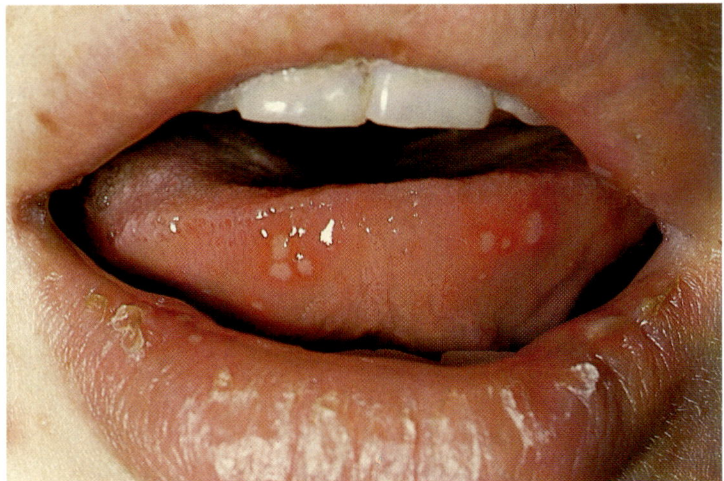

Figure 327 Aphthae of the tongue in a patient with viral aphthoid stomatitis.

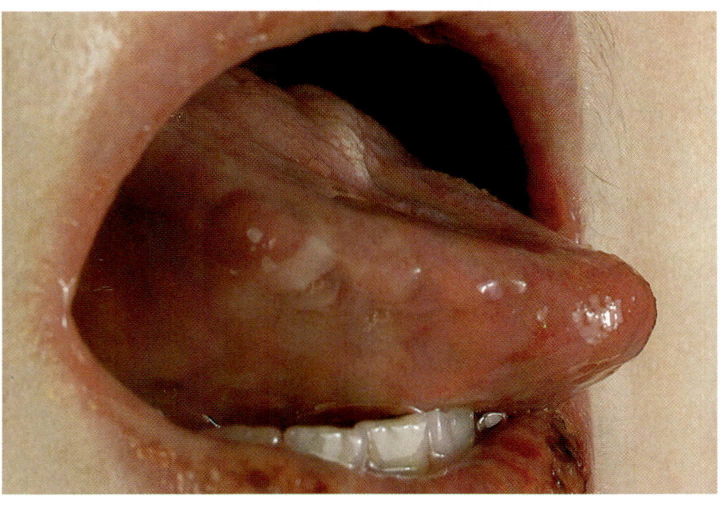

Figure 328 Erosive-ulcerative glossitis in a patient with drug-induced inflammation of the oral mucous membranes.

D. Median Rhomboid Glossitis

This is a depression or elevation in the midline of the tongue that usually appears in midlife or old age. It is assumed that the condition is a developmental defect, a persisting tuberculum impar (median tongue bud).

Clinical Features

1. The characteristic lesion is a smooth, rhomboid area, approximately 1 x 2 cm in size, without papillae, located in the long axis of the tongue. It can be either depressed or elevated in an irregular, nodular fashion. The area can develop a leukoplakia-like aspect secondarily.
2. The changes are located in the midline at the junction between the posterior and middle third of the tongue.
3. There are no subjective symptoms. The patients consult a physician because they are afraid they have cancer.

Therapy

No effective treatment exists for this harmless developmental anomaly. In some cases, the condition responds to antimycotic therapy (e.g., nystatin suspension), probably because of secondary infection with *Candida albicans*.

E. Increased Coating of the Tongue

A coated tongue appears to be discolored white on the dorsal surface. It is due to a temporary increase in keratinization of the filiform papillae and can be caused by inflammation or by decreased desquamation. Increased coating of the tongue is seen in conditions with high fever, such as upper respiratory infections. Desquamation is decreased when no solid food is eaten, for example, in patients on parenteral nutrition. The increased coating normally seen in the morning is caused by reduced desquamation since the tongue moves less during sleep. A coat is found more often in the posterior parts of the tongue because movement and abrasion are less there than on the tip or margins.

II. Sexually Transmitted Diseases and Non-Venereal Genital Diseases

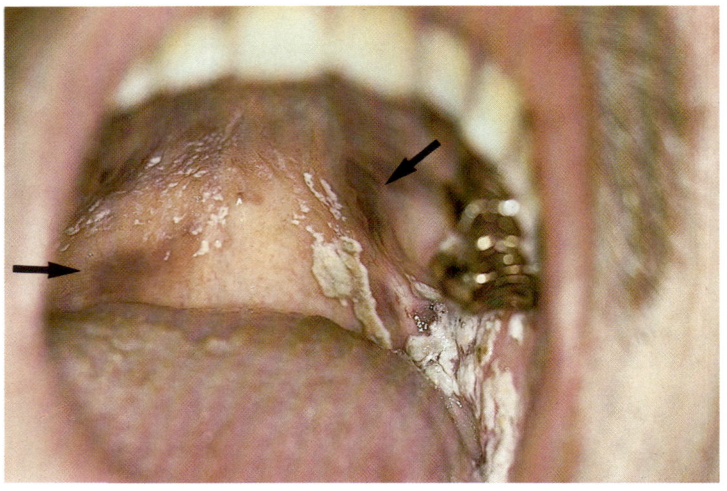

Figure 329 AIDS. Kaposi's sarcomas (→) and thick white coatings caused by marked candidiasis.

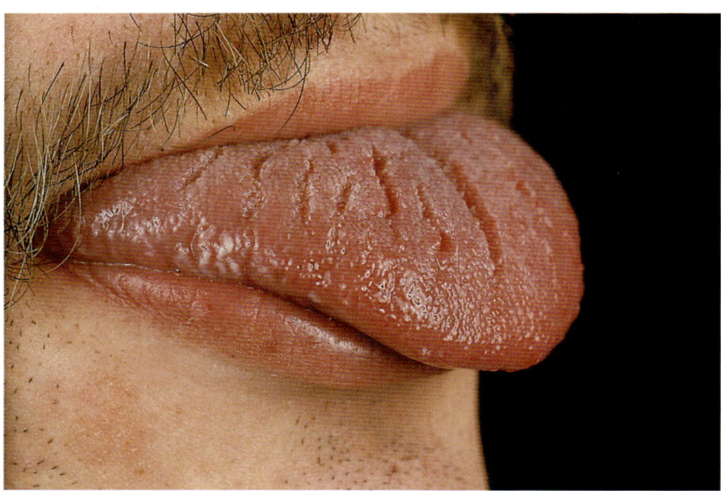

Figure 330 AIDS. Oral hairy leukoplakia with washboard-like, vertical fluting on the lateral, posterior border of the tongue.

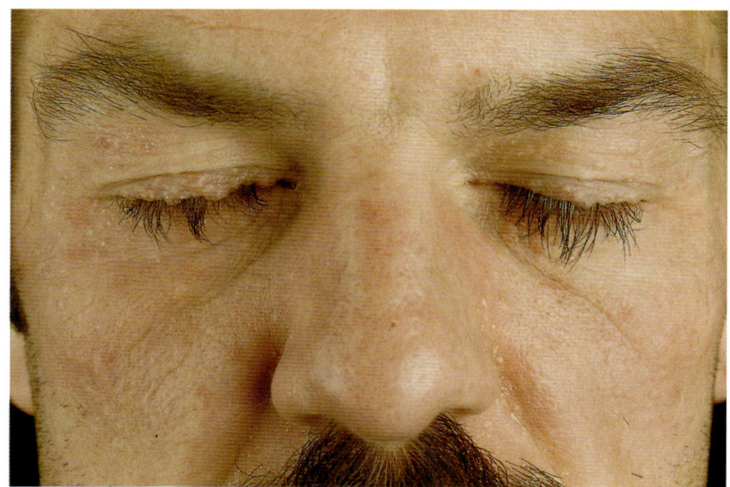

Figure 331 AIDS. Mollusca contagiosa on the eyelids.

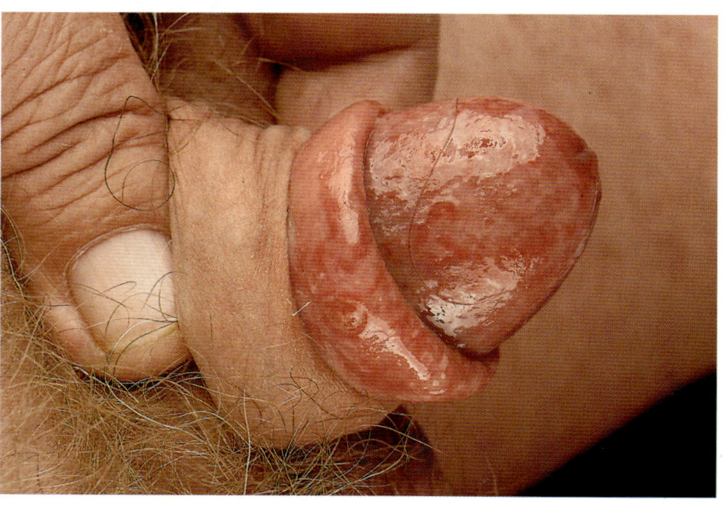

Figure 332 Syphilis. Primary lesion on the foreskin and distinct thrush balanitis. Diagnostic work-up disclosed HIV infection.

AIDS, HIV Infection

The acquired immunodeficiency syndrome (AIDS) is the result of an HIV infection (human immunodeficiency virus) and presents itself in the form of secondary immune defects. The infection is transmitted by bodily secretions containing the causative organism, e.g., from sexual intercourse, blood (transfusions, contaminated syringes, scalpels or minor skin injuries), organ transplants and pregnancy.

Two types of HIV organisms are known. HIV-1 occurs mainly in Central Africa, Europe, North and South America. HIV-2 is responsible for infections in West Africa but is seen with increasing frequency in other countries and continents.

Both virus types belong to the lentiviruses, a subgroup of the retroviruses.

They are able to infect T4 lymphocytes (T cells, CD4+ cells) as well as macrophages. The HIV infection develops from a symptom-free latent phase into a chronic lymphadenopathy and then into a manifest T-cell defect with severe opportunistic diseases.

Even in our regions, the number of AIDS cases is expected to increase further. This makes thorough knowledge of the symptomatology as well as the skin changes very important.

Transmission of the material containing the virus occurs through homosexual (where injuries occur frequently) or bisexual intercourse, in drug addicts who use the same contaminated needles, and in rare cases through transfusion of infected blood. The groups at risk are promiscuous male homosexuals, bisexual men who change their male partners frequently, heterosexual partners of infected individuals, persons addicted to intravenous drugs, hemophiliacs and newborn babies of infected mothers. Male homosexuals are mainly affected, but the disease also occurs in other men, women and children. The number of infected heterosexual individuals has increased significantly in recent years.

The patients can be categorized into 4 stages, depending on the progression of the disease caused by the virus-induced reduction in the number of CD4+ cells:

Stage I is the acute retroviral (primary) HIV infection; stage II represents the asymptomatic early phase of the disease; stage III is the early symptomatic disease; stage IVa is the late symptomatic phase of the disease and stage IVb is the advanced phase of the disease. The acute retroviral infection occurs either without symptoms or in the form of a short, mononucleosis-like disease (approximately 1–2 weeks, 1000–500 CD4+ cells). In the asymptomatic, early infection there can be enlarged lymph nodes, but usually no other symptoms (up to 10 years or more, 750–500 CD4+ cells). The early symptomatic phase is characterized by infections which are not life-threatening and chronic or intermittent illness (duration: 0–5 years, 500-100 CD4+ cells). The late symptomatic disease is characterized clinically by increasingly more severe symptoms such as life-threatening infections and malignant tumors (duration: 0–3 years, 500-100 CD4+ cells). The advanced stage is characterized by opportunistic infections and an increasing number of life-threatening infections, as well as symptoms of the central nervous system (duration: 1–2 years; 50-0 CD4+ cells).

Exact immunologic work-up is elaborate and should be done at an AIDS clinic. The prognosis of the disease is extremely poor; most patients with manifest symptoms of AIDS die within a few years.

Clinical Features

1. The acute infection usually runs a subclinical course and is asymptomatic; clinical diagnosis is difficult. Less frequently, fever and swollen lymph nodes are seen after an incubation period of 3–6 weeks, similar to influenza or mononucleosis, in rare cases with symptoms of aseptic meningitis. Occasionally, an exanthema develops with papulosquamous eruptions that is similar to that of secondary syphilis or mononucleosis.
2. The early disease is characterized by enlarged lymph nodes, but is otherwise symptom-free. Its duration varies; it can last up to 10 years or more.
   The early symptomatic disease (stage III) occurs with further reduction of the CD4+ cells. It is characterized by persistent or intermittent fever, fatigue, anorexia and weight loss (> 10%) without recognizable cause, nausea, diarrhea of more than one week's duration, as well as increased sweating, night sweats and various skin infections. This stage can last for several months or years.

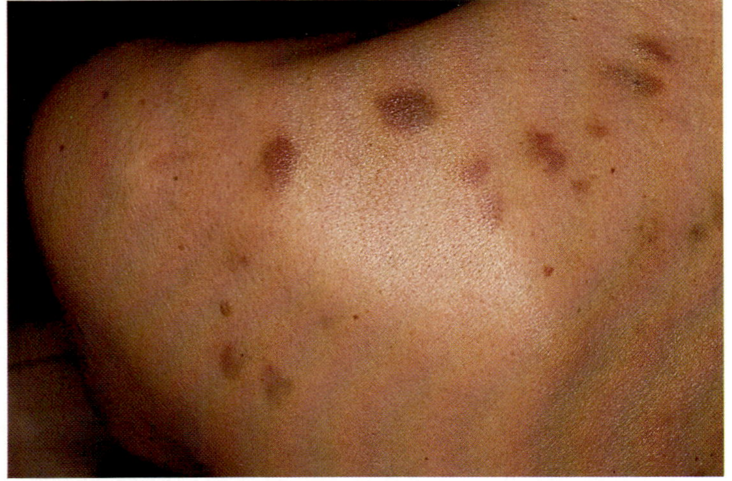

Figure 333 Kaposi's sarcomas in a patient with AIDS. Disseminated, red-brown tumors on the shoulder.

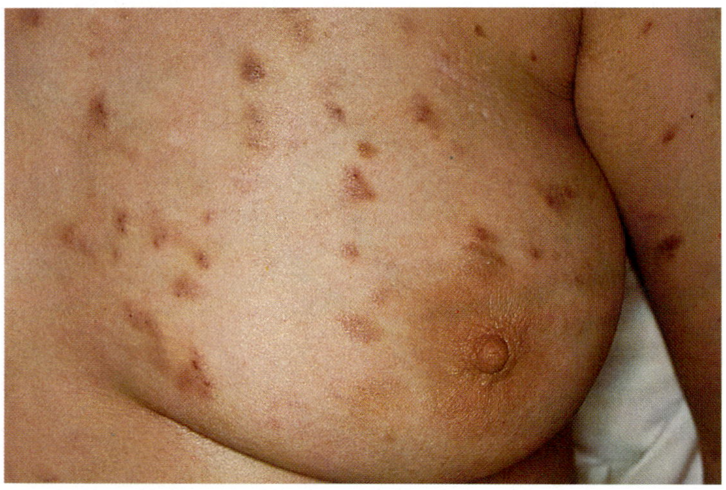

Figure 334 Kaposi's sarcomas in a patient with AIDS simulating prurigo.

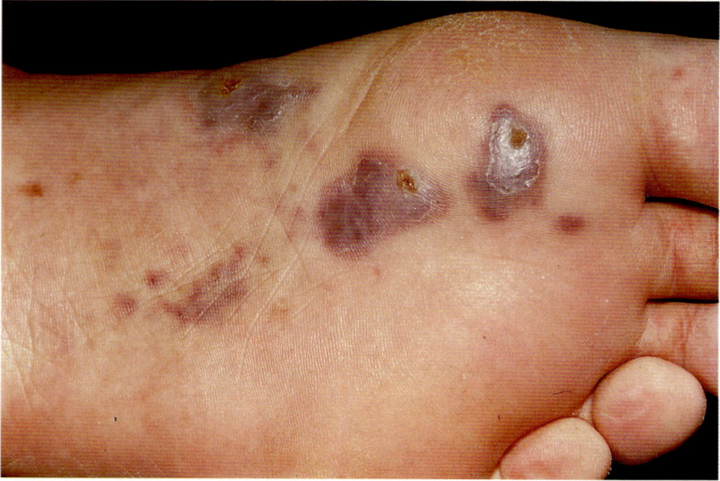

Figure 335 Kaposi's sarcomas on the sole of the foot in a patient with AIDS.

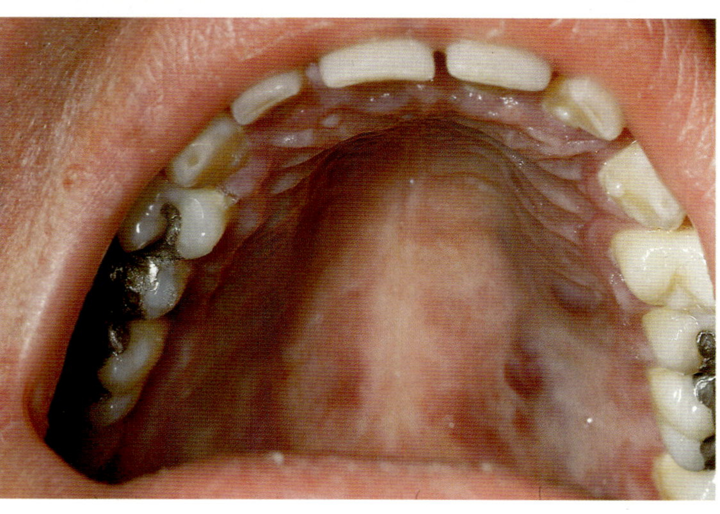

Figure 336 Kaposi's sarcomas on the upper jaw in a patient with AIDS.

3. As the immune system continues to be suppressed (stage IVa – the late asymptomatic disease), life-threatening infections, such as pneumonia caused by *Pneumocystis carinii* and persistent infections with cytomegalovirus, herpes simplex virus and *Toxoplasma* become more frequent. Candidal infections of skin and oral mucosa that are resistant to therapy are regularly seen, especially accompanied by angular cheilitis (perlèche: see page 99).
4. Kaposi's sarcoma of the skin, an angiosarcoma, is one of the symptoms of advanced AIDS. The clinical features include disseminated purple to dark-red or blue to brown-red vascular tumors that are often oval and are oriented along the cleavage lines of the skin. On the legs, the brownish discoloration of the Kaposi's sarcomas predominates as a result of increased hemosiderin deposits. They are also found on the mucous membranes and their transitional zones in the mouth, nose, eyes and rectum. Most patients regard Kaposi's sarcomas only as cosmetic problems.
5. Oral hairy leukoplakia is one of the most frequent and specific symptoms of HIV infection. It is caused by the Epstein-Barr virus and is usually a unilateral, occasionally bilateral, slightly raised thickening of the mucosa of the middle or posterior third of the tongue. It is up to 3 mm in size and has a papillomatous or hair-like surface. A corrugation running perpendicularly (washboard-like) along the side of the tongue is especially characteristic. Spotted forms also occur.
6. Skin infections, especially viral, are seen frequently. They include mollusca contagiosa, common warts, herpes zoster, herpes simplex as well as diseases caused by cytomegalovirus. The course of the disease is often more serious and more prolonged than it is in patients with an intact immune system.
7. Acute and chronic bacterial diseases are also seen, e.g., acute necrotizing ulcerative gingivostomatitis or tuberculosis.
8. Other unspecific skin symptoms such as seborrheic dermatitis of the face, persistent folliculitis, acne or erythema of the shoulder are seen less frequently.

Therapy

1. Effective causal therapy for HIV infection does not exist at the present time. Zidovudine (Retrovir) and other antiretroviral agents can delay progression of the disease and prolong survival. They can reduce the incidence of opportunistic infections or mitigate their course. Otherwise, therapy is mainly symptomatic.
2. Discrete Kaposi's sarcomas can be camouflaged cosmetically. Fractionated treatment with soft x-rays is effective, as is treatment with an argon laser. Intralesional and systemically applied cytostatic drugs can be helpful. Individual lesions can be excised.
3. Oral hairy leukoplakia requires treatment only when it causes symptoms. Topical treatment consists of podophyllin, the combination of vitamin A-acid gel and systemic acyclovir.
4. For oral thrush, some of the newer triazole preparations, such as fluconazole (100–400 mg per day orally) and itraconazole (200–400 mg per day orally) are given. Duration of treatment is 1–2 weeks. Recurrent oral candidiasis with a low CD4+ cell count requires long-term prophylaxis with fluconazole or similar medications. Exclusive topical therapy with nystatin solution, amphotericin lozenges or miconazole alone is usually not sufficient in HIV-infected patients.
5. Skin infections are often more severe in HIV-infected patients. Such infections may be life-threatening in these patients, and appropriate therapy for herpes simplex or herpes zoster should be given in higher doses and for longer periods of time.

Prophylaxis

Blood donations should not be accepted from a member of risk groups. Frequent change of sexual partners should be avoided; condoms must be used. The sexual partners, attending physicians and dentists (risk of infection from operations) should be informed of positive results of HIV tests. Members of the health professions must observe the same guidelines for prophylaxis against infection and disposal of infectious material as those being taken against hepatitis B. Observation of these guidelines in communities where a person with HIV infection lives should do much to minimize the danger of infection. The HIV virus is very susceptible to usual disinfectant materials and to desiccation.

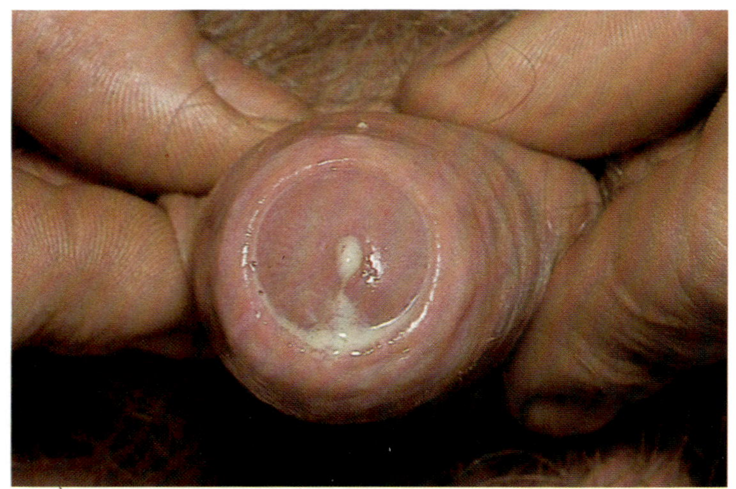

Figure 337 Typical appearance of acute gonorrhea with purulent discharge in a man.

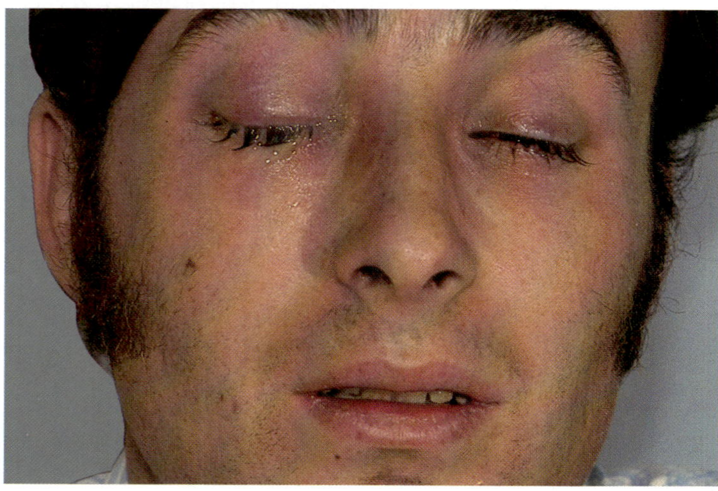

Figure 338 Gonoblennorrhea. Gonorrheic conjunctivitis caused by contact infection.

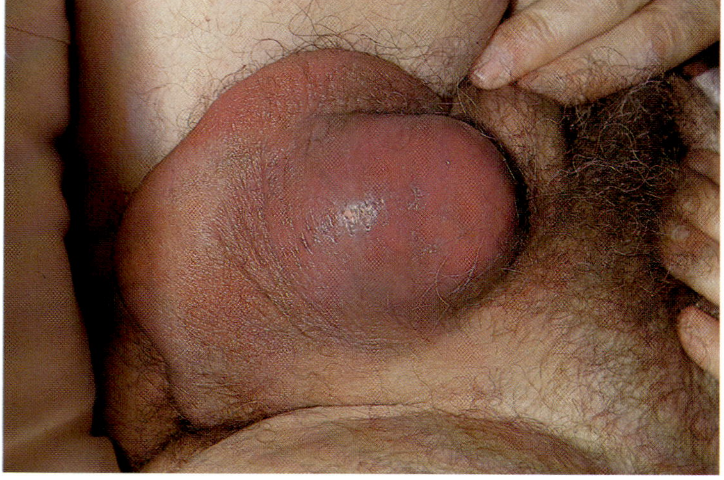

Figure 339 Gonorrhea. Extensive inflammatory conglomerate tumor in the area of the left adnexae caused by gonorrheic orchiepididymitis.

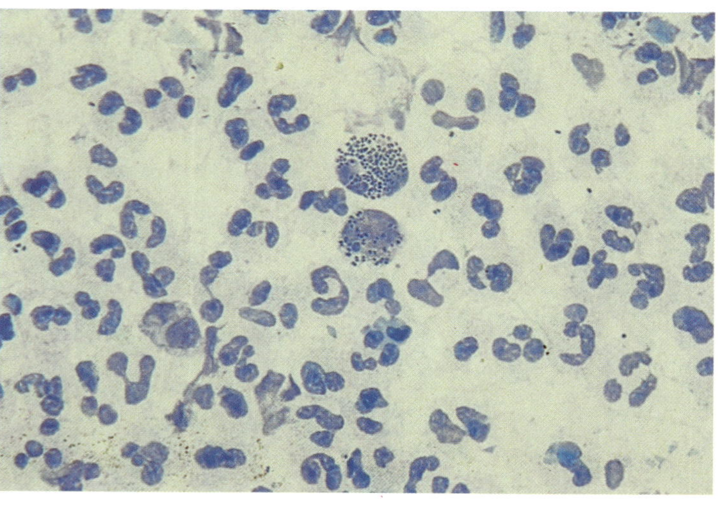

Figure 340 *Neisseria gonorrhoeae.* Typical appearance of intracellular organisms in a methylene blue-stained smear (630x).

Gonorrhea

Gonorrhea is one of the most common bacterial infectious diseases. Transmission of the disease is possible only through sexual intercourse because the organism is highly sensitive to oxygen and desiccation. Changes in sexual and recreational behavior allow more and more penicillin- and streptomycin-resistant organisms to be introduced from Southeast Asia. This makes eradication of the disease in future years very questionable. A smear stained with a relatively simple methylene blue or Gram's stain can be used as a screening test. The causative organisms appear as gram-negative diplococci, usually located within leukocytes. However, the diagnostic value of this method is not very specific because of the similar morphology of other Neisseria strains and because there are fewer organisms present in patients with chronic gonorrhea. In persons who change their sexual partners frequently, in sex tourists and in patients suspected of having chronic gonorrhea, the organisms should be identified by culture with subsequent sensitivity studies. The smear can be taken in the physician's office and sent to a laboratory in an appropriate medium (e.g., Transgrow).

Clinical Features

a) Gonorrhea in the Male

1. Following an incubation period of 3 (1–14) days, an acute inflammation of the anterior parts of the urethra occurs with a purulent discharge that is increased in the morning.
2. The patient complains of marked burning with urination.
3. During the subsequent course of the disease, the posterior urethra, the prostate (chronic prostatitis) and the epididymis (acute epididymitis) may become involved. The patient then complains of severe pain, swelling, and malaise.
4. Homosexuals may develop rectal or pharyngeal infections with *Neisseria*.

b) Gonorrhea in the Female

Clinical manifestations of the disease differ, depending on the location of the infection.

1. Gonorrheal urethritis shows the clinical signs of acute urethritis (dysuria, frequency, etc.).
2. Cervicitis may be present. There is increased vaginal discharge but no other symptoms.
3. Infection of Bartholin's glands with abscess formation is often accompanied by marked swelling of the external genitals, erythema and pain.
4. Rectal and pharyngeal infections are also possible.
5. Chronic infection of the fallopian tubes can lead to adhesions in the tubes and subsequent sterility.
   Rarely, a disseminated infection can occur with fever and septic pustules.

Therapy

The penicillin therapy used in the past had to be abandoned due to an increase in the strains of gonococci resistant to therapy.

1. Spectinomycin **(R. 53)** 2 g i.m. is given as a one-time dose, or ceftriaxone **(R. 50)** 1 g i.m. as a one-time dose.
2. Oral treatment with a one-time dose of 500 mg ciprofloxacin **(R. 54)** or 400 mg of cefixime. Unfortunately, the one-time dose sufficient for treatment of gonorrhea is not available as a commercial package.
3. For complicated and disseminated infection the above medications should be given for a period of at least 7 days.
4. The patient should be clinically examined to confirm therapeutical success. Should symptoms persist, a microbiological control may be necessary.
5. The patients should always be evaluated for other genital infections, especially syphilis.
6. The diagnosis "gonorrhea resistant to treatment" can mask an infection with *Chlamydia, Mycoplasma* or *Trichomonas*.
7. The legal reporting regulations must be observed (see page 177).

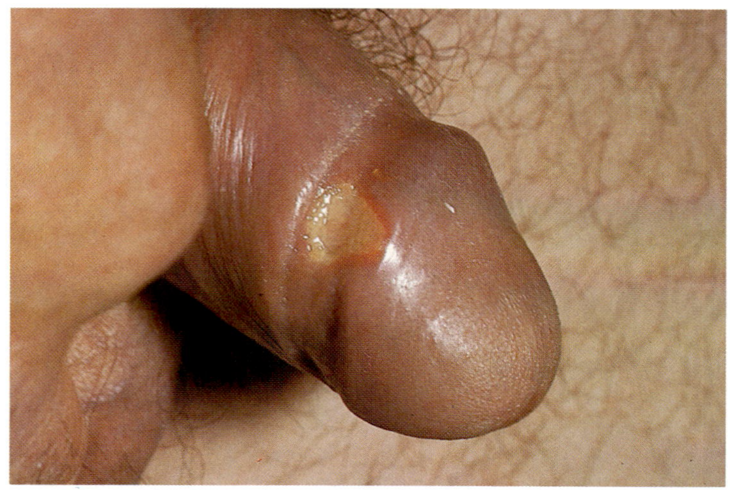

Figure 341 Syphilis I. Primary lesion. Firm fibrin-covered ulcer with reddened margin.

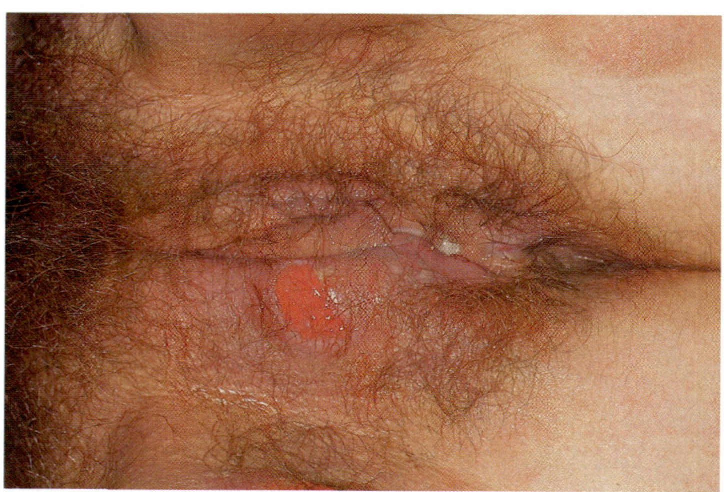

Figure 342 Syphilis I. Primary lesion. Ulcer with ham-colored floor.

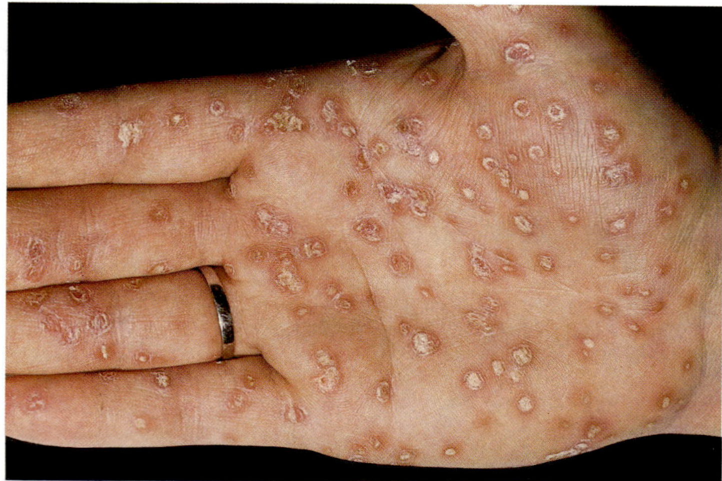

Figure 343 Syphilis II. Lenticular, psoriasiform, scaling papules on the palm of the hand.

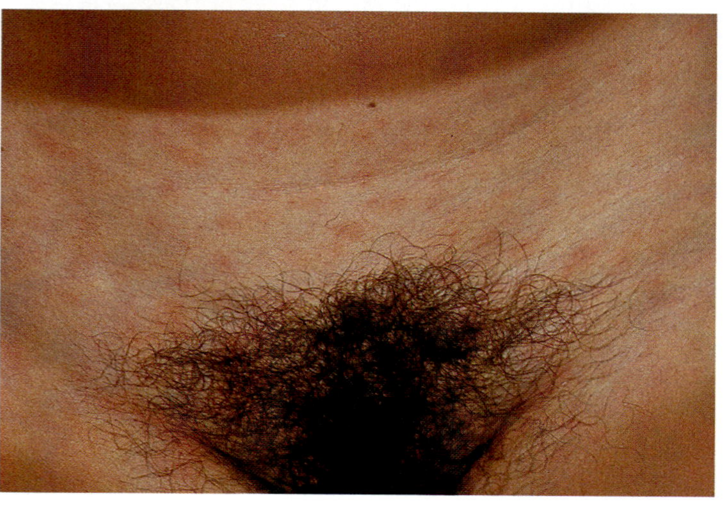

Figure 344 Syphilis II. Pale, macular exanthema, in this case, visible only in nontanned areas. So-called roseola syphilitica.

Syphilis

Syphilis is still one of the most common venereal diseases. It is usually transmitted by sexual intercourse, but infection is also possible through contact with secretions and blood that contain the organisms. In addition, an infected mother can transmit the disease to her fetus during gestation. Untreated syphilis can lead to death through organ complications in the tertiary stage, especially through cardiovascular syphilis. The morphology of syphilitic skin changes is manifold, especially in the secondary stage, and should always be considered in the differential diagnosis of exanthematous skin changes. Diagnostic work-up for syphilis should include the clinical presentation, identification of the causative organism (Treponema pallidum) in the tissue fluid, and the demonstration of specific antibodies with different serologic methods (TPHA test, VDRL test, FTA-ABS test). At least two of these three diagnostic tests must be positive to confirm a diagnosis of syphilis.

The course of the disease can be divided into 4 stages.

Primary Stage: Stage of the primary lesion (hard chancre) with subsequent swelling of the regional lymph nodes.

Secondary Stage: Stage of generalization. This stage begins approximately 7 weeks after infection and lasts approximately 2 years.

Tertiary Stage: So-called organ syphilis occurs after 3–10 years.

Quaternary Stage: Neurosyphilis with tabes dorsalis and progressive paralysis, manifest after 15–30 years.

Clinical Features

a) Primary Stage

1. A small painless nodule develops at the site of inoculation 10–14 days after infection and is often overlooked. It develops into the primary lesion, an eroded, painless, weeping, indurated ulcer. The causative organism can usually be demonstrated by dark-field microscopy in the serum from the primary lesion.
2. Since the disease is transmitted by sexual intercourse, approximately 90% of all syphilitic primary lesions are found in the genital area, in men on the glans penis, on the sulcus coronarius, or on the shaft of the penis. In women, primary lesions are observed less frequently. They usually appear on the labia majora or minora, occasionally in the vagina or on the cervix. Depending on the patient's sexual practices, perianal or oral chancres can also be found. Multiple primary lesions are also possible.
3. The accompanying unilateral (rarely bilateral) painless enlargement of the lymph nodes that occurs approximately 1 week after the primary lesion is typical for the disease.

b) Secondary Stage

1. Skin manifestations of the secondary stage appear approximately 6–12 weeks after the infection. At this time, the chancre has often not healed yet or is visible as a fresh scar. The early symptoms of the secondary stage consist of a pale macular exanthema primarily on the trunk (so-called syphilitic roseola). Later, new crops of eruptions appear, and the maculae gradually change into papules. In the genital and perianal regions, as well as other moist areas (e.g., the interdigital spaces of the toes), these pale to dark red papules may form weeping lesions (condylomata lata). The secretions from these lesions are full of treponemes and are highly infectious. Palms and soles are often affected; here, the exanthema frequently resembles psoriasis. Sometimes hair is lost in a diffuse, spotty distribution (moth-eaten).
2. In immunosuppressed patients, a so-called lues maligna can develop with weeping, erosive-ulcerative, destructive infiltrates covered with crusts.
3. Disseminated lesions on the oral mucosa show rapid ulcerative destruction (mucous plaques).
4. Generalized indurated and painless swelling of the lymph nodes is present during the secondary stage of syphilis.
5. Systemic manifestations can be transient fever, shin pain, pharyngitis and hepatitis.

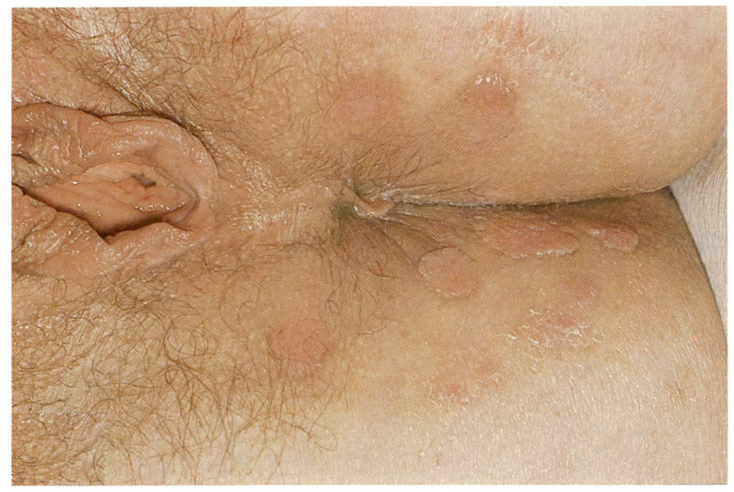

Figure 345 Syphilis II. Condylomata lata. Wide, soft, superficially weeping, highly infectious papules.

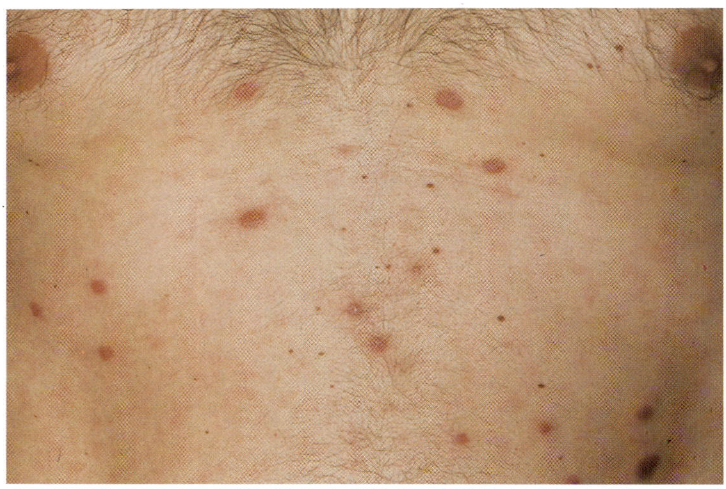

Figure 346 Syphilis II. Lenticular, brownish papules and pale brownish, macular exanthema.

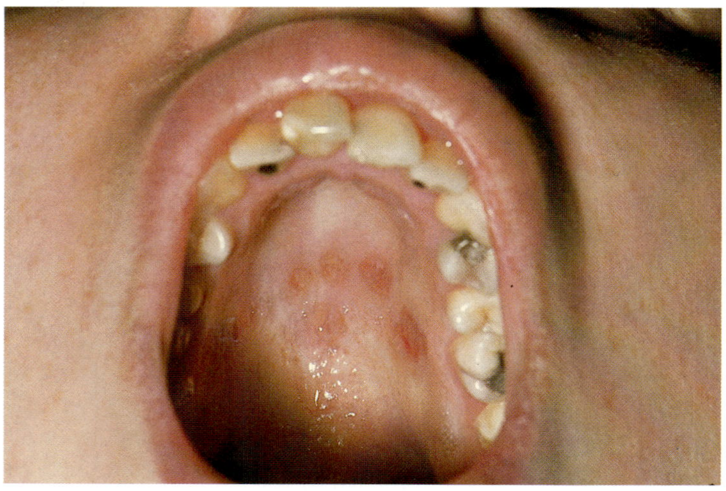

Figure 347 Syphilis II. Involvement of the mucous membranes of the mouth. Sharply demarcated erosions on the hard palate.

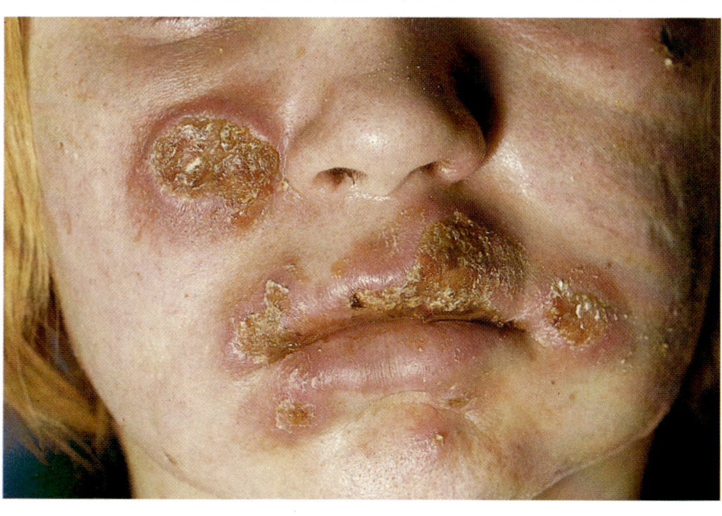

Figure 348 Syphilis II. So-called lues maligna. Pronounced inflammatory reaction with crusty and weeping infiltrates.

c) Tertiary Syphilis

Tertiary syphilis is seen very rarely today. It is characterized by circumscribed serpiginous foci that consist of small individual nodules and continue to enlarge peripherally (tuberoserpiginous syphilid) over months or even years. Circumscribed granulomas (gummas) in the subcutis frequently become necrotic with central ulceration or perforation (for instance on the hard palate). Cardiovascular syphilis can be life-threatening if an aortic aneurysm develops.

d) Neurosyphilis

Tabes dorsalis and progressive paralysis are rarely seen by the practitioner today. A positive history of syphilis and a positive serologic reaction in connection with neurologic or psychiatric symptoms (ataxia, loss of position sensation, absent patellar and Achilles tendon reflexes) are indicative of tabes dorsalis. Psychiatric disorders, such as progressive dementia, manic depressive symptoms, or paranoia and hallucinations are typical of progressive paralysis. The patient should be referred to a neurologist or a psychiatrist for confirmation of the diagnosis.

Therapy

1. In Germany, generally a treatment with clemizole penicillin is preferred. In the early stage (primary stage and secondary stage until one year after infection), 1 million units should be applied daily for 14 days, for neurosyphilis, 1 million units for 21 days. Because of the possibility of anaphylactic shock, Hoigné syndrome or a Jarisch-Herxheimer reaction, the necessary precautions must be taken. Prophylaxis for a Jarisch-Herxheimer reaction is 50–100 mg prednisolone given parenterally with the first injection of penicillin G. For treatment of neurosyphilis, 6 x 5 million units of aqueous penicillin G daily should be given for 10 days, followed by 1 million units of clemizole penicillin daily for 21 days or, alternately, by benzathine penicillin at a dose of 2.4 million units given i.m. once weekly for 3 successive weeks.
2. In the U.S., benzathine penicillin remains the drug of choice, as it provides effective treatment in a single visit. Patients should be treated with a one-time dose of 2.4 million units of benzathine penicillin (Bicillin L-A) for early syphilis and 2.4 million units of benzathine penicillin one time per week for 3 weeks for late syphilis.
3. As an alternative in patients allergic to penicillin, doxycycline 2 x 100 mg per day should be given orally for 15 days.
4. After termination of treatment, serologic checkups are necessary at regular intervals to insure success of treatment: in early syphilis, every 3 months for 1 year, in late syphilis, every 3 months for at least 3 years. Treponema-specific IgG antibodies that can be demonstrated by FTA-ABS and TPHA tests are usually present for the rest of the patient's life, yet they do not protect against reinfection. IgM-FTA titers and VDRL titers (reagin test) decrease significantly with therapy and can even become negative.
5. When treating patients with syphilis, public health regulations including reporting must be observed. Careful documentation of patient data, physical findings and therapeutic measures and results is absolutely necessary. It is important to advise the patient that he or she must abstain from sexual relations until treatment is completed and that he or she must inform any sexual partners about the venereal disease and urge them to seek medical help.

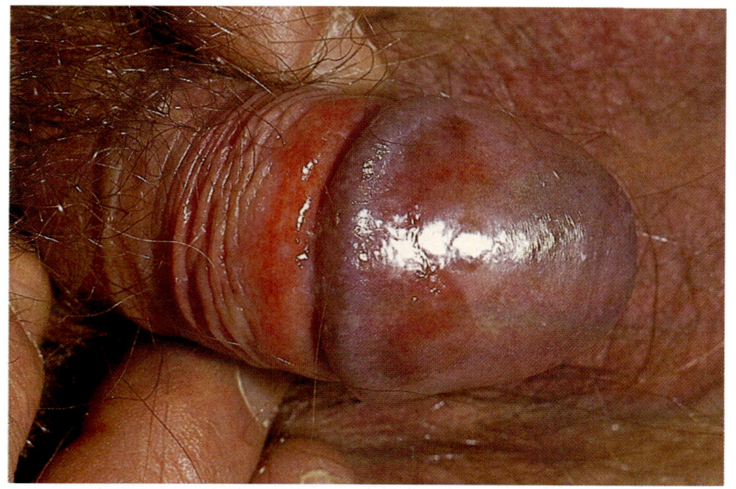

Figure 349 Balanitis simplex. Acute inflammation with erythematous weeping lesions on glans penis and prepuce.

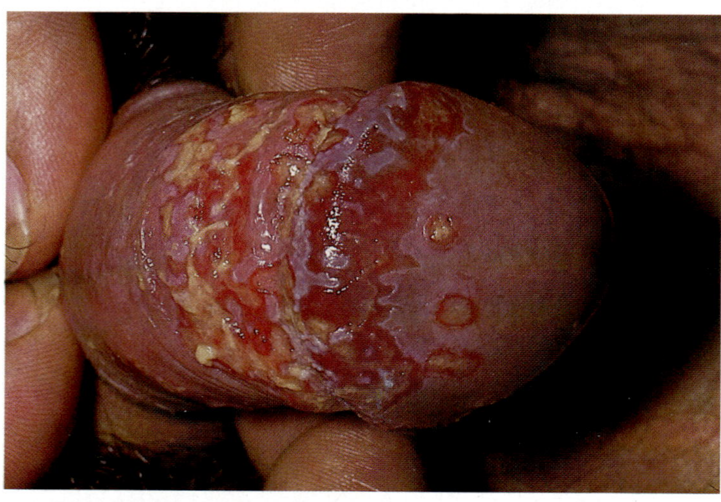

Figure 350 Genital herpes. Painful erosions that are often arranged in a clover leaf fashion as a sequel of the pre-existing vesicles.

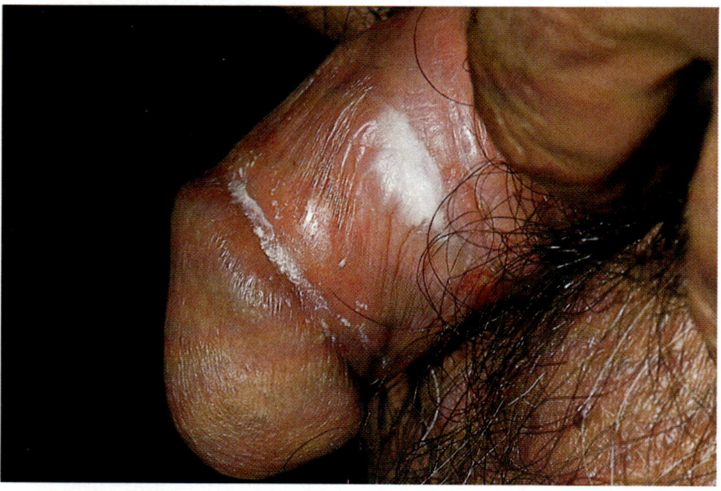

Figure 351 Kraurosis penis. Planar atrophy with erosions and leukoplakia.

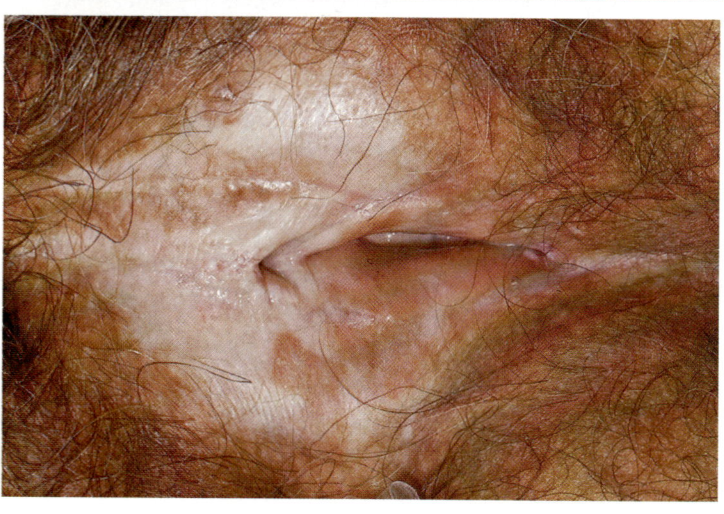

Figure 352 Kraurosis vulvae. Extensive atrophy with marked flattening of the external female genital. Distinct whitish discoloration of the atrophic area.

Non-Venereal Genital Diseases

A. Balanitis

This is an inflammation of the glans penis, while balanoposthitis is an inflammation of the glans penis with involvement of the internal mucous lining of the foreskin. The anatomy of the preputial space predisposes to inflammation from bacteria, yeast or irritating agents (spermicides, aphrodisiacs, medications), especially when genital hygiene is either poor or excessive. Generalized infections, excessive coffee consumption, and insufficient sleep can also promote an acute balanitis.

Clinical Features

1. Initially, there is only erythema and a foul smelling, watery secretion.
2. Longer lasting inflammations or phimosis can lead to retention of secretions and maceration followed by ulceration with purulent discharge.
3. Secondary candidiasis develops frequently.
4. Chronic balanitis is often seen in patients with diabetes mellitus.

Therapy

1. The penis should be soaked in disinfectant solutions or detergents ($KMnO_4$ solution 1:10,000).
2. Wet dressings, provided the foreskin can be reduced, are helpful. Otherwise, the preputial space should be irrigated with a syringe fixed with a bulb-headed cannula.
3. Candida infection is almost always present and is treated with nystatin paste **(R. 31).**
4. The causes must be eliminated to avoid a recurrence.

B. Vulvovaginitis

Acute vulvovaginitis is usually infectious (gonorrhea, herpes, candidiasis, trichomoniasis, syphilis). It can also be caused by a contact dermatitis. Chronic vulvovaginitis is frequently due to candidiasis in patients with diabetes mellitus.

Clinical Features

1. Inflammatory erythema and swelling of the external genitals with erosions and increased vaginal discharge are characteristic. The vaginal mucosa is often involved.
2. The main subjective symptoms are pruritus and occasionally moderate to severe pain.

Therapy

The cause should be eliminated if at all possible. Symptomatic treatment includes sitz baths with disinfectant solutions (**R. 4**), moist dressings (**R. 1**), zinc oil or zinc lotion (**R. 20**) and dabbing with a dye solution (0.1–0.5% watery solution) (**R. 14a**). Ointments should be avoided; they frequently cause an exacerbation.

C. Kraurosis Penis, Kraurosis Vulvae

This is a progressive phimosis and atrophy of the glans penis and foreskin in men and a progressive atrophy of the vulva in women. Most frequently, the condition is due to lichen sclerosus et atrophicus, a connective tissue disease with primary location in the genital area. Genital kraurosis can lead to leukoplakia (see page 231), a precancerous lesion.

Clinical Features

1. Whitish atrophic lesions with parchment-like shriveling of the skin are characteristic. In lichen sclerosus, one also sees small keratotic flakes associated with the follicles. Extensive atrophy of the external genitals develops with advancing disease.
2. The vulva is affected in women, foreskin and glans penis in men.
3. The disorder can occasionally cause obliteration of the urethral orifice with severe impairment of urination.
4. There is often severe pruritus, and constant scratching causes inflammation with further increase of pruritus.

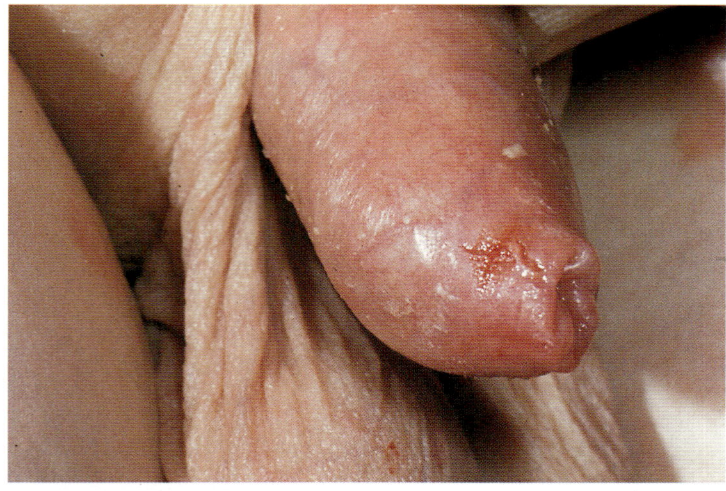

Figure 353 Phimosis.

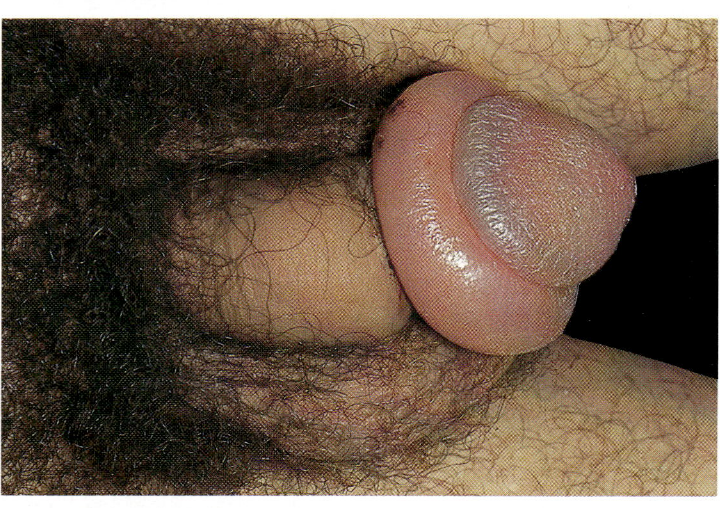

Figure 354 Paraphimosis (appearance of a "Spanish collar"). Massive circular edema of the foreskin after retraction of phimotic foreskin.

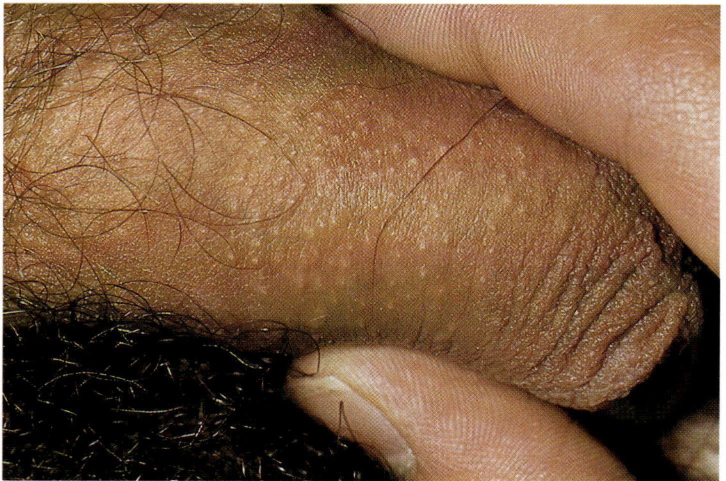

Figure 355 Ectopic sebaceous glands on the shaft of the penis. This is a frequent and harmless finding.

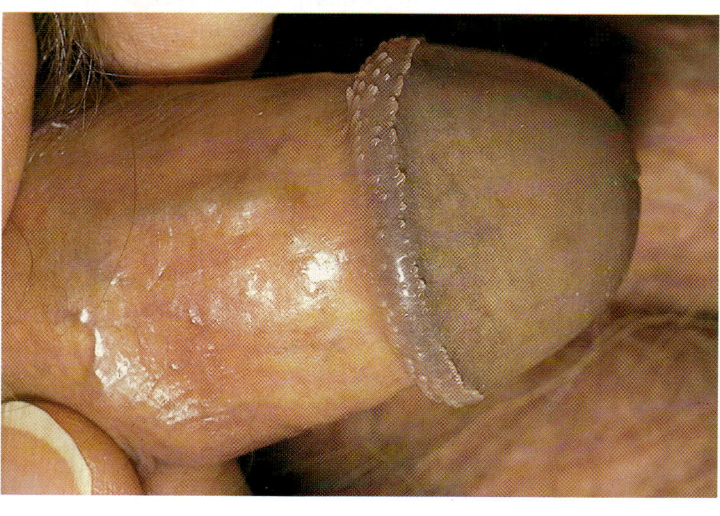

Figure 356 Pearly penile papules. Filiform papillomata on the junction between glans penis and sulcus coronarius. Harmless variation of the norm.

Atheromas, Retention Cysts, Pilar Cysts

An atheroma (wen) is a cyst that occurs mainly on the scalp and originates from the epithelium of the hair follicle. It is also known as a trichilemmal cyst. These lesions show an autosomally dominant inheritance. They occur as solitary lesions in approximately 30% of all patients, but in most patients, they occur as multiple lesions.
Retention cysts (epidermal cysts) occur much more frequently and are difficult to distinguish from atheromas. They originate from the orifice of the follicle and occur predominantly in men.

Clinical Features

a) Atheroma (trichilemmal cyst, pilar cyst)

1. This is a globular, tense-elastic tumor, reaching the size of a plum, which is mobile and covered with atrophic, thin skin. The robust cysts have a thick wall and are filled with a white, pasty keratinous material, produced by the epithelium of the hair follicle. They are often easier to palpate than to see. There is no external opening, such as that often found in retention cysts.

2. Atheromas are found almost exclusively on the scalp. The skin over the larger cysts is usually bald due to damage from the pressure on the follicular apparatus.

3. Trauma rarely causes inflammation or proliferation of the lesion; malignant degeneration is almost never seen.

b) Retention cysts (epidermal cysts)

1. These are cutaneous or subcutaneous tumors of pinhead to plum size, depending on their developmental stage.

2. Areas of predilection are the face and trunk, but they can occur in all areas where hair follicles are present.

3. The cysts are ruptured easily by manipulation; the keratinous material can be pressed into the surrounding tissue, where it acts as a foreign body and can cause the development of a granuloma. Secondary bacterial infection can lead to abscess formation.

4. The expanded gland duct of retention cysts is frequently open, and the foul-smelling contents (rancid lipids and debris) can be evacuated. The cysts refill after some time because the cyst's wall remains intact.

Therapy

Repeated inflammation, proliferation and other complications are indications for surgical removal. Inflammation must be allowed to subside before surgery. The cyst is removed by blunt enucleation with an attached spindle-shaped piece of skin. It is important not to leave remnants of the cyst, because a recurrence originates from these remnants. Scars from prior inflammations can make enucleation difficult.

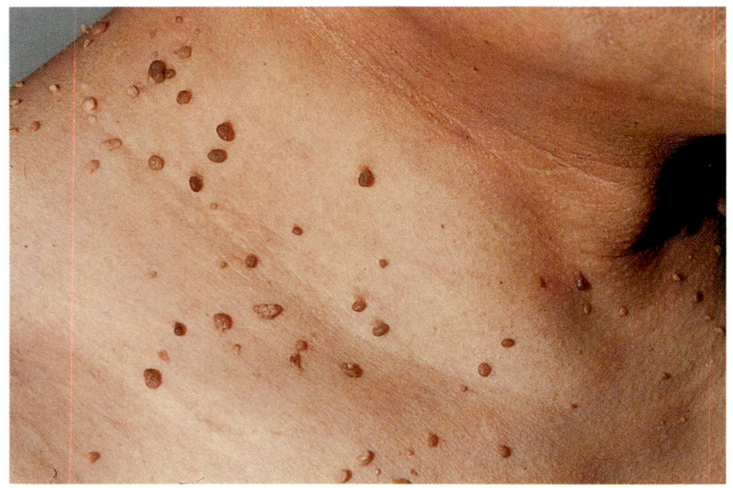

Figure 361 Soft fibromas (skin tags). Soft, pedunculated, often pigmented tumors on the neck.

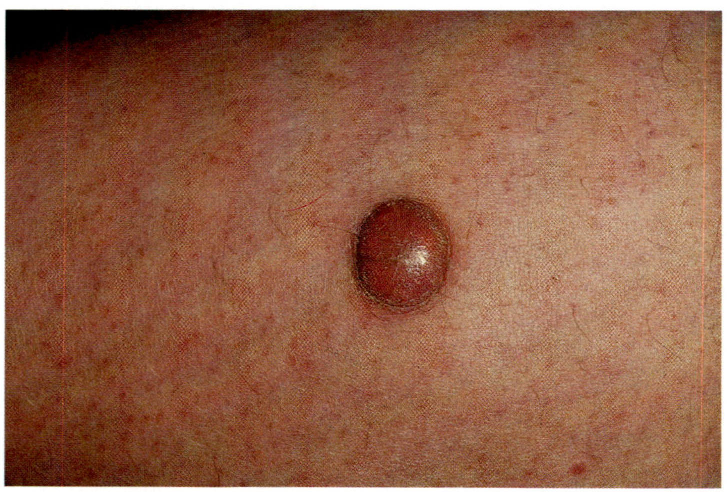

Figure 362 Histiocytoma. Early form. Lentil-sized, firm, slightly pigmented tumor.

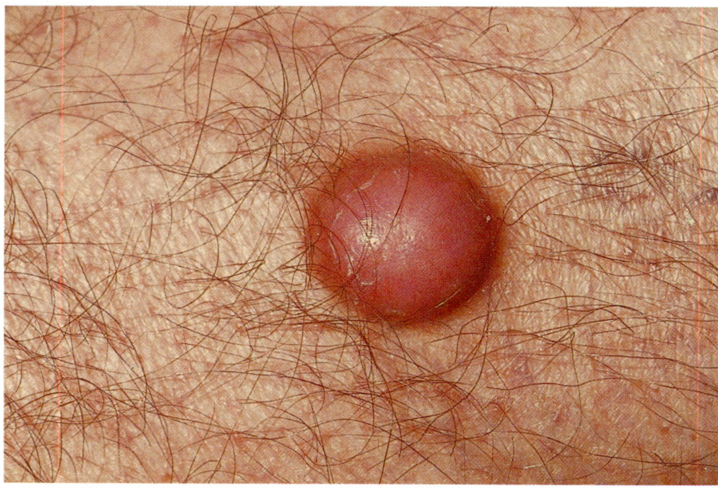

Figure 363 Histiocytoma. Early form. Typical appearance of the hemispheric, firm tumor with brownish margin (hemosiderin storage).

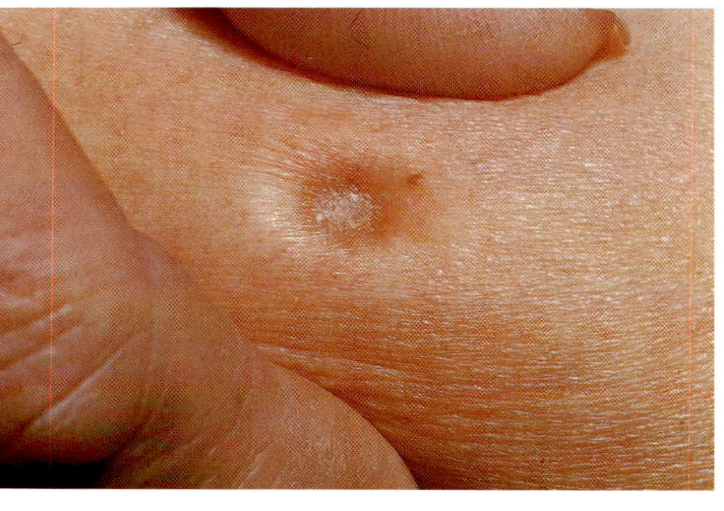

Figure 364 Histiocytoma. Advanced stage. Firm tumor deeply embedded in the skin with depression of the overlying layers of the skin following tangential pressure.

Fibromas

Fibromas are common, benign neoplasms. They can be classified as soft pedunculated fibromas (fibroma molle, fibroma pendulans) and hard fibromas, such as histiocytomas or dermatofibromas. Histiocytomas occur mainly in young adults, especially on the extremities, and persist during the patient's entire lifetime without ever causing any symptoms. There is no malignant degeneration of histiocytomas; they are reactive changes. The patients often report insect bites or folliculitis prior to development of the tumor.

A. Fibroma Molle (Skin Tags)

Clinical Features

1. Soft fibromas are usually small, lentil-sized, pedunculated, skin-colored tumors. In rare cases, they can grow to the size of a tangerine.
2. Fibroma pendulans is often found on the lateral aspects of the neck, on the shoulders, in the axillary and submammary regions, and occasionally in the inguinal region.
3. They often occur as multiple lesions. Obesity and hyperhidrosis predispose to the development of pendulous fibromas.
4. Fibromas are found mainly in adults and can show a familial disposition.
5. Soft fibromas occasionally become inflamed or show hemorrhagic infarction after torsion of the pedicle.

Therapy

Surgical removal can be performed by electrocautery sling or with scissors. The removal of large fibromas may be accompanied by considerable bleeding and require several sutures to close the wound.

B. Histiocytoma, Dermatofibroma

Clinical Features

1. These are hard, singular or multiple, hemispherical or disc-shaped nodules which are mobile and rarely grow to more than 2-3 cm in size. Their color can be reddish or skin-colored, although sometimes one sees a brownish discoloration caused by hemosiderin deposits. Histiocytomas that have been present for a longer period of time are no longer raised above the level of the skin, but are visible as slightly depressed lesions that can be palpated as thickened areas.
2. Areas of predilection are the extremities; the legs are more often affected than the arms.

Therapy

Treatment of these slow-growing tumors is usually not necessary as long as the diagnosis has been confirmed. Tumors that cause cosmetic or diagnostic difficulties should be excised.

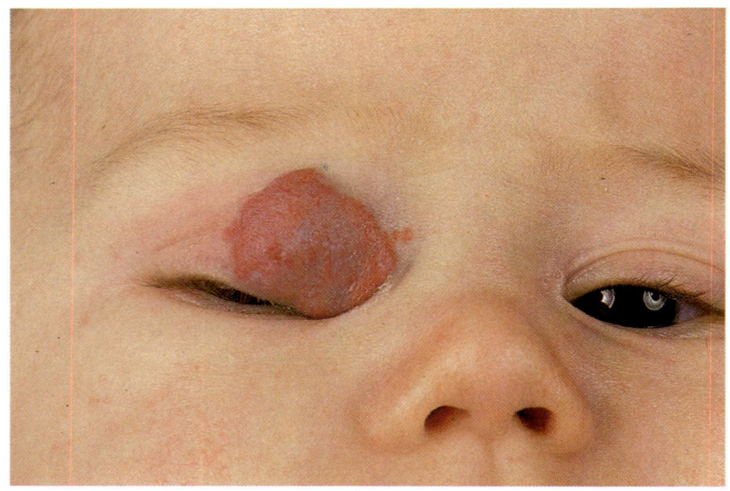

Figure 365 Capillary hemangioma of the upper eyelid.

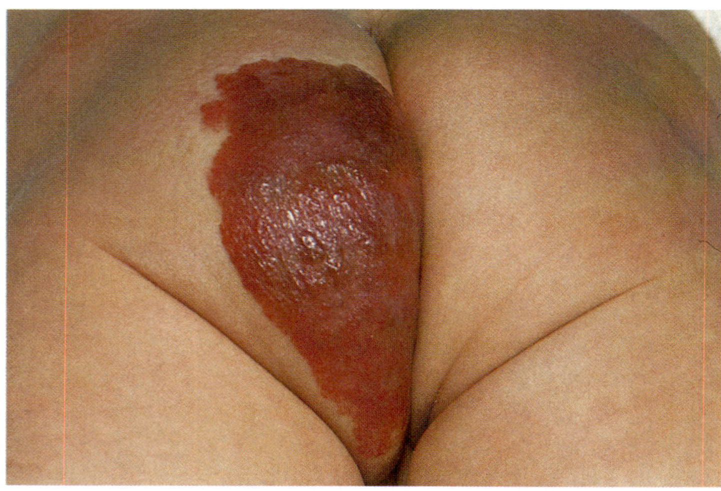

Figure 366 Capillary hemangioma in the gluteal area. Strawberry-like color and surface.

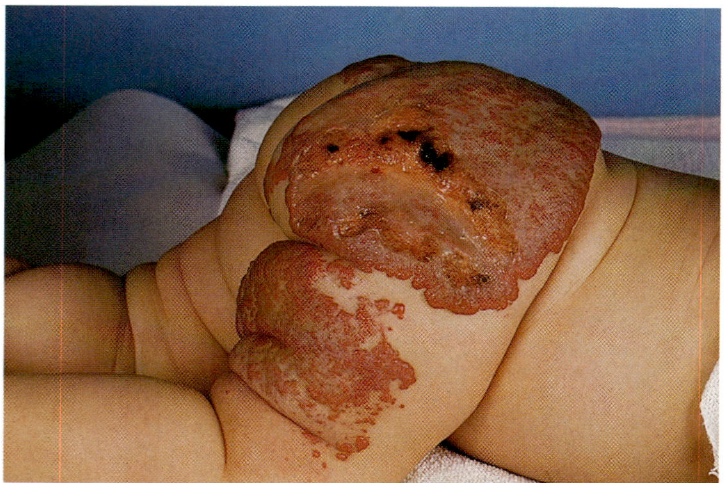

Figure 367 Capillary hemangioma. Ulceration and grayish discoloration as signs of beginning involution.

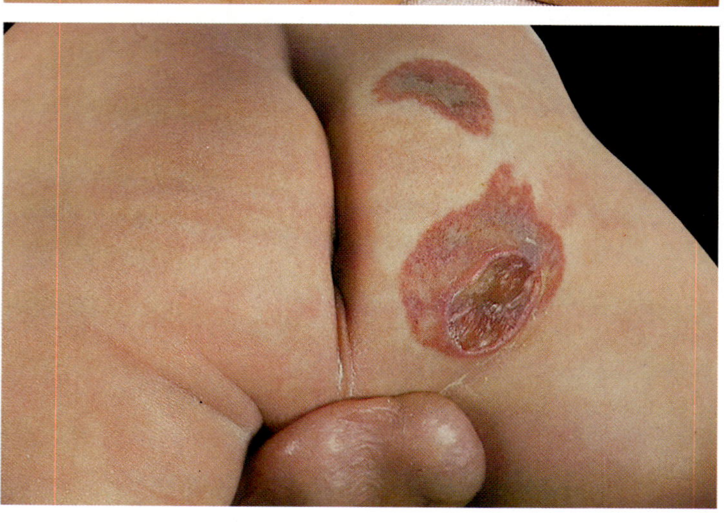

Figure 368 Capillary hemangiomas. Advanced involution with grayish discoloration and decrease of the tumors.

Hemangiomas

Vascular tumors are among the most frequent benign tumors of the skin. They can be distinguished on the basis of their clinical appearance and can be diagnosed without difficulty. Treatment depends on the type of the tumor.

A. Capillary Hemangioma (Strawberry Hemangioma)

Capillary hemangioma occurs almost exclusively in children (approximately 10% of all children; two thirds girls, one third boys) and is rarely seen in adults. Practically all capillary hemangiomas involute spontaneously within a period of years, usually during childhood. The deep lesions involute later than the superficial ones do. Radical therapy should be avoided, if at all possible, since the tumors disappear spontaneously in almost all cases. In the past, capillary hemangiomas in children were often treated with x-rays or radioactive substances such as thorium X paint or strontium platelets. Occasionally, one still sees the sequelae: radiation scars (chronic radiation damage) with or without trophic ulcers, occasionally atrophy of bone, hypoplasia of the breast, etc. (see page 137).

Clinical Features

1. A capillary hemangioma appears as a hemispherical or flat tumor that is bright-red in color. Occasionally, the tumors can show through the skin with a bluish color. Deep-seated lesions can be palpated as soft tissue masses; the overlying skin may have normal color. The tumors can occur as single or multiple lesions.
2. Larger hemangiomas can occasionally cause atrophy of the underlying bone.
3. Some capillary hemangiomas can ulcerate and are then covered with crusts. Serious bleeding fom capillary hemangiomas is very rare.
4. These tumors can be located anywhere on the skin, including the face.
5. As the tumor involutes, its color gradually changes to gray. Eventually, only a flaccid sac remains that also involutes slowly.

Therapy

1. Treatment should be delayed as long as possible to await probable spontaneous involution of the lesion.
2. For unproblematic capillary hemangiomas, the most important (and frequently difficult) therapeutic measure is to convince the parents that this is a harmless, cosmetic alteration that involutes spontaneously and that they should resist various recommendations for therapy (cryotherapy, laser therapy, etc.). Thus, it might be possible to save the parents unnecessary worry. Otherwise they tend to misinterpret the capillary hemangioma as a flaw which they allow or even seek to be unnecessarily treated, perhaps due to misguided cosmetic conceptions, perhaps also due to impatience.
3. Operative treatment is indicated for tumors that impair breathing, eating or other vital functions.
4. Large, erosive capillary hemangiomas with a tendency to hemorrhage may require treatment with a neodymium-YAG laser.
5. Other invasive therapeutic measures such as cryotherapy, laser therapy, intralesional or even systemic corticosteroid therapy may be indicated in exceptional cases. If so, an experienced dermatologist should be consulted before such treatment is attempted.

B. Nevus Flammeus, Port-Wine Stain

Two different forms of this angiectatic abnormality can be distinguished.

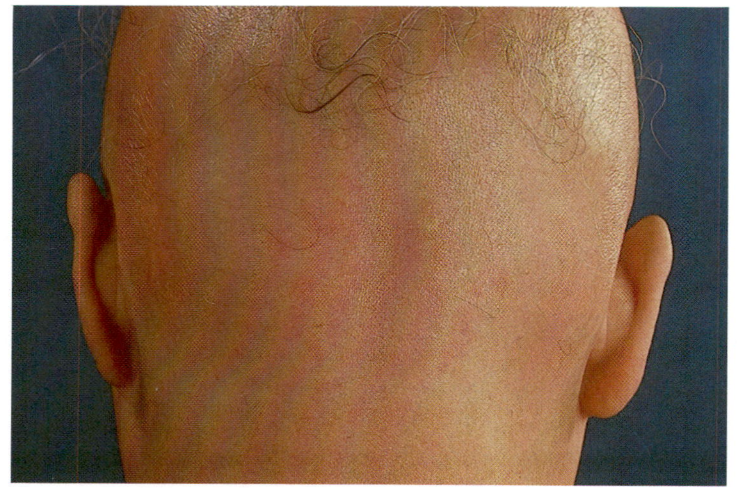

Figure 369 Median nevus flammeus of the neck. So-called "storkbite".

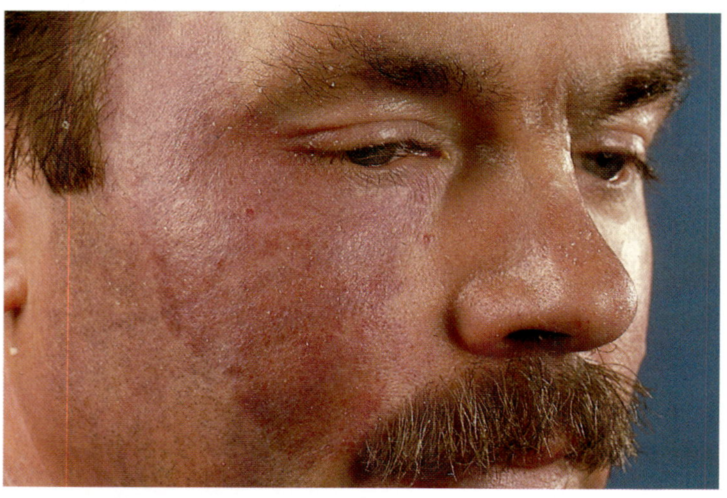

Figure 370 Lateral nevus flammeus in the distribution of the second trigeminus branch on the right.

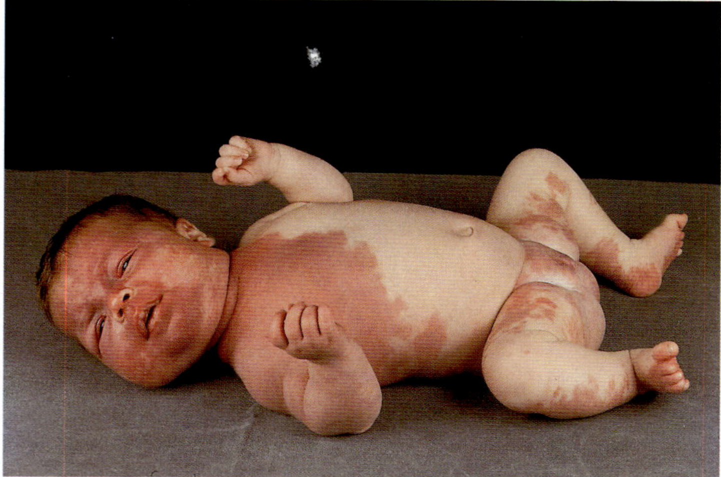

Figure 371 Extensive nevus flammeus.

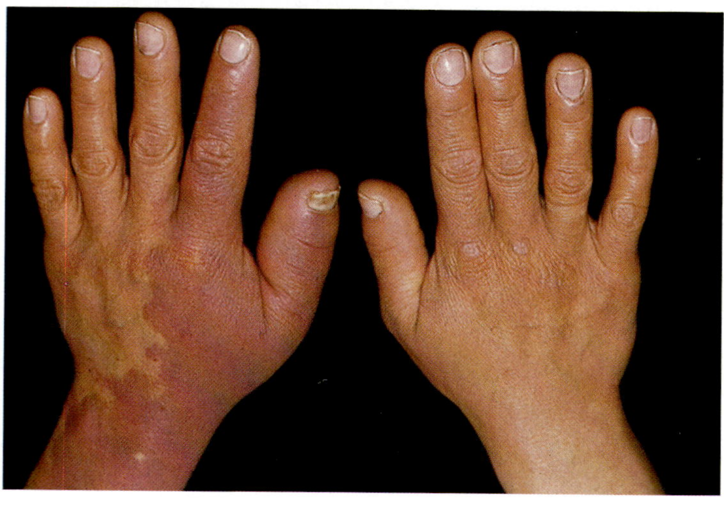

Figure 372 Nevus flammeus. Hypertrophy of thumb and index finger are clearly visible.

a) Median Nevus Flammeus

Discrete median or symmetrical nevi flammei are present at birth in two thirds of all children; the lesions disappear within the first year with a few exceptions (Unna-Pollitzer nevus nuchae, "stork bite").

Clinical Features

1. These are pale-pink lesions in which telangiectasias are often clearly visible.
2. The lesions are always found in a median symmetric location, especially on the neck, the middle of the forehead, the glabellar region and the eyelids.

Therapy

Treatment is not necessary. The lesion either disappears or regresses significantly during the first year of life.

b) Lateral Nevus Flammeus

This is the more striking form of nevus flammeus. It is present at birth and persists during the patient's entire life.

Clinical Features

1. The laterally located purple or dep red lesions can be only a few millimeters in size or cover a large area of skin. The surface is usually smooth.
2. These nevi flammei are usually unilateral. They can be irregular or show a segmental arrangement. They are seen most often on the face and the upper trunk.
3. The oral mucosa can be affected, especially with segmental involvement of the second and third divisions of the trigeminal nerve.
4. In middle-aged or older patients, nevus flammeus can undergo cavernous alteration, so that those segments of the tumor can become quite prominent.
5. Lateral nevi flammei can be associated with other developmental anomalies:
   - Sturge-Weber syndrome (nevus flammeus in one or two segments of the trigeminal nerve, occasionally associated with glaucoma, amaurosis, convulsions, oligophrenia and mental disorders),
   - Klippel-Feil-Trenaunay syndrome (nevus flammeus, usually involving an entire extremity with bone and soft tissue hypertrophy and varicosities),
   - von Hippel-Lindau syndrome (nevus flammeus with cerebral, ocular and many other symptoms).

Therapy

Treatment of these conditions is still disappointing, although the development of the pulsed dye laser has produced significant progress. However, in many cases no treatment is necessary.

1. The pulsed dye laser is quite effective cosmetically. Principle: The pigment of the blood absorbs the energy of the dye laser, leading to selective obliteration of the enlarged blood vessels. This treatment can be performed in babies, children and adults. The late cosmetic results are best when treatment is performed as early as possible. Duration of treatment can be several weeks to several months, depending on the extent of the nevus flammeus. The laser treatment causes local pallor with edema, then the skin becomes hemorrhagic, but the surface does not develop erosions. Complete removal of the nevus flammeus is not always possible; however, it usually becomes significantly lighter in color. The tissue hypertrophy that is occasionally associated with this condition remains unchanged. In Europe, this laser treatment is performed in departments of dermatology, by practicing dermatologists, in so-called laser centers, by pediatric surgeons and by plastic surgeons, and is usually covered by insurance.
2. As an alternative treatment, camouflage of the lesion with a water-insoluble make-up in the color of the surrounding skin can be tried. The make-up adheres to the skin for several days.
3. Attempts to obliterate the enlarged blood vessels with diathermy or injection of sclerosing solutions have produced disappointing results.

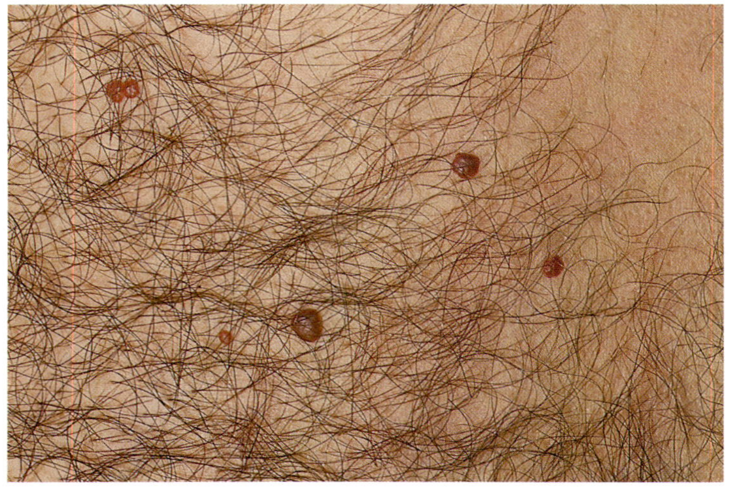
Figure 373 Senile angiomas (cherry angiomas). Medium to dark red, approximately lentil-sized tumors. Normal finding of senile skin.

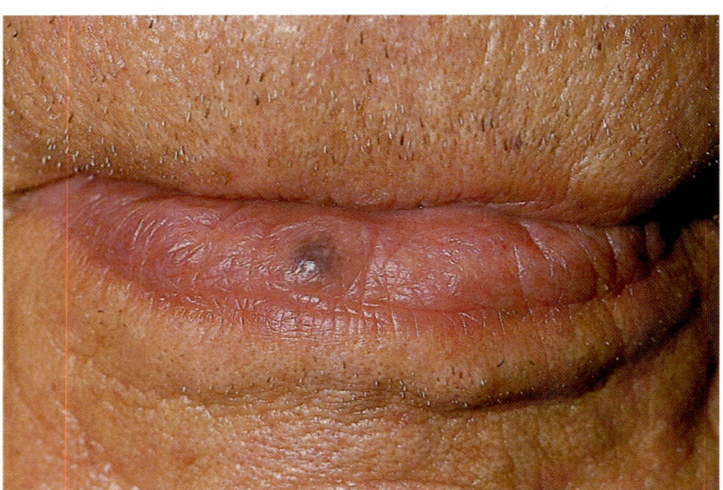
Figure 374 Venous angioma of the lip (venous lake).

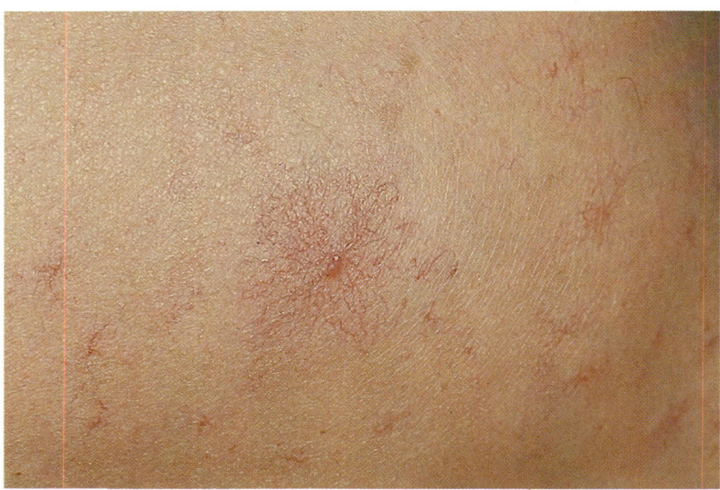
Figure 375 Spider nevi. Central, occasionally pulsating prominence with stellate-shaped dilatation of the efferent blood vessels.

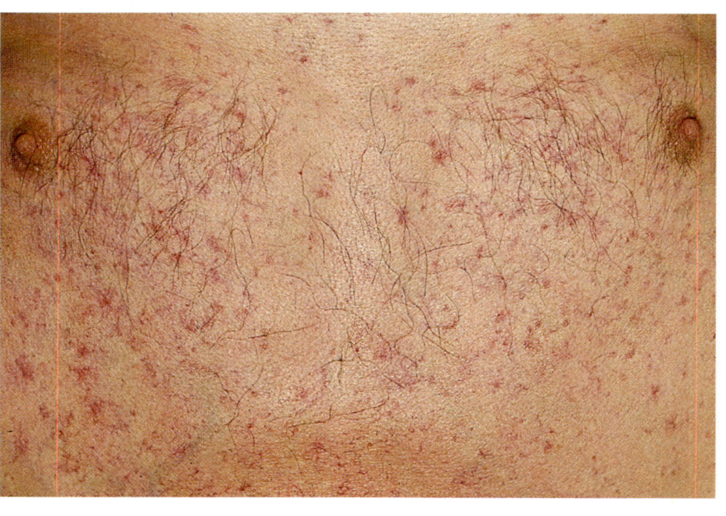
Figure 376 Multiple spider nevi in a patient with cirrhosis of the liver.

C. Senile Angiomas

These are benign tumors consisting of aggregates of ectatic blood vessels. They are normal findings in the skin of the elderly.

Clinical Features

1. Pinhead to pea-sized, light to dark-red tumors that never bleed are characteristic.
2. The lesions are found primarily on the trunk, but also on the extremities and the face.

Therapy

Different types of lasers can be used to remove these lesions. Electrocaustic needling is also effective.

D. Venous Angioma of the Lips (Venous Lake)

This is a blue or blue-red vascular tumor that is found almost exclusively on the lower lip of older persons, more frequently in men than in women. It can be evacuated easily by pressure. The tumor consists of ectatic venous vessels. No treatment is necessary. The lesion can be removed for cosmetic reasons by excision or laser.

E. Spider Nevi (Nevus Araneus, Eppinger Stars)

Spider nevi are found in healthy persons, in patients with chronic liver disease, with estrogen therapy, and during pregnancy.

Clinical Features

1. A pulsating central arteriole (which can be demonstrated by magnifying glass and pressure with a glass spatula) with stellate, efferent blood-filled capillaries is typical for the lesion.
2. Spider nevi are located mainly in the face, the chest, the upper back, and less often on the back of the neck or the dorsum of the hand.
3. Palmar erythema can be an associated symptom, with or without liver disease.
4. In patients with cirrhosis of the liver, spider nevi can occasionally grow to penny size with a very prominent central arteriole. Abrupt arterial bleeding, either spontaneously or from minimal trauma, can rarely occur with these lesions.

Therapy

Spider nevi that develop during pregnancy involute spontaneously. The rest can involute partially, yet most of them persist. Therapy can be indicated for cosmetic reasons.

1. Needling or cautery with a diathermy needle is an elegant and very effective method, but the central arteriole must be obliterated. If unsuccessful, cautery must be repeated after several weeks. Local anesthesia is not always necessary.
2. The lesions can also be removed with different types of lasers.

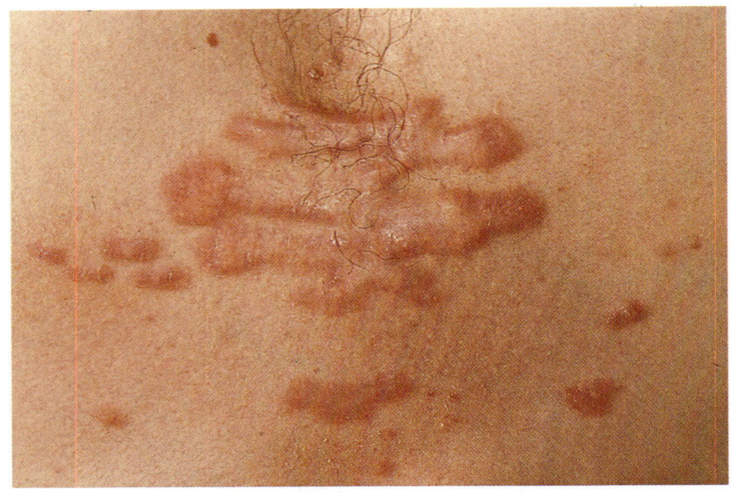

Figure 377 Keloids. So-called spontaneous keloids in the center of the chest as a sequel of acne vulgaris.

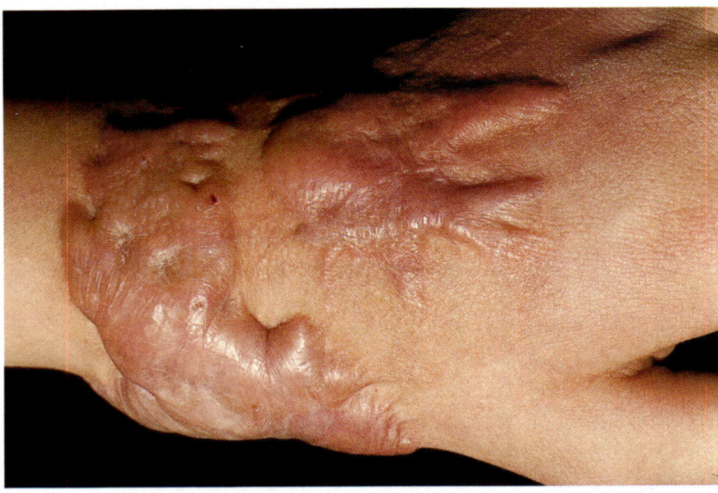

Figure 378 Burn keloids.

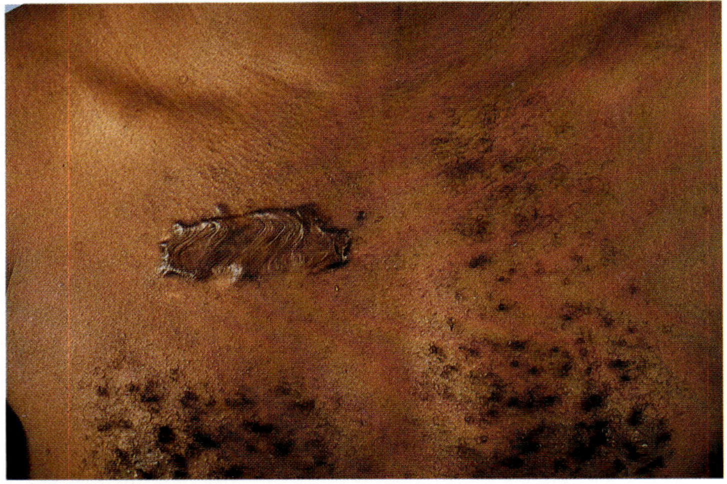

Figure 379 Pigmented keloid in a black patient. Racial disposition. Partial involution after treatment with a pressure pad.

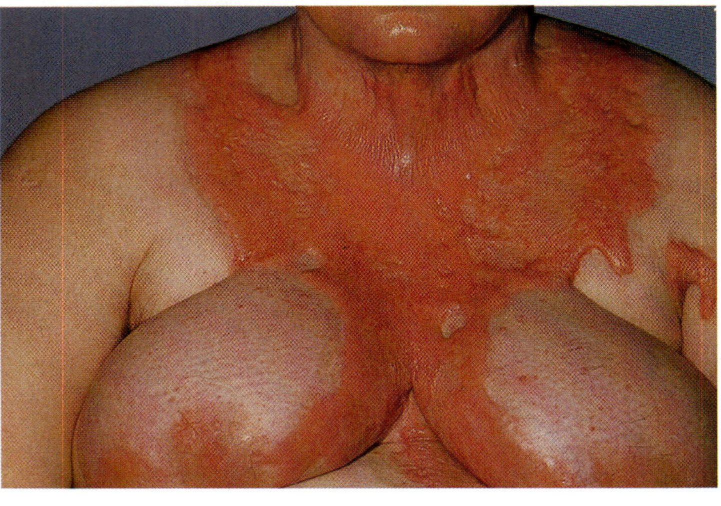

Figure 380 Extensive keloid formation in burn scars. There is also distinct scar contracture in the neck area.

Keloids

Keloids are circumscribed, benign proliferations of connective tissue. They usually occur after injuries, especially after thermal and chemical burns. Spontaneous keloids can develop without preceding trauma. There appears to be a genetic disposition for keloid formation. Keloids are known to have a familial tendency, and they occur more frequently in blacks and in Asians. Certain skin diseases, especially acne, also represent a predisposition for keloids. Hypertrophic scars must be distinguished from keloids, even though they have a similar appearance clinically and histologically. These scars develop without special predisposition after injuries or in surgical scars that do not lie in the cleavage lines of the skin.

Clinical Features

1. Keloids are sharply delineated, firm fibrous tissue excrescences of reddish color that can develop at the site of a preceding injury or spontaneously. Telangiectatic, enlarged blood vessels are visible occasionally. The overlying skin is often atrophic and thin without follicle openings or hairs.
2. Keloids are found most often on the upper body, in particular on the face, the neck, and the upper part of the trunk, here especially in the presternal region.
3. The lesions are tender, hyperesthetic or pruritic.

Therapy

There is no known effective systemic treatment for keloids.

1. Regression of fresh keloids can be achieved with topical corticosteroid treatment under an occlusive foil **(R. 38c),** or, even better, with intralesional injections of a corticosteroid crystal suspension **(R. 46),** in addition to repeated sessions of cryotherapy with liquid nitrogen.
2. Circumscribed, firm keloid strands can be softened by frequent massages with bland ointments.
3. If the location allows it, a pressure pad worn like a truss can cause some regression of the keloid.
4. Surgical procedures should be used only in selected cases; a new keloid often forms after excision of the lesion. However, one can try to suppress this renewed keloid formation by immediate injection of a corticosteroid crystal suspension (or with radiation therapy).

Hypertrophic scars represent a different situation. Excision of the hypertrophic scar, followed by revision of the incision (Z-plasty, continuous W-plasty, etc.) often produces a satisfactory cosmetic result.

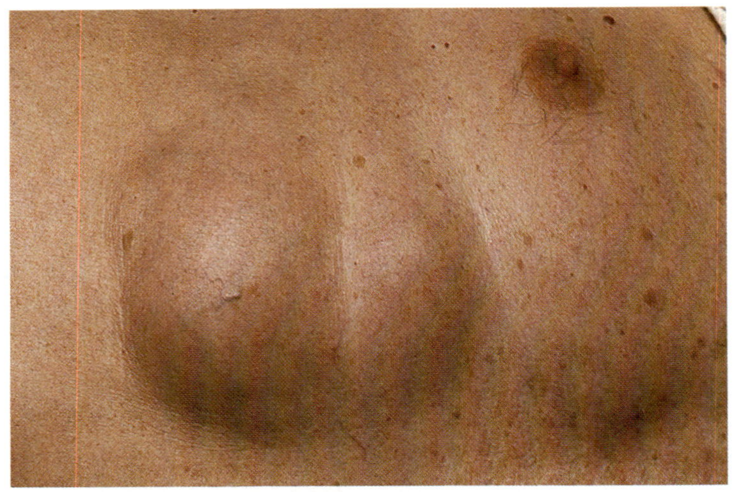

Figure 381 Lipoma. Soft, subcutaneous tumor, here with septum formation.

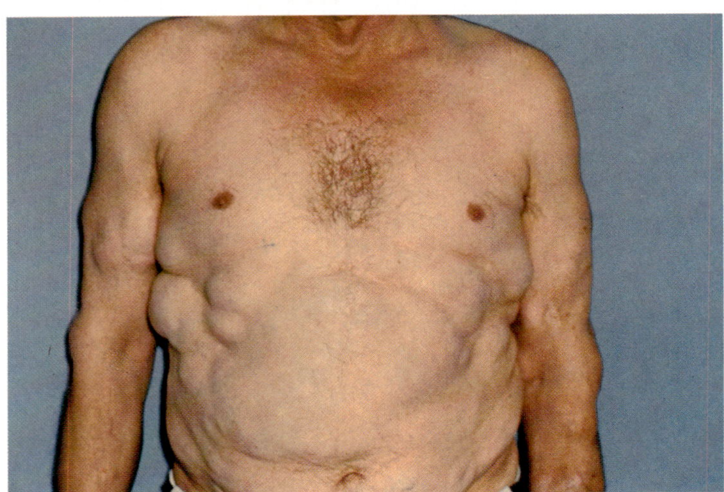

Figure 382 Benign symmetric lipomatosis. Multiple lipomas with largely symmetric arrangement.

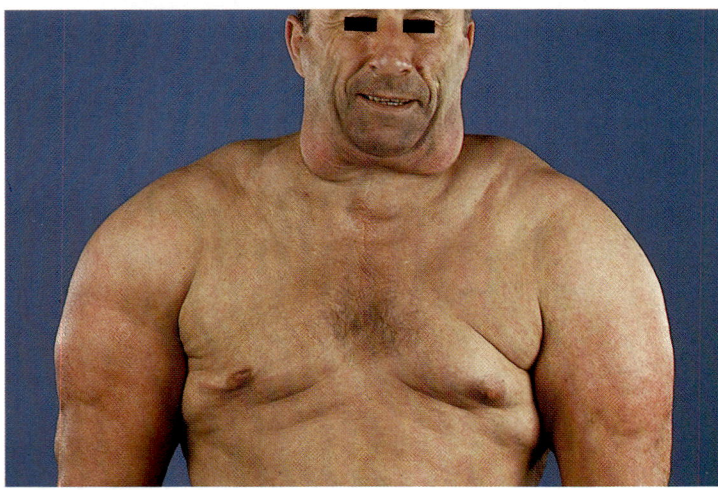

Figure 383 Benign symmetric lipomatosis with a so-called Madelung's fat neck. Multiple extensive symmetric lipomas simulate an athletic habitus.

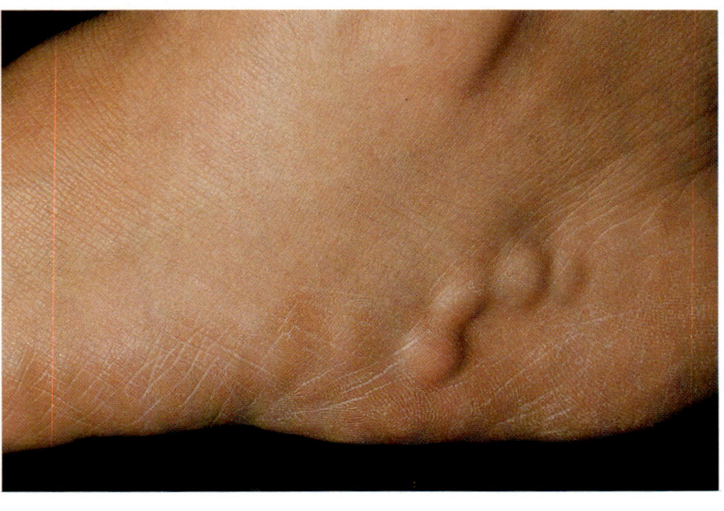

Figure 384 Painful piezogenic pedal papules (PPPP). Small, occasionally painful, fat hernias on the heel.

Lipomas, Lipomatosis

Lipomas can occur as solitary or multiple lipomas, without other symptoms or as part of other diseases, especially benign symmetric lipomatosis, occasionally in Gardner's syndrome, and in neurofibromatosis (von Recklinghausen's disease).

A. Solitary or Multiple Lipomas

Lipomas are benign tumors of fatty tissue that can occur as solitary or multiple lesions (multiple in 7% of all lipoma patients). Multiple lipomas can appear as a few or as numerous lesions in an irregular, asymmetric distribution. They can be diffuse or limited to certain regions without showing a defined syndrome to which a particular lipomatosis can be classified. These multiple lipomas or solitary lipomas have no sexual preference. The cause of the disorder is not known.

Clinical Features

1. This is a slowly developing, soft, smooth, flat tumor.
2. These tumors can be found in any region of the body that contains fatty tissue, including the oral mucosa. However, lipomas are seen most frequently in areas containing much subcutaneous fat, especially the trunk and the extremities. Solitary and multiple lipomas occur in an irregular and disseminated fashion, in contrast to benign symmetric lipomatosis.
3. Any lipoma can be painful during a growth spurt, especially individual or numerous lipomas of a lipomatosis. Solitary lipomas are rarely painful. Angiolipomas, however, often cause pain.

Therapy

No therapy is necessary when the diagnosis is confirmed. Surgical excision may be necessary because of size and/or location (e.g., face).

B. Benign Symmetric Lipomatosis (Madelung's Syndrome)

Multiple lipomas are the leading symptom of benign symmetric lipomatosis, a rare, nonhereditary disease that affects men five times more than women. The disease usually occurs between the thirtieth and sixtieth year of life.

Clinical Features

1. Multiple soft or firm, symmetrically arranged lipomas with a typical distribution are characteristic.
2. Lipomas are located most often in the neck or posterior neck region, creating the typical appearance of Madelung's fat neck or buffalo neck. Other lipomas are frequently found on the head, the upper trunk and the proximal parts of the upper extremities.
3. Lipomas can remain unchanged for many years and then grow rapidly for some time, during which they can be painful, either spontaneously or upon pressure. As part of any lipomatosis, even the benign, symmetrical form, lipomas can develop in the respiratory, the gastrointestinal and the urogenital tracts, but very rarely in other organs.
4. Some of these patients have pathologic changes of the liver from alcohol abuse. Hyperuricemia and rheumatoid joint pains can also exist.

Therapy

Causal therapy can only be directed against an underlying disease. In most cases, no treatment is possible. Impairment of vital functions (e.g., narrowing of the airways) can be an indication for surgical removal.

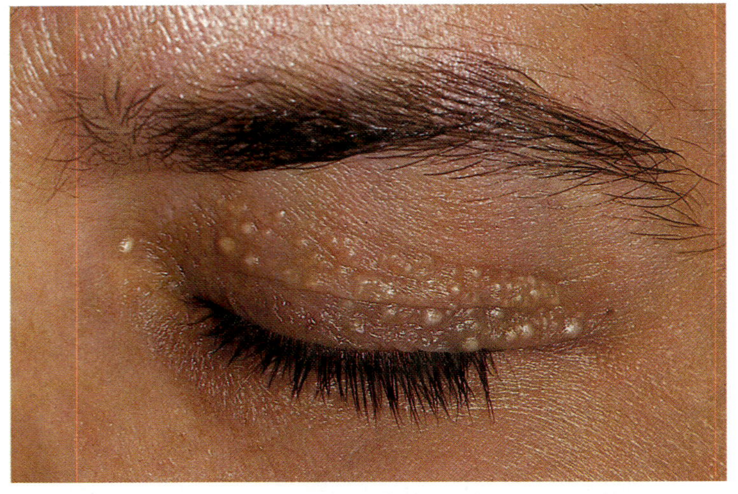

Figure 385 Milia of the upper eyelid. Whitish, non-inflammatory keratin cysts.

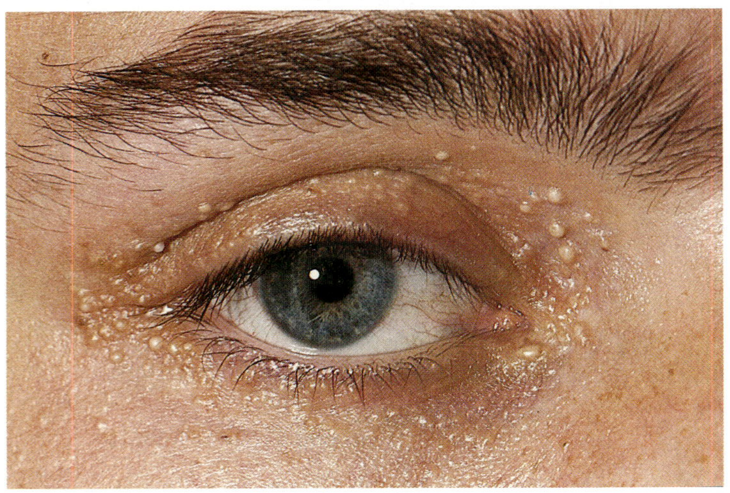

Figure 386 Milia. Extensive involvement around the eye.

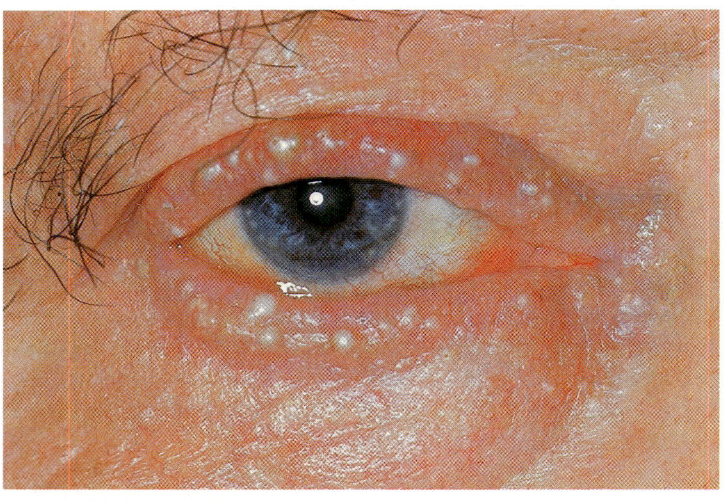

Figure 387 Extensive milia involvement in a patient with mycosis fungoides.

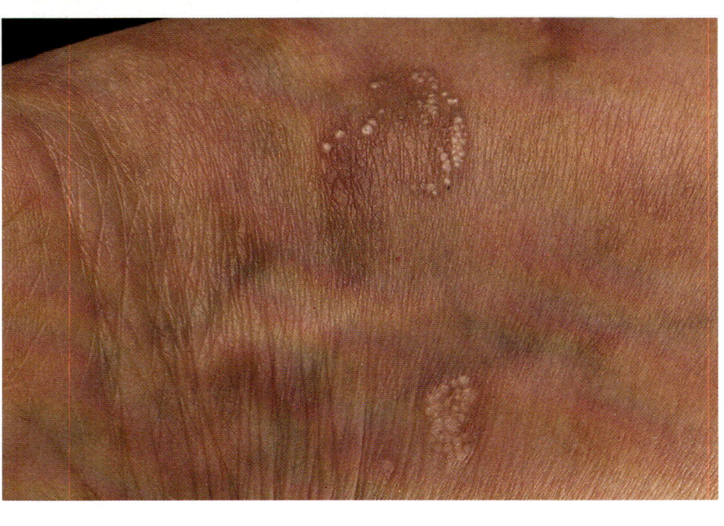

Figure 388 So-called post-inflammatory milia, here as a sequel of bullous pemphigoid.

Milia

Milia are small, subepidermal keratin cysts. They occur from childhood to old age, are common and mainly of cosmetic significance. Occasionally, milia are the result of excessive exposure to sunlight. Milia can develop rapidly and in large numbers, in an eruptive manner, especially in young women. They can also be the result of subepidermal blister formation, e.g., after burns, in porphyria cutanea tarda, bullous pemphigoid or epidermolysis bullosa. Occasionally, milia are found in patients with mycosis fungoides, cortisone-induced atrophy of the skin and after radiation therapy.

Clinical Features

1. White or yellow flat tumors, 1 to 2 mm in size, are characteristic.
2. They are usually located in the face, especially around the eyes, on the eyelids and on the cheeks.

Therapy

Incision of the epidermis over the milium with a lancet, needle or scalpel and subsequent expression of the cyst is a simple and effective treatment.

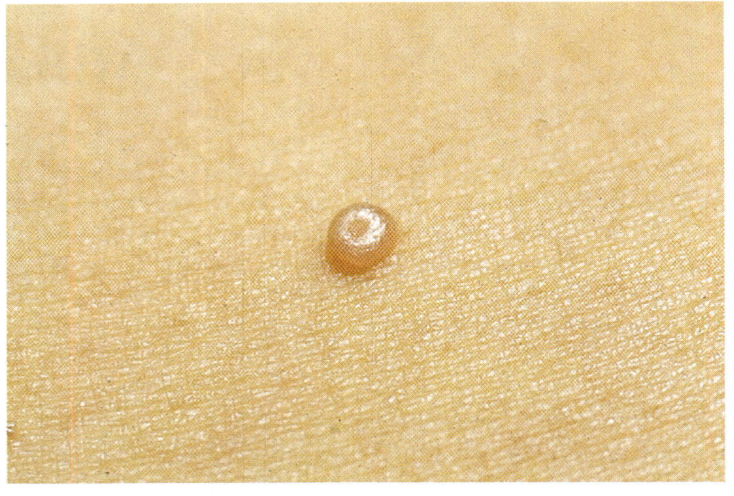

Figure 389 Molluscum contagiosum. Glassy, pitted nodule.

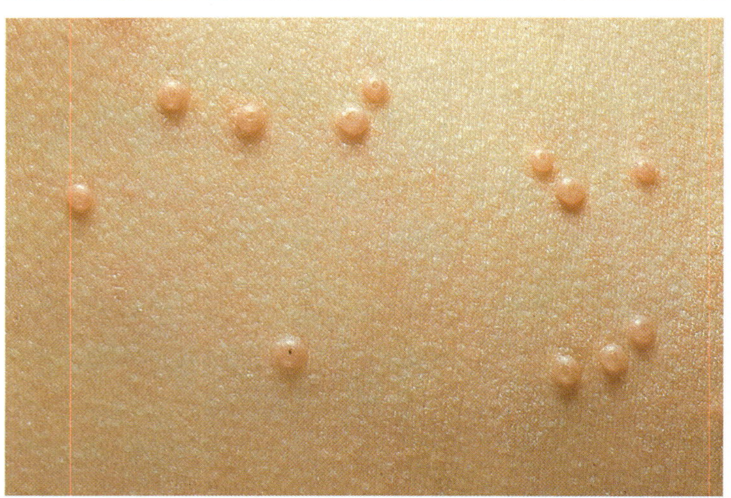

Figure 390 Mollusca contagiosa. Dissemination of glassy, in some cases pitted, nodules without inflammatory reaction.

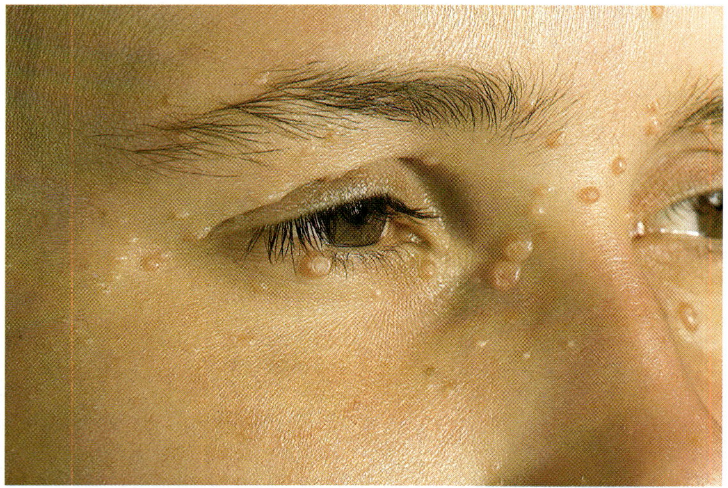

Figure 391 Mollusca contagiosa. Dense involvement with mostly pitted, round tumors of varying sizes.

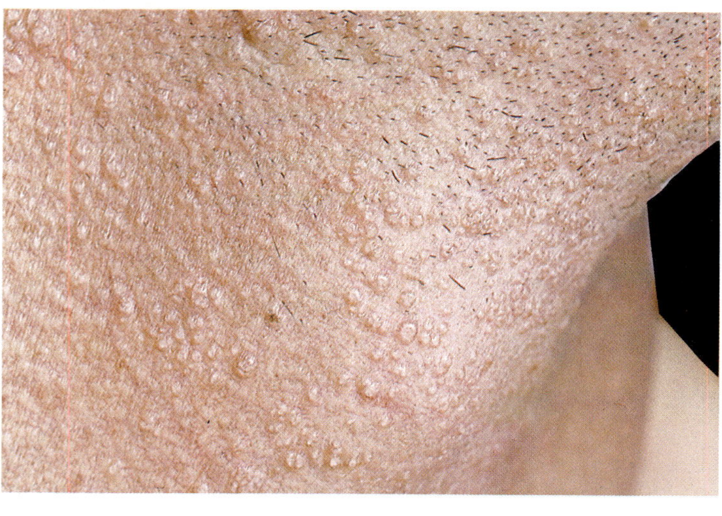

Figure 392 Mollusca contagiosa. Exanthematous dissemination on skin that had been treated with cortisone.

Molluscum Contagiosum

Mollusca contagiosa are seen most frequently in children, but are not uncommon in adults. They are a form of warts caused by a virus and are spread by infection. In contrast to other infectious warts, they are not caused by papilloma virus, but are caused by a pox virus.
Children with atopic dermatitis and patients with immunodeficiency from corticosteroid or cytostatic therapy and patients with AIDS are especially susceptible. In most cases, however, the patients are otherwise completely healthy. Mollusca conagiosa can be expected to heal spontaneously approximately 6 months to 3 years after the eruptions begin.
The infection is transmitted by direct contact; in adults, it can be transmitted by sexual intercourse. Incubation is 2–3 weeks. The disease often spreads by autoinoculation.

Clinical Features

1. Skin-colored or pearly white, waxy, dome-shaped or umbilicated tumors, 2 to 10 mm in size, appear in large numbers or at least as multiple lesions. The pitted tumors are distributed on the skin asymmetrically, often in groups or disseminated. They do not show increased keratinization like common warts.
2. Areas of predilection are the neck, the trunk, and especially the axillary and genital regions, but all locations are possible, including the lips, tongue and oral mucosa.
3. Inflammatory erythema, pustules and crusts can develop spontaneously or after scratching, especially where solitary or only a few mollusca contagiosa are present. This can make diagnosis difficult, especially for solitary lesions. Otherwise they are easy to diagnose (typical appearance, multiple lesions).

Therapy

The disease is harmless and usually heals spontaneously. Only those treatment methods that do not result in scars should be employed.

1. When only a few mollusca are present, they can be removed with a curette under local anesthesia or freezing with ethyl chloride. In children, this can be done more gently with a topical anesthetic (lidocaine cream, effective for approximately 30 minutes).
2. Incision of the epidermis overlying the molluscum and expression of the whitish contents is another successful treatment method.
3. For widespread involvement, treatment with vitamin A acid can be tried, for sensitive skin as a cream **(R. 44b),** in all other cases as a gel **(R. 25b)** or as a solution.
4. Only in cases where these methods are unsuccessful, general anesthesia could be necessary in small children and with widespread involvement in order to remove the lesions.

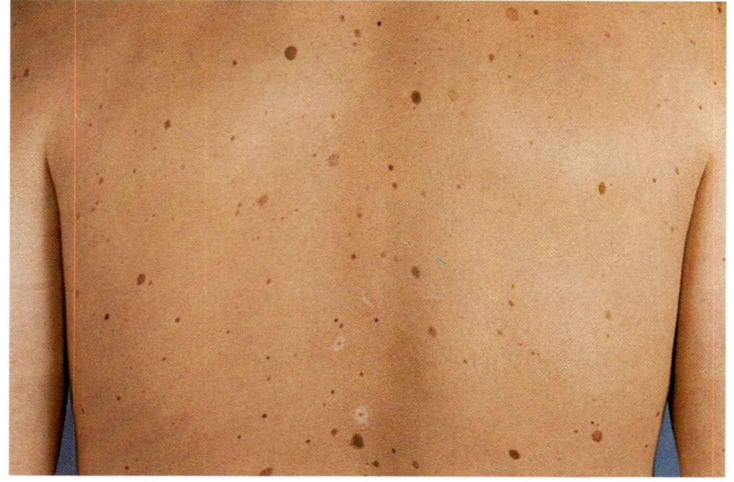

Figure 393 Nevomelanocytic nevi. Normal spectrum of pigmented nevi.

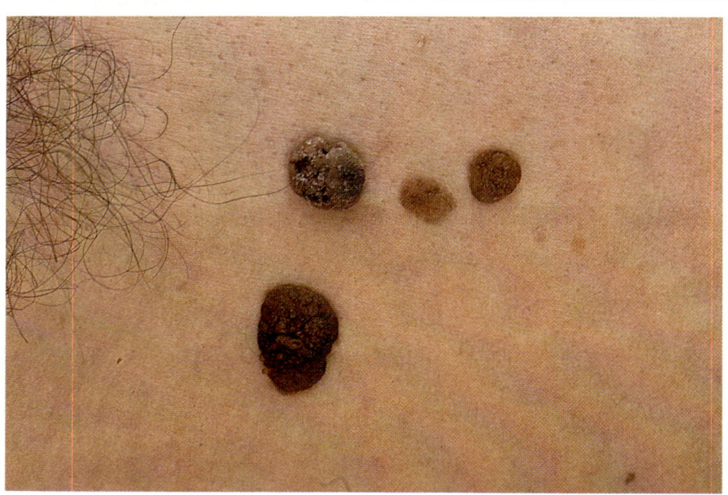

Figure 394 Nevomelanocytic nevi. Mulberry-shaped, exophytically growing pigmented nevi. Normal findings.

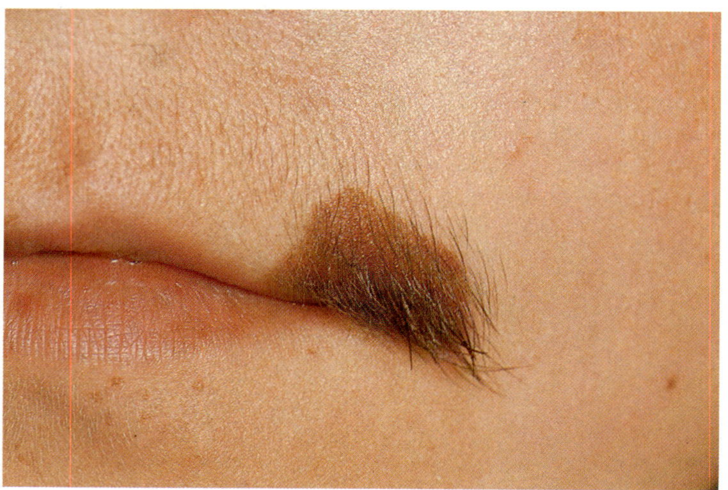

Figure 395 Nevomelanocytic nevus. Nevus pigmentosus et pilosus with increased hair growth. This occurs frequently in large nevomelanocytic nevi.

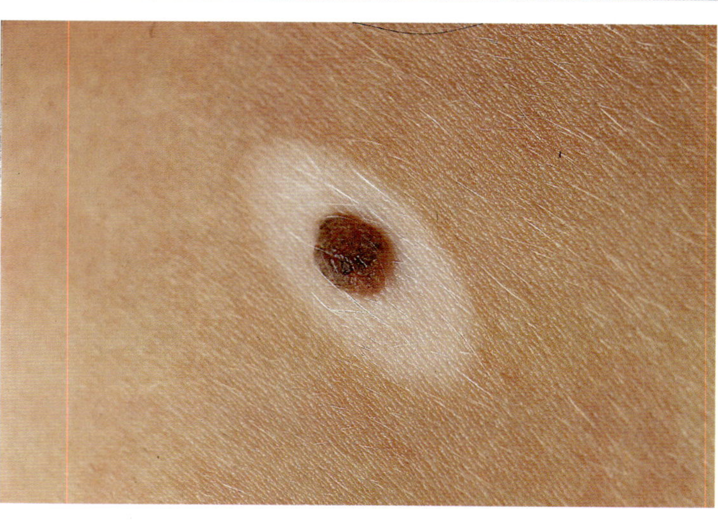

Figure 396 Sutton's nevus. Nevomelanocytic nevus with sharply demarcated, depigmented halo.

Pigmented Nevi

A. Common Acquired Nevomelanocytic Nevus

Nevomelanocytic nevi are benign tumors of normal skin caused by proliferation of nevomelanocytes. They are found in practically all people. At birth, none or only a few individual nevomelanocytic nevi are present; they increase in number in the first years of life and reach a maximum of 30 to 50 nevomelanocytic nevi in the third and fourth decade. After that, their numbers gradually decrease, partly with loss of pigment and formation of fibrous tissue. A few isolated nevomelanocytic nevi can appear in old age. Nevomelanocytic nevi must be distinguished from malignant melanomas. Visibly rapid growth, change in color or weeping, bleeding and pruritus should make one suspect malignancy. Early stages of malignant melanoma (see below) are difficult to distinguish from nevomelanocytic nevus. A dermatologist with experience in dermatologic oncology should be consulted in these cases.

Clinical Features

1. Nevomelanocytic nevi develop very slowly. Almost all stages of development can be seen, from light to dark-brown, from flat, round tumors of 1 to 2 mm in size to soft, more prominent tumors in all shades of brown. Nevomelanocytic nevi are often hairy, with thick brown hair.
2. The lesions are usually distributed over the entire skin in an irregular fashion.
3. Nevomelanocytic nevi do not occur on the oral mucosa. Nevi on the red of the lips are almost always nevus spilus and not nevomelanocytic nevi.

Therapy

Nevomelanocytic nevi usually do not require removal. Exceptions are: a) Nevi with a history of rapid growth, or nevomelanocytic nevi with suspicious clinical morphology. These should be excised to confirm the diagnosis. b) Congenital nevomelanocytic nevi (see below). Offensive nevomelanocytic nevi can occasionally be removed for cosmetic reasons. Incomplete removal usually results in a recurrence, but this case is no different from trauma to a nevomelanocytic nevus, i.e., there is no subsequent risk of developing a malignant melanoma.

B. Sutton's Nevus, Halo Nevomelanocytic Nevus

This is a special form of nevomelanocytic nevus characterized by a depigmented halo surrounding a pigmented or non-pigmented nevomelanocytic nevus. Later, the central nevomelanocytic nevus can disappear, and only the round leukodermic area remains. Eventually, this too can disappear through repigmentation.

C. Congenital Nevomelanocytic Nevus

Congenital nevomelanocytic nevi are present at birth. They grow with the child and do not regress. Nevomelanocytic nevi, usually the hairy type, can grow to a significant size (giant nevus, animal skin nevus, bathing trunk nevus). Degeneration of a congenital nevomelanocytic nevus into melanoma is definitely possible, but there is controversy regarding the frequency of this occurrence. Congenital nevomelanocytic nevi of diameters exceeding 1.5 cm are at a greater risk of transforming into malignant melanoma after the 18th year of life. The histologic appearance of a congenital nevomelanocytic nevus can be remarkably similar to that of a malignant melanoma.

Clinical Features

1. The tumor is usually dark brown, but sometimes lighter colored and soft. Its surface is large and can be smooth or irregular in texture and in some cases creased or even papillomatous. The tumors are often covered by thick black-brown hairs that often form a vortex.
2. The size of the tumors varies significantly from penny size to tumors that cover large areas of the body or an entire extremity.
3. All areas of the body can be affected.

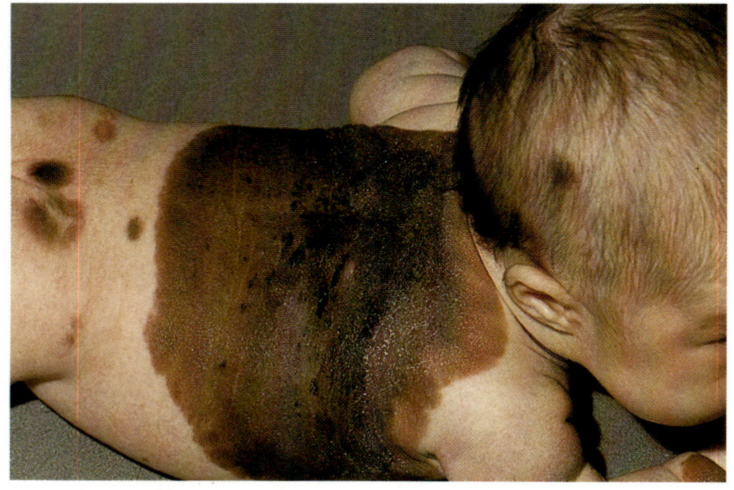

Figure 397 Congenital nevomelanocytic nevus. Multiple, extensive nevomelanocytic nevi with varying pigmentation.

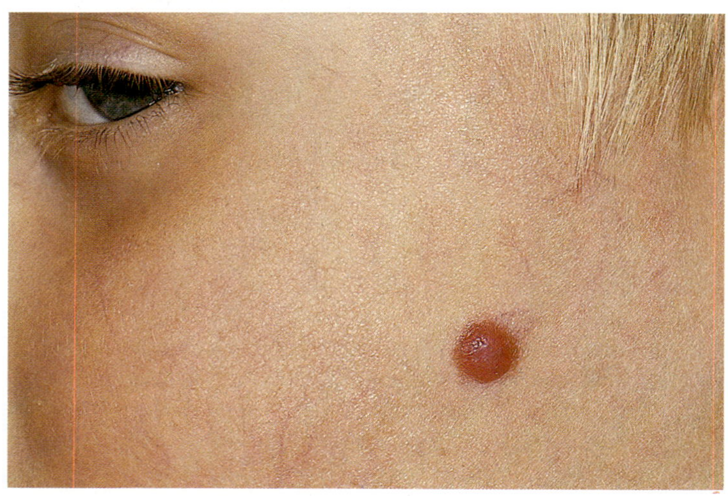

Figure 398 Spindle cell nevomelanocytic nevus (Spitz nevus). Reddened, hemispheric tumor with smooth surface.

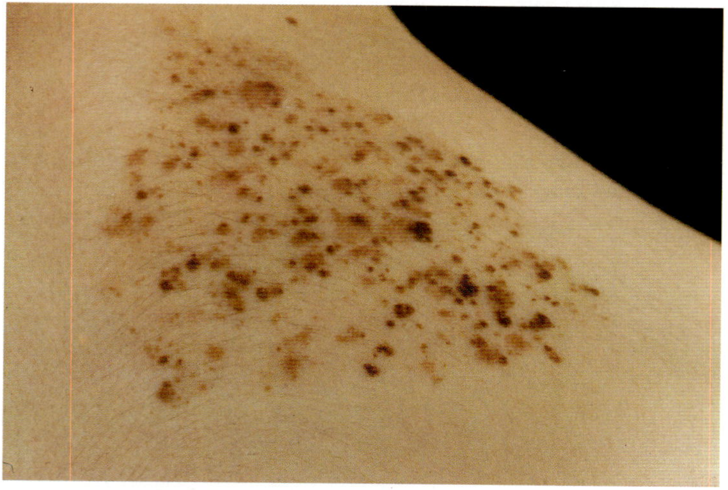

Figure 399 Nevus spilus. Extensive, sharply demarcated light-brown discoloration with enclosed nevomelanocytic nevi.

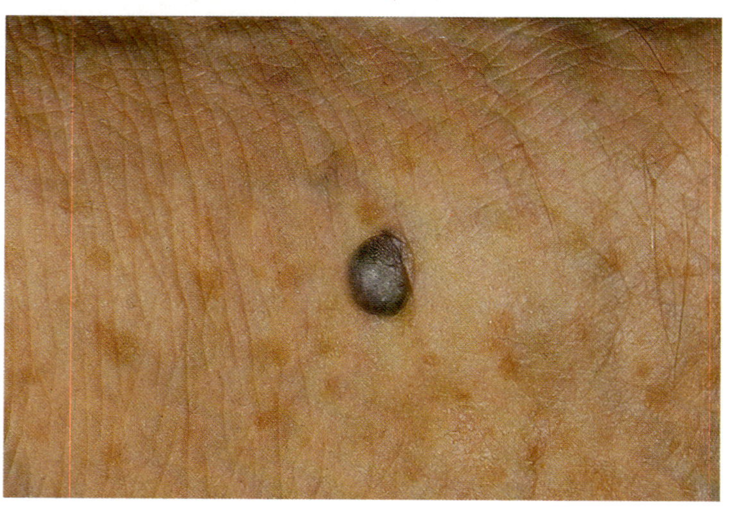

Figure 400 Blue nevus. Firm, blue-black tumor.

Therapy

1. Opinions vary whether all congenital nevomelanocytic nevi should be excised, even the small ones. In any case, large congenital nevomelanocytic nevi are at risk of transforming into a melanoma and should be excised as soon as the patient's growth is completed (if necessary, excision can be performed in several sittings, followed by plastic coverage of the defect). Complete excision of large congenital nevomelanocytic nevi may not always be possible. In such cases, one may have to be satisfied with regular control examinations and excision of suspicious areas.
2. Dermabrasion should only be considered during the first few weeks of life. The patient must be hospitalized and the procedure performed under general anesthesia. It may not be possible to remove deeper parts of the tumor, so that the risk of malignant transformation to melanoma persists. Recurrences are frequent and the cosmetic result cannot be predicted, which is the case with all tissue-destructive procedures.

D. Spindle Cell Nevomelanocytic Nevus, Spitz Nevus

This tumor is always benign and often lacks pigment (originally erroneously called juvenile melanoma). It occurs mainly in children and only rarely in adults. It represents a special form of nevomelanocytic nevus, and its histologic appearance can be bizarre enough to resemble a malignant melanoma.

Clinical Features

This round, hemispheric or cone-shaped tumor usually develops in early childhood. It is well vascularized, which gives it a red, reddish-brown, or, rarely, a brown color. Its maximal size is 1 to 2 cm in diameter. The surface is sometimes fragile and crusty; minimal trauma can cause bleeding. The face is the most frequent location, especially the cheeks, followed by the legs and other areas of the skin.

Therapy

Surgical excision of the entire tumor is the treatment of choice. Conservative excision is sufficient.

E. Nevus Spilus

Clinical Features

Nevus spilus is a sharply delineated, light-brown pigmentation that may or may not be speckled with lentigines or nevomelanocytic nevi. It occurs frequently as a harmless solitary lesion. Multiple nevi spili are found as café au lait macules in neurofibromatosis von Recklinghausen.

Therapy

Removal of nevi spili is usually not necessary. They can be removed with a ruby laser.

F. Blue Nevus

These are very slowly growing, blue or blue-black tumors consisting of pigmented melanocytes. They are located deep in the dermis, which causes their blue color. Blue nevi can be present at birth or develop later in life.

Clinical Features

The tumors are usually flat, occasionally elevated in a nodular fashion and with a smooth surface. They are dark-blue, sometimes with a grey or whitish center, and rarely more than 1 cm in diameter. Blue nevi are found mainly on the extremities, the back of the hands, the feet, the buttocks and the face.

Therapy

Surgical removal is not necessary as long as one is sure of the diagnosis. Excisional biopsy should include the subcutaneous tissue, because blue nevi often extend into the subcutis.

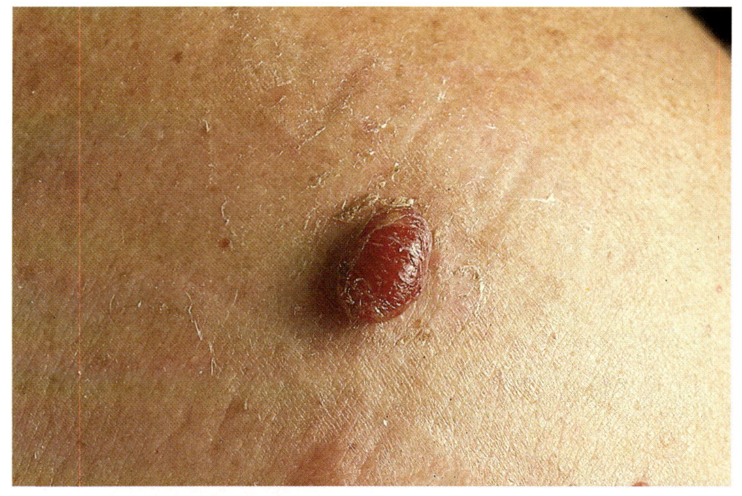

Figure 401 Pyogenic granuloma. Intensively reddened, soft tumor with surrounding raised and scaling margin. The surface is very friable.

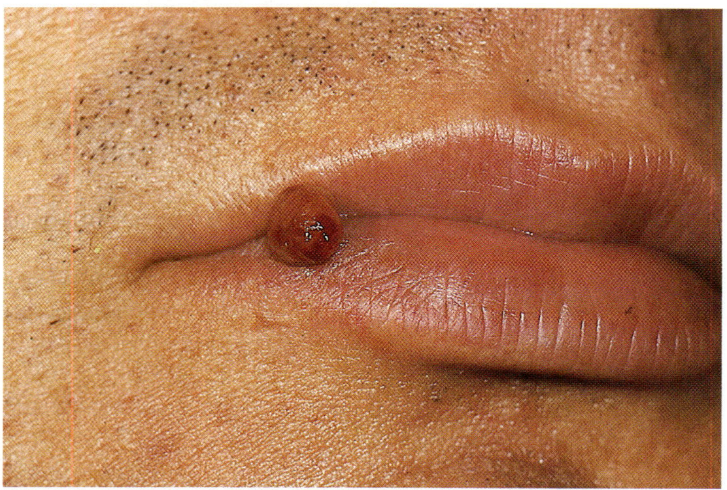

Figure 402 Pyogenic granuloma. Slightly hemorrhagic, erosive, pedunculate tumor on the lower lip.

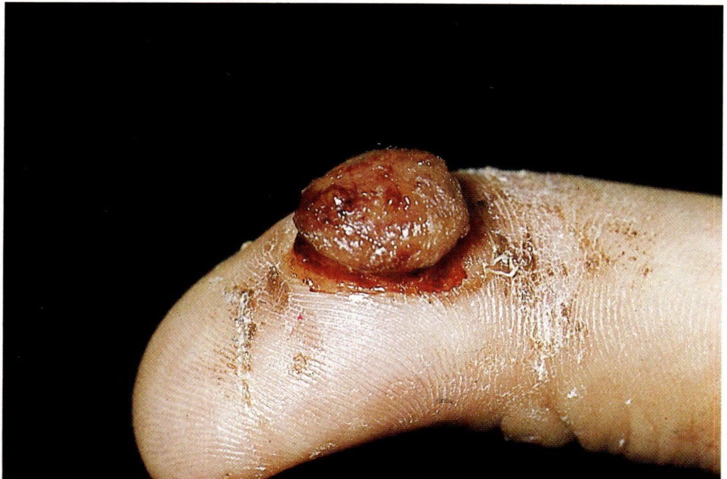

Figure 403 Pyogenic granuloma. Superficially eroded tumor with small base that developed rapidly after an injury.

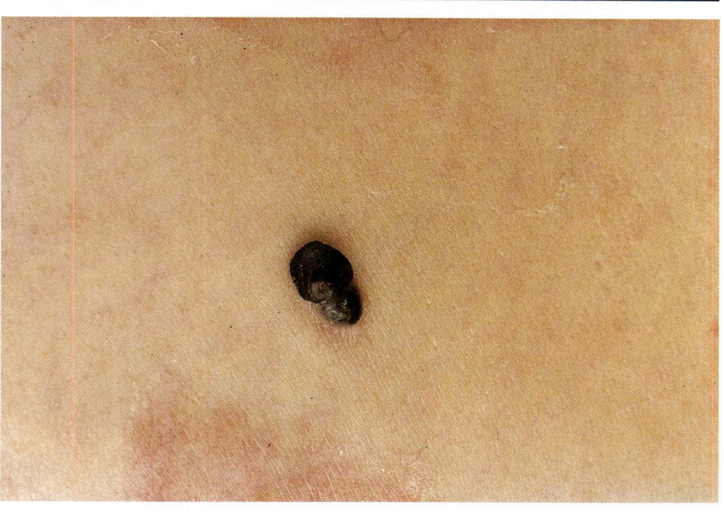

Figure 404 Pyogenic granuloma. Black tumor caused by hemorrhagic infarction. The tumor simulates a malignant melanoma.

Pyogenic Granuloma

These are tumor-like growths of well vascularized granulation tissue that develop a few weeks after minor injuries or folliculitis. They are not infectious, despite their misleading name. Since they grow rapidly, weep and bleed easily, they are often mistaken for malignant lesions, especially malignant melanoma. Pyogenic granulomas (granuloma telangiectaticum, granuloma pediculatum) occasionally show a tendency for more severe bleeding. These inflammatory tumors occur somewhat more frequently in children, in young adults and during pregnancy. Diagnosis is based on the rapid growth and the clinical appearance of a well vascularized, friable tumor. Histologic examination is absolutely necessary, because clinical diagnosis is often false.

Differential diagnoses include seborrheic warts with inflammatory changes, nevomelanocytic nevi, mollusca contagiosa and angiomas, as well as the above-mentioned malignant melanoma.

Clinical Features

1. Pyogenic granulomas are red, occasionally red-brown or blue-black, soft, non-tender tumors that can be sessile with a broad base or pedunculated. They measure 5 to 10 mm in diameter and are surrounded by an epithelial wreath. The surface can be smooth or erosive, occasionally weeping or bleeding, or they can be covered by a yellowish layer of fibrin. Spontaneous involution occurs rarely when the hemorrhagic black tumor dries up.
2. The most frequent locations are the hands, especially the fingers (toes), the lips, the head and the trunk.
3. The oral mucosa, especially the gingiva, can also be involved (epulis telangiectatica, "epulis of pregnancy").

Therapy

1. Complete excision is the treatment of choice; remnants often lead to a recurrence. The excised tissue should always be examined histologically.
2. The tumor can also be removed with a curette or by electrocoagulation.

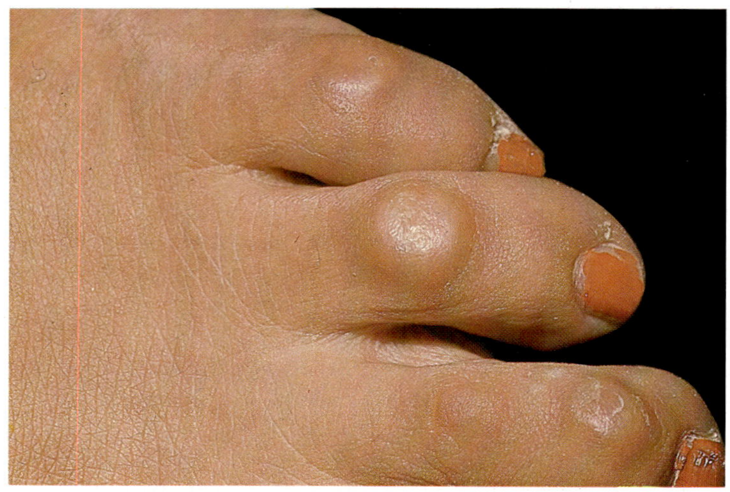

Figure 405 Clavi, corns. Round, painful calluses on the toes.

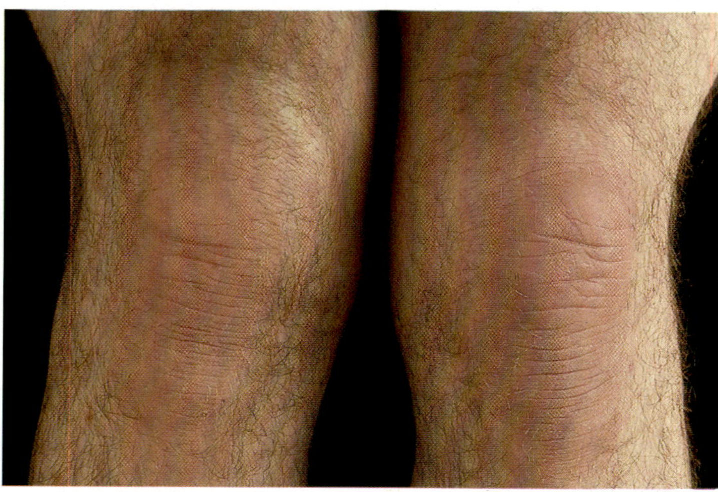

Figure 406 Floor-layer's knee. Chronic inflammation and thickening of the skin from prolonged kneeling.

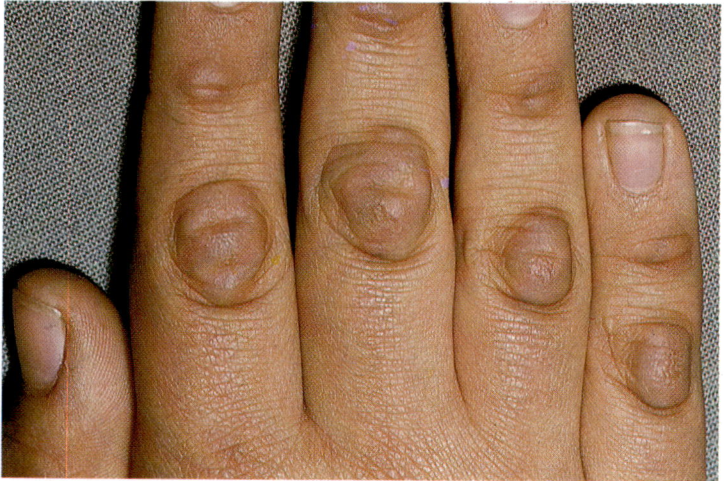

Figure 407 Knuckle pads. Circumscribed, callus-like thickening of the skin over the finger joints.

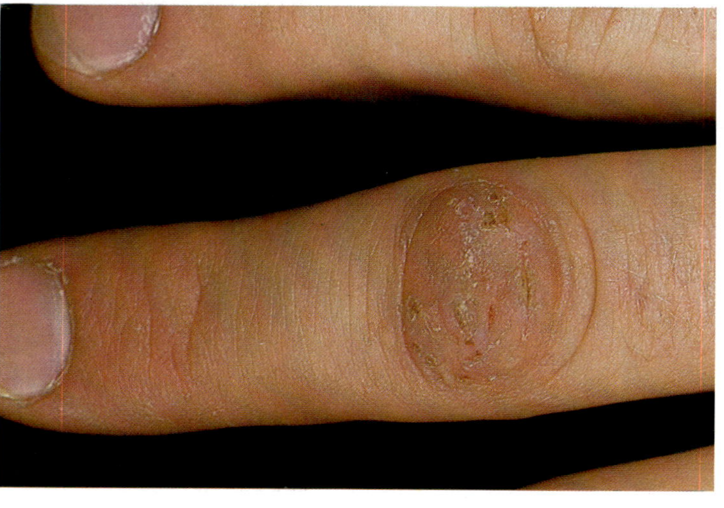

Figure 408 Callus caused by chewing. Circumscribed inflammation and reactive callus formation caused by habitual chewing on the knuckle.

Calluses

These circumscribed hyperkeratoses are reactions of the skin to chronic intermittent mechanical irritation. The tendency to form calluses varies significantly among individuals. Location of the callus is often an indication of a special activity or occupation, but calluses can also be stigmata of bad habits (chewing, sucking). Callus formation is a protective mechanism of the skin and only rarely the symptom of a disease.

Clinical Features

1. Circumscribed hyperkeratosis in the area of the increased pressure is characteristic.
2. Calluses form mainly on the palms of the hands and on the soles of the feet. They may develop in other locations as stigmata of certain occupations (tile layer's knee, trumpeter's lip).
3. Calluses are not tender. They disappear completely after cessation of the pressure.

Several special forms can be differentiated according to the characteristic clinical appearance and the typical causes.

A. Clavi

Clavi (corns) are round hyperkeratoses with central keratinous cores. They develop over bony prominences on the feet from friction or pressure, especially when inappropriate shoes are worn or abnormalities of the foot skeleton are present. Irritation of the underlying dermis causes inflammation and irritation of sensory nerves, resulting in marked tenderness.

B. Lip Calluses

Lip calluses are primarily an increase of the connective tissue and epithelial reactive changes of the lips, caused by frequent and prolonged mechanical pressure. Lip calluses are found in persons who are exposed to increased mechanical pressure from their occupational activity such as trumpeters (trumpeter's lip) and other players of wind instruments like clarinetists and oboists. They can also be found in glass blowers. This increase of connective tissue results in a decrease in the intensity of the red of the lips. The lips become paler and the border between the red of the lips and the skin becomes less distinct. The lips become more firm, which can produce difficulties for musicians playing wind instruments. Initially, the condition produces an opaqueness in the epithelium of the involved part of the lips. Later, a distinct leukoplakial, white, but otherwise reactionless lip callus can develop.

C. Lip Callus of the Nursing Infant

The lip callus of the nursing infant is usually visible in the middle of the upper lip. It is a protrusion of the red of the lip in the region of the philtrum. Keratotic changes can be present. The lip callus is symmetrical, sharply delineated and slightly raised. This is a harmless normal finding which involutes spontaneously after a few months.

D. Fiddler's Neck

A "fiddler's neck" is seen frequently in violinists and viola players. It is located where the greatest pressure is applied to the chin by the chin rest. The callus is found on the left side of the neck caudally and slightly medial to the angle of the mandible. The symptoms vary initially. Often, only hyperpigmentation (light brown to medium brown) develops in the beginning. Later, the skin can thicken. In other cases, a soft thickening of the skin develops. The tissue in that area becomes firmer with time and assumes an edema-like, nodular appearance with or without erythema. Pigmentation of the region develops later. In extreme cases, prominent, soft, large fibromatous lesions develop. Complications can be folliculitis, especially in juveniles and young adults in the "acne age", and scars can develop. In most cases, the condition is caused by the placement of the violin between the jaw, the neck and the shoulder. The technique of holding the violin with too much pressure, as well as anatomic variations in these areas probably play a major role. Other causes can be friction and sweating. In rare cases, a poorly fitting chin rest can be the cause of the "fiddler's neck". Treatment depends on the severity of the symptoms,

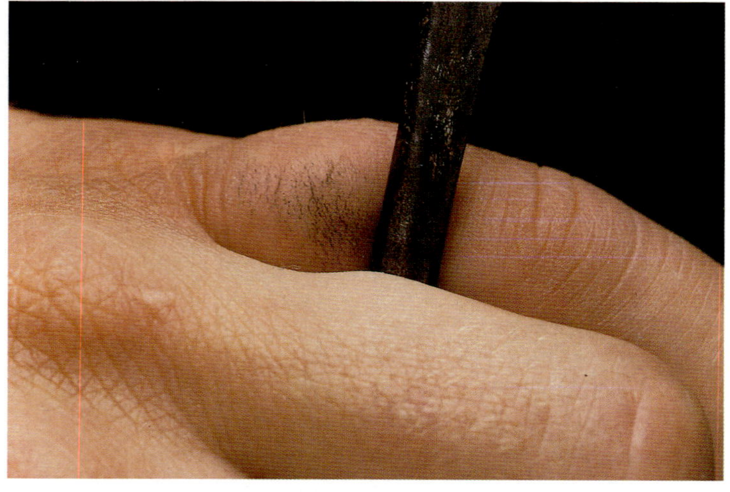

Figure 409 Typical occupational callus of a stone mason.

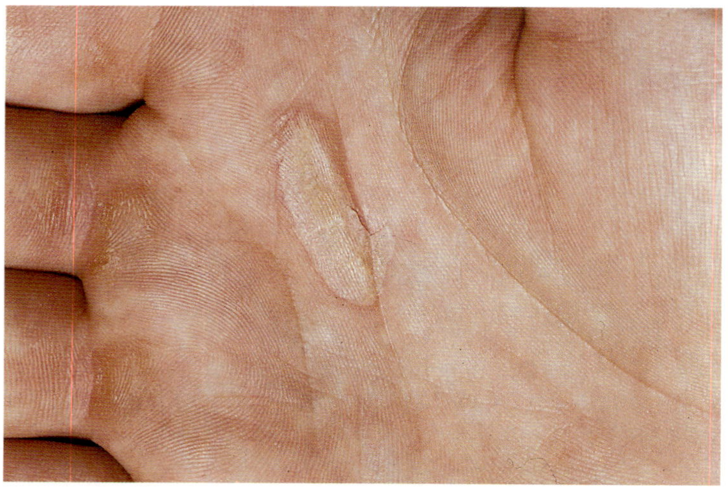

Figure 410 Callus caused by a tennis racket.

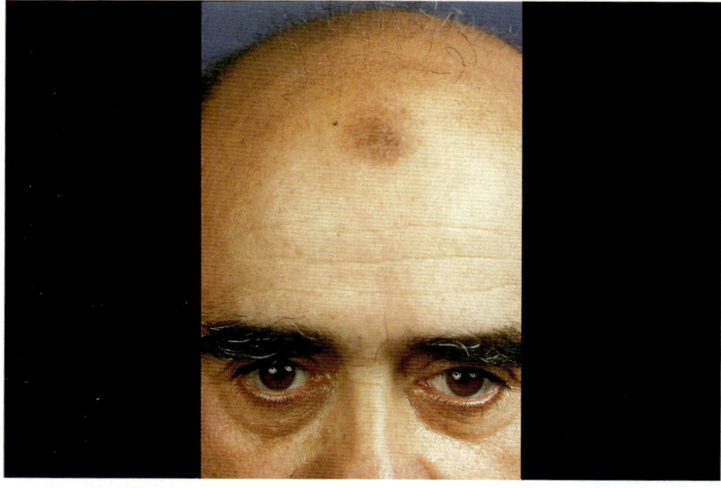

Figure 411 Pigmented pressure callus in a Muslim, caused by frequent praying.

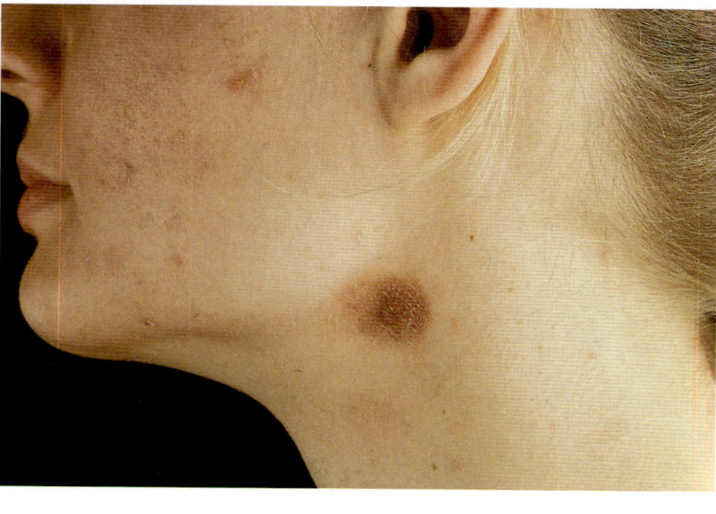

Figure 412 "Fiddler's neck". Pigmented callus caused by the chin rest.

which are minor in most cases. Frequently, this is only a cosmetic problem. When more severe inflammatory changes are present, relief of pressure on the involved area (e.g., change of the chin rest or the shoulder support) and local therapy such as that recommended for acne may be indicated. Occasionally, a period of rest from playing the instrument may be necessary. The use of a cloth over the chin rest may be helpful.

E. Occupational Callus

Physical labor exposes the palms of the hands to significant mechanical pressure. Calluses on the hands were seen in many occupations in the past and were often typical for many jobs. Occupational calluses develop as a result of pressure and also following prolonged friction. Today, occupational calluses are seen less frequently as a result of increasing automation of hard manual labor, with help from machines, better protection against mechanical pressure through the use of work gloves and also from shorter work hours. Occupational calluses on typical locations are so-called "occupational stigmata" that are caused by the individual's occupation. These include the calluses on ring and little finger of stone masons, calluses on the lips of musicians, calluses on the finger tips of violinists and harpists, calluses on the knees of tile layers and cleaning personnel (rarer today) and calluses on the fingers of clothes cutters caused by large scissors.

F. Plantar Callus

Plantar calluses are seen frequently following increased mechanical pressure on the soles of the feet, e.g., through inappropriate shoes, or as heel calluses from wooden sandals. Plantar calluses are seen most frequently as circumscribed keratoses of the forefoot. Orthopedic shoes and orthopedic consultation are often necessary, since all therapeutic measures must take the total biomechanics of the foot into consideration.

G. Prayer Callus

Prayer calluses are found in the middle of the forehead in Moslems as a result of repeatedly touching the ground with the forehead during prayer. They can also occur as knee calluses from long-lasting and frequent praying in a kneeling position.

H. Masticatory Welt

Chewing and biting of the fingers and the resulting masticatory welts are often seen in children and young adults who are under emotional stress. Masticatory welts are most often found over the carpometacarpal joint of the thumb and the middle joint of the index finger.

Therapy

Ordinarily calluses do not require treatment. Within normal limits, they are a desirable protective reaction of the skin against increased mechanical pressure. Calluses that are the result of "bad habits" usually disappear when the activities are eliminated.

Therapy of calluses consists of softening the hyperkeratotic tissue with adhesive bandages containing salicylic acid or a corresponding solution (salicylic acid solution, lactic acid solution). The hyperkeratotic tissue can then be removed easily after a hot foot bath. After removal, the most important task is the prevention of a recurrent callus. The patient must be advised to wear proper, comfortably fitting shoes and to relieve pressure on the areas exposed to mechanical pressure by felt donuts or rings. Patients with foot deformities should be referred to an orthopedist for evaluation and correction of these deformities. Procedures with scalpel or curette should be avoided in patients with diabetes or occlusive artery disease. Even minimal trauma can cause gangrene or malum perforans in these patients.

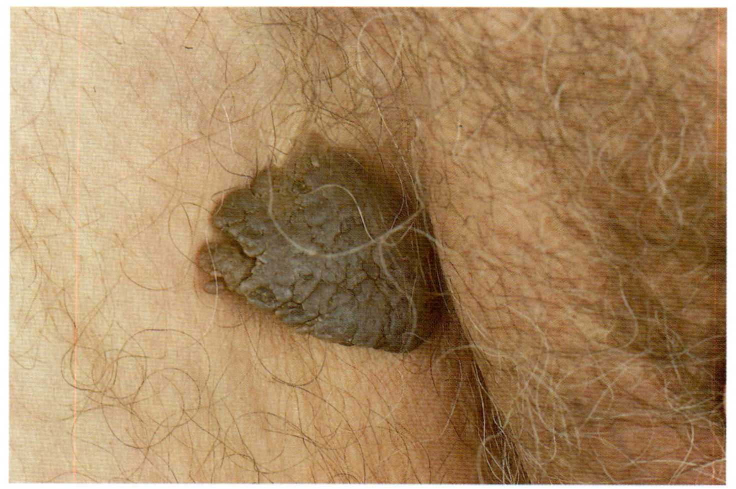

Figure 413 Seborrheic keratosis. Pigmented tumor with fissured surface.

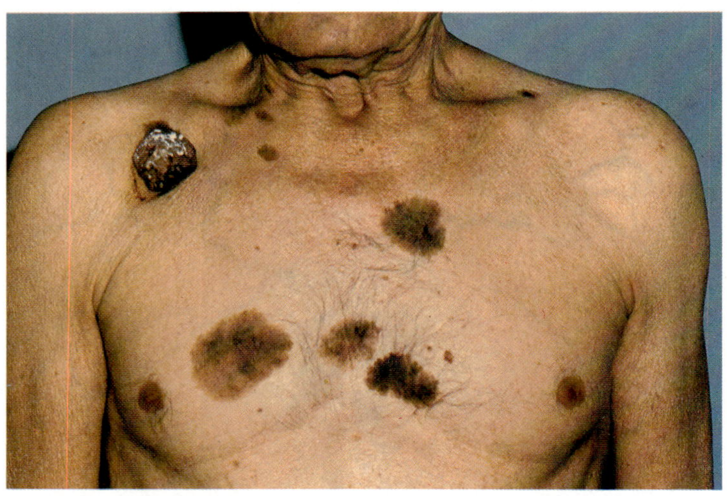

Figure 414 Seborrheic keratoses. Several unusually large tumors with varying pigmentation.

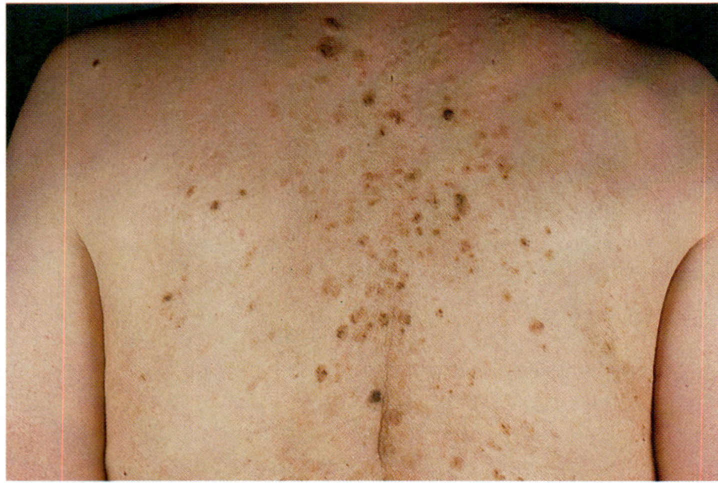

Figure 415 Multiple seborrheic keratoses on the patient's back.

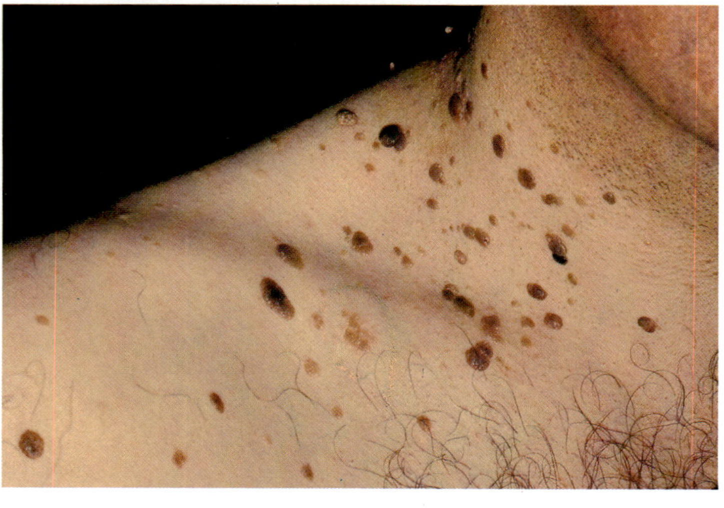

Figure 416 Multiple small seborrheic keratoses on the lateral aspect of the neck.

Seborrheic Keratoses

Seborrheic keratoses or senile warts are seen very frequently. The patients are not greatly affected by them and often accept them as inevitable stigmata of aging. Men and women are affected equally. There is often a familial tendency. Typical seborrheic keratoses are rarely found before the fifth decade of life. Since pigmented spots are biopsied and examined histologically more often today, the early stages of seborrheic keratoses are frequently diagnosed in the third or fourth decade. In most cases, seborrheic keratoses are harmless symptoms of aging. Rarely, the sudden appearance of multiple seborrheic keratoses may be associated with a malignant tumor. Malignant degeneration of seborrheic keratoses has not been reported.

Clinical Features

1. Seborrheic keratoses are sharply demarcated, initially flat, lentil- to coin-size areas with brown pigmentation. With time, they develop into papillomatous, hemispherically raised tumors with dark brown to black pigmentation. They are soft with a crumbly and seborrheic surface. On close examination, one can distinguish horny cores in the follicle openings.

2. Seborrheic keratoses can occur in any area with sebaceous glands, most frequently on the trunk and in the face. They are never seen on the soles or the palms.
Large, flat, "granulated" seborrheic keratoses are seen mainly in the face and on the scalp.

3. Irritation can cause crust formation on the surface and inflammation at the base, which may make differentiation from a squamous cell carcinoma or a malignant melanoma difficult.

Therapy

Seborrheic keratoses are harmless, and their removal is not necessary as long as one is sure of the diagnosis. They should be removed if a malignant tumor such as basal cell carcinoma or malignant melanoma cannot be excluded. Other indications for removal are frequent or severe irritation or for cosmetic reasons. Other than by excision, other methods of removal are with a diathermy sling or a curette, or with CO_2 laser. These are tissue-destructive procedures and should be used only when the diagnosis is confirmed.

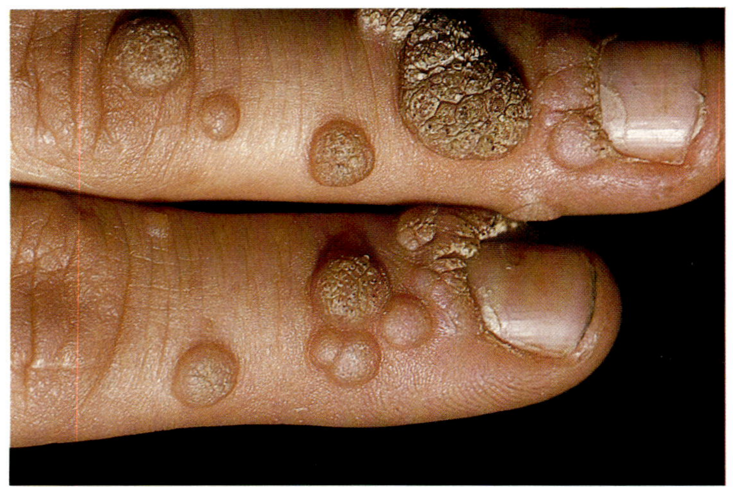

Figure 417 Common warts. Tumors of varying keratinization, especially on the groove of the nail.

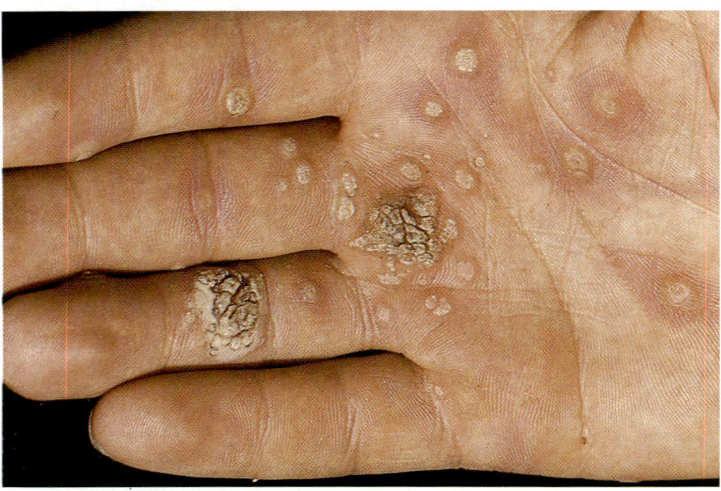

Figure 418 Multiple common warts on the palm of the hand.

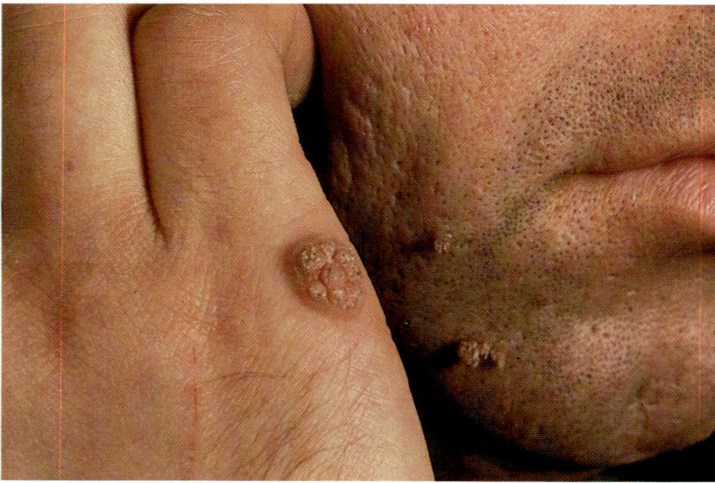

Figure 419 Filiform warts in the face, transmitted through contact with the hand.

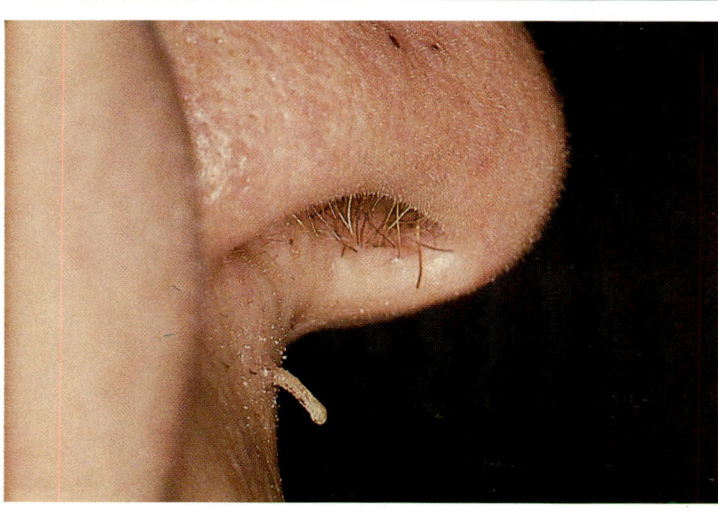

Figure 420 Filiform wart below the nose.

Infectious Warts

Infectious warts are papules induced on skin and mucous membranes by human papillomavirus. They can be classified according to clinical, histologic, and virologic criteria. For practical purposes, the clinical classification is most useful. It distinguishes between common warts (verrucae vulgares), plantar warts (verrucae plantares), flat warts (verrucae planae juveniles), verruciform epidermodysplasia and condylomata acuminata. The time of incubation is several weeks to months. The clinical manifestations after contact with the infectious organism are determined by the patient's disposition. These predisposing factors include cool, moist acra and impairment of the immune system (malignant tumors, congenital or aquired immune defects, immunosuppressive therapy). In immunosuppressed patients, multiple common warts often occur in a dissemintated fashion.

A. Common Warts (Verrucae vulgares)

Clinical Features

1. Common warts are firm nodules with keratinous, rough surfaces. They range in size from pinhead to pea size and can coalesce to form extensive beds of warts.
2. They are mainly located on the dorsum of hands and fingers but can occur on any part of the body. Common warts occur mainly in children.
3. Common warts usually dissapear spontaneously in children generally after 6 to 12 months, in adults after 12 to 24 months. They do not leave scars. Pressure from warts near the nailbed can cause permanent deformities of nail growth.

Therapy

Aggressive therapeutic measures should be avoided, since common warts heal without scars after a relatively limited period of time. A more intensive treatment may be indicated for widespread involvement of hands and to prevent further dissemination of the warts. Therapeutic measures in use today are based on physical or chemical destruction of the warts.

1. Adhesive bandages containing salicylic acid or other film-forming solutions are used to soften the hyperkeratotic material.
2. Two or three days later, the hyperkeratotic tissue is removed with a curette after a hot bath. The procedure may have to be repeated several times.
3. Freezing with liquid nitrogen is an alternative. The wart can be removed together with the blister caused by the freezing. This method is very effective, but it is not very economical to keep a supply of liquid nitrogen in the physician's office. Cryotherapy is effective in 50% of the patients but may be painful when used for treatment of periungual and plantar warts, thus requiring local anesthesia.
4. Removal of the wart with a CO_2 laser is effective; the evaporated material is potentially infectious and must be removed by suction.
5. For chemical treatment, 5-fluorouracil in dimethyl sulfoxide is available in Germany. This drug must be applied to the affected areas regularly up to three times daily for several weeks. As long as the treated areas are small, there will be no systemic effects. Caustic treatment has a similar effect.
6. Contrast baths stimulate circulation.
7. Excision of warts with the scalpel cannot be recommended. It results in scar formation and is plagued by recurrences.
8. Radiation therapy of common warts is obsolete.
9. Scratching, biting and chewing promotes spread of common warts (autoinoculation) and should be avoided.

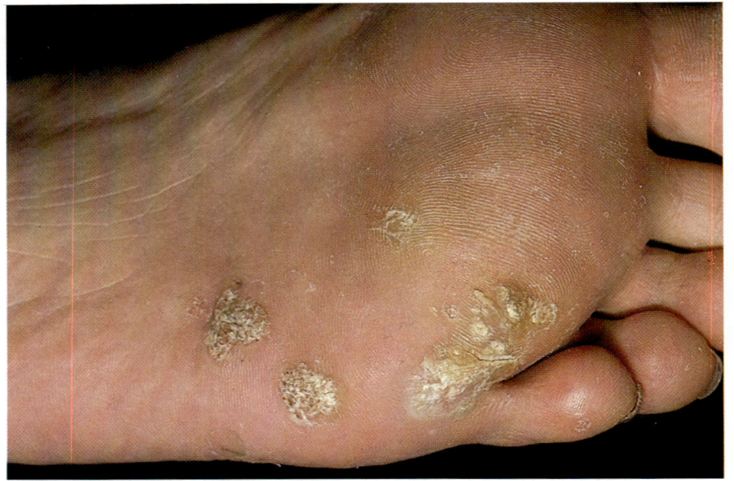

Figure 421 Plantar warts. Aggregated, very painful, keratotic tumors, which are not very exophytic due to the constant pressure.

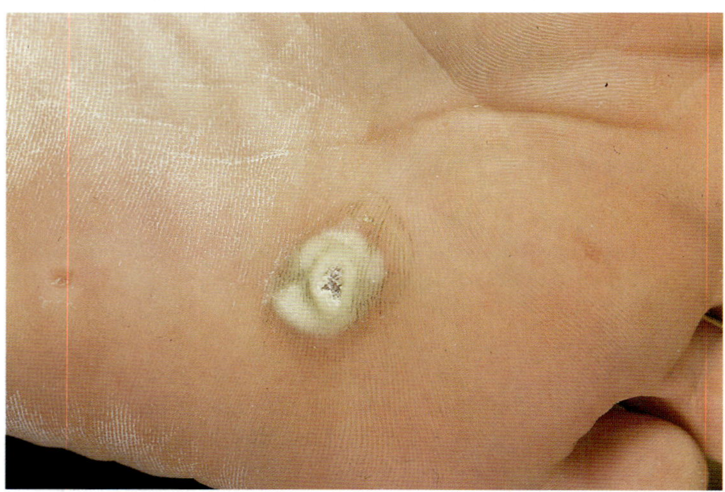

Figure 422 Plantar warts. White discoloration caused by corn pad.

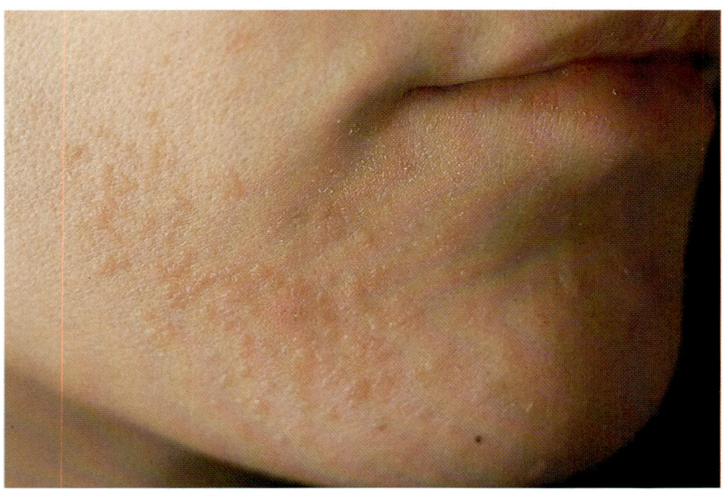

Figure 423 Flat warts. Slightly raised, skin-colored to slightly brownish, usually multiple tumors that are frequently located on the face, as in this case.

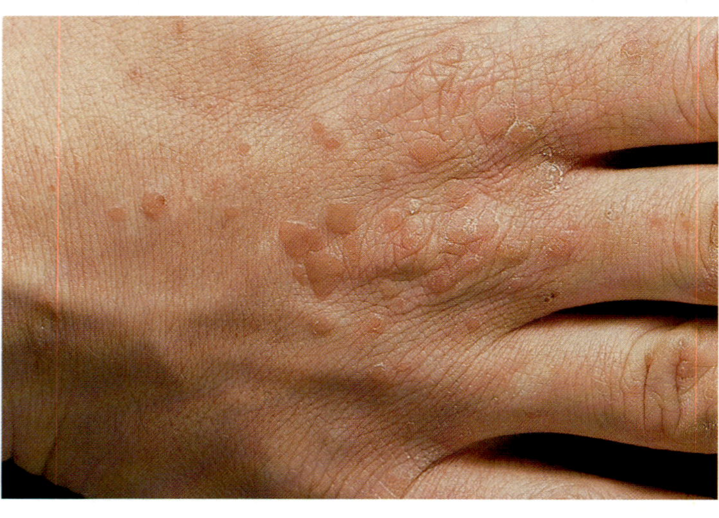

Figure 424 Flat warts. Multiple, slightly raised, skin colored to slightly reddened tumors.

B. Plantar Warts

Clinical Features

Warts on the soles of the feet have a distinctive appearance caused by the constant mechanical pressure. Multiple flat warts may be arranged in patches and are called mosaic warts. Circumscribed solitary warts with cone-shaped extensions in the deep tissue are called thorny warts. The constant pressure on the soles forces the keratinous material into the deeper tissues. The cone-shaped extension is usually covered by a callus. These lesions are very painful.

Therapy

1. Topical therapy is the same as that described above for common warts.
2. Pressure on the lesion should be relieved by wearing felt rings and shoe inserts that allow the wart to grow outward. This also brings significant pain relief.
3. For persistent plantar warts that continue to recur at the same site, orthopedic consultation to exclude a possible skeletal deformation of the foot may be indicated.
4. Patients who are prone to develop plantar warts should avoid going barefoot in places where plantar warts are easily acquired, such as swimming pools and washrooms.
5. There should never be any radiation therapy of the soles (or palms) (see page 137).

C. Flat Warts

Clinical Features

1. Soft, flat or slightly raised, skin-colored to light yellow nodules are characteristic. They are often visible only with a magnifying glass in oblique light.
2. Areas of predilection are the face (they may be spread by shaving) and the dorsum of the hand.
3. These warts frequently develop primarily as multiple lesions. They can persist for a long time and respond poorly to therapeutic measures. They generally disappear spontaneously after 6–24 months.

Therapy

1. In men, warts in appropriate locations can be hidden by a beard until they heal spontaneously.
2. Lesions that are not too extensive can be treated with topical applications of preparations containing lactic acid plus salicylic acid (DuoFilm, Tiflex) or fluorouracil (Efudex, Fluoroplex).
3. The skin can be peeled with a vitamin A preparation, for sensitive skin as a cream **(R. 44b)**, or as a gel **(R. 25b)**. Therapy may have to be interrupted temporarily if the skin becomes too irritated.

D. Condylomata Acuminata

These are a clinical variety of virus-induced warts that occur only in the anogenital area. They are sexually transmitted and have an incubation period of up to 8 months. Condylomata acuminata can disappear spontaneously within months or several years. Whenever condylomata acuminata are present, the diagnostic work-up should always include other venereal diseases (gonorrhea, syphilis, trichomoniasis and chlamydial infections). Localization of condylomata acuminata in the anal region can be an indication of special sexual practices with increased risk of HIV infection. Condylomata acuminata in children may point to sexual abuse.

Clinical Features

1. The initial lesion is a pinhead-sized, pink to whitish nodule. As the disease progresses, the typical morphology develops with beds of warts and cauliflower-like masses that can eventually involve the entire anogenital region through autoinoculation.
2. In women, condylomata acuminata are found mostly on the labia majora et minora but can be spread into the vagina and cervix uteri. In men, the main locations are the sulcus coronarius and the mucous membrane of the foreskin. Involvement of the urethra is also possible. Condylomata acuminata of the perianal region may involve the mucous membrane of the anus, and a recurrence often originates from these lesions.
3. The accumulation of secretions in the intertriginous spaces leads to maceration and necrotic decomposition of the surface with the formation of malodorous material.

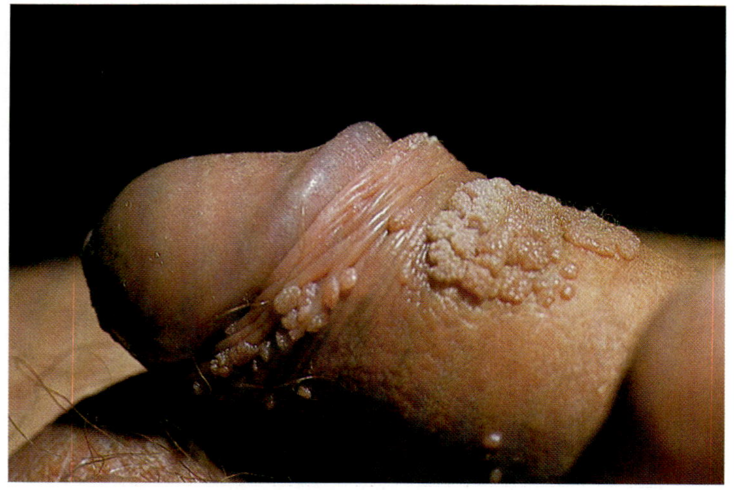

Figure 425 Condylomata acuminata. Soft, skin-colored to slightly whitish virus papillomata in a grape-like aggregation.

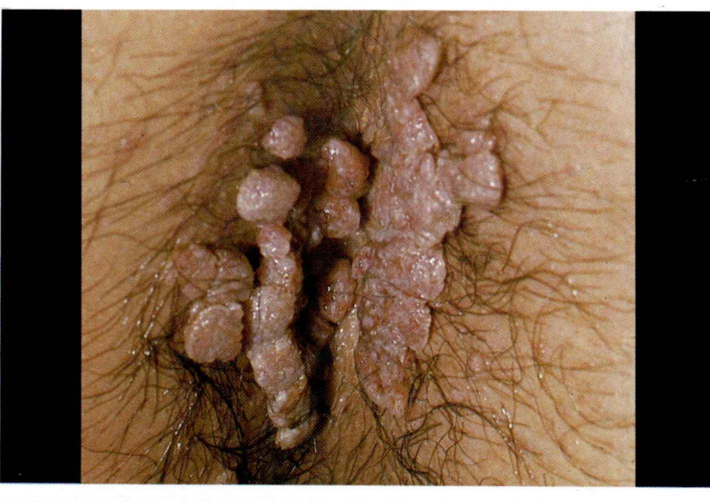

Figure 426 Condylomata acuminata. Weeping condyloma aggregation in the perianal area.

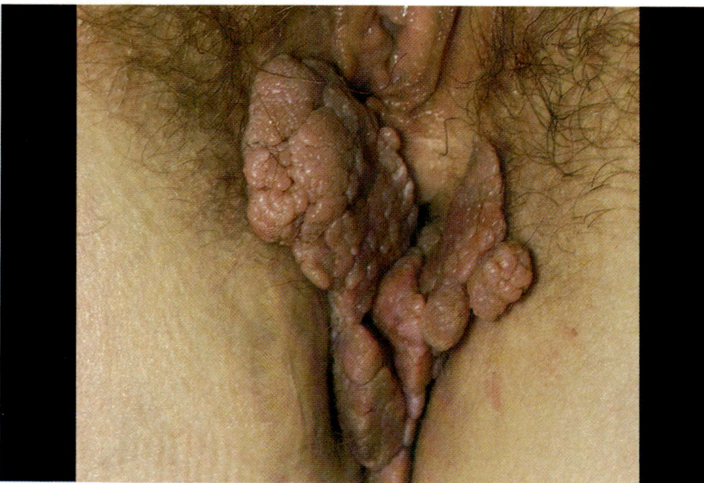

Figure 427 Condylomata acuminata. Extensive involvement of papillomatous tumors, partly flattened by compression.

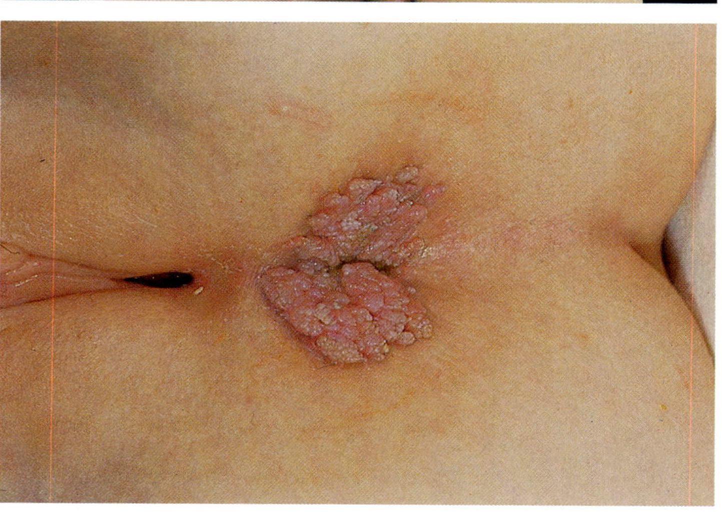

Figure 428 Perianal condylomata acuminata in a 5-year-old girl.

4. Malignant degeneration of condylomata acuminata is extremely rare (giant condylomata Buschke-Löwenstein).

Therapy

1. Podophyllum resin (25%) in alcoholic solution (Pod-Ben-25, Podofin) is helpful. The affected areas of the skin are dabbed with this solution 1 to 2 times per week. The healthy skin is covered with zinc paste to avoid irritation. The medication is removed in a sitz bath after 30 minutes (vulva, foreskin) or after 2–4 hours (penis, perianal region). Not more than 1 to 2 ml of this solution per day should be used to avoid podophyllum resin toxicity. Podophyllum resin should not be used during pregnancy.
2. Large clusters of genital warts can be removed by electrocautery, cryosurgery or with a CO_2 laser. This may require general anesthesia.
3. The sexual partner should always be examined and treated if necessary to avoid ping-pong infection.

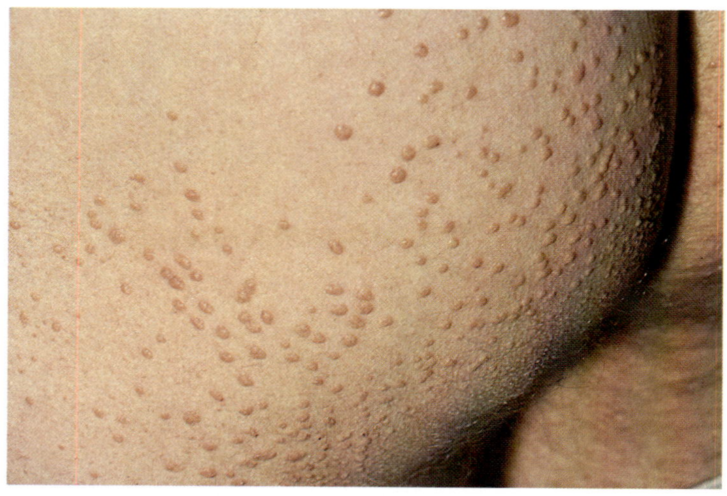

Figure 429 Eruptive xanthomas. Rapidly developing, yellowish to reddish lenticular tumors in the gluteal region.

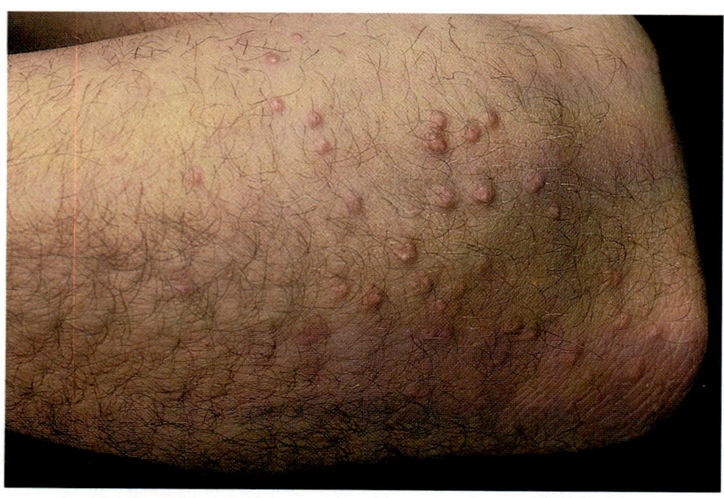

Figure 430 Eruptive xanthomas near the elbow.

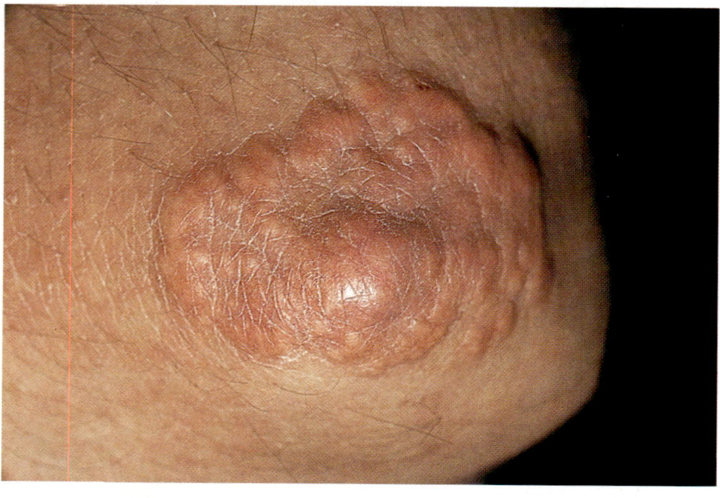

Figure 431 Tuberous xanthoma. Plate-like tumor composed of yellowish nodules at the elbow.

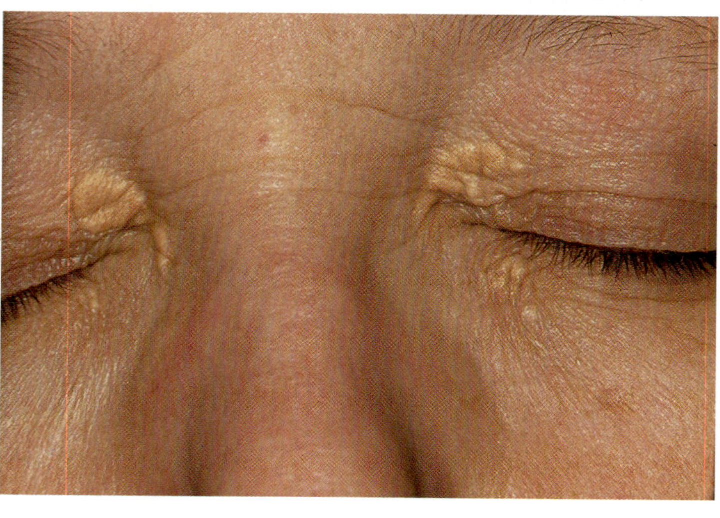

Figure 432 Xanthelasma palpebrarum. Slightly raised, yellow to yellow-brown tumors at the medial canthus.

Xanthoma, Xanthelasma

A. Eruptive Xanthoma

This genetically fixed, familial disturbance of fat metabolism (hyperlipidemia type I and IV and occasionally type V according to Frederickson) causes a dissemination of fat-storing tumors. The serum triglycerides are always extremely high. Lipid electrophoresis is necessary for exact classification into Frederickson's categories.

Clinical Features

1. Pinhead to pea-sized yellow nodules with an at least initially distinctly reddened base are disseminated in large numbers. Nodules over the buttocks or the elbows occasionally coalesce.
2. The buttocks, chest, abdomen, back, arms and face are mainly involved, rarely the oral mucosa (type I).
3. Frequent associated symptoms are hepatosplenomegaly and retinal lipemia (type I), or obesity, atherosclerosis, recurrent pancreatitis and again retinal lipemia (type IV).

Therapy

Dietary measures are usually sufficient. Alcohol should be avoided, and physical activity and weight reduction should be encouraged. Drug therapy is usually not necessary.

B. Tuberous Xanthomas

They are rare and belong to hyperlipidemia of type II and occasionally types III and IV. They are often associated with hypercholesterolemia.

Clinical Features

1. Firm yellow or orange-red nodules with a diameter of 0.5 to 2.5 cm and occasionally larger are characteristic. These nodules are often surrounded by a red halo. They do not cause any discomfort.
2. The knees and elbows are mainly affected; tumors are also found on the buttocks, heels and palms.
3. Associated symptoms are xanthelasma palpebrarum and xanthomas of the tendons and fasciae. The cardiovascular system is frequently affected with myocardial infarction, intermittent claudication, occlusive artery disease, cerebral hemorrhages, etc. Involvement of the liver can lead to biliary cirrhosis. The gallbladder often contains cholesterol stones. Arcus cornealis ("arcus senilis") is sometimes a diagnostic sign of hypercholesterolemia.

Therapy

A low-calorie, low cholesterol diet is helpful. Lipid-lowering medications such as Atromid-S, etc. are not always effective. Large xanthomas may require surgical removal.

C. Xanthelasma Palpebrarum

Clinical Features

1. These frequent, easily recognizable changes in older individuals consist of soft, occasionally velvet-like yellow nodules or plaques on the eyelids. They usually occur bilaterally and approximately symmetrically.
2. Xanthelasma is often found on the upper lid and on the inner canthus. They are also seen on the lower lid, and in extreme cases they involve the entire upper and lower lids.
3. In rare cases, a simultaneous hyperlipidemia exists with tuberous or eruptive xanthomas.

Therapy

Treatment of choice is excision under local anesthesia, usually for cosmetic reasons. This is not a causal therapy and relapses occur frequently.

IV. Malignant and Potentially Malignant Tumors

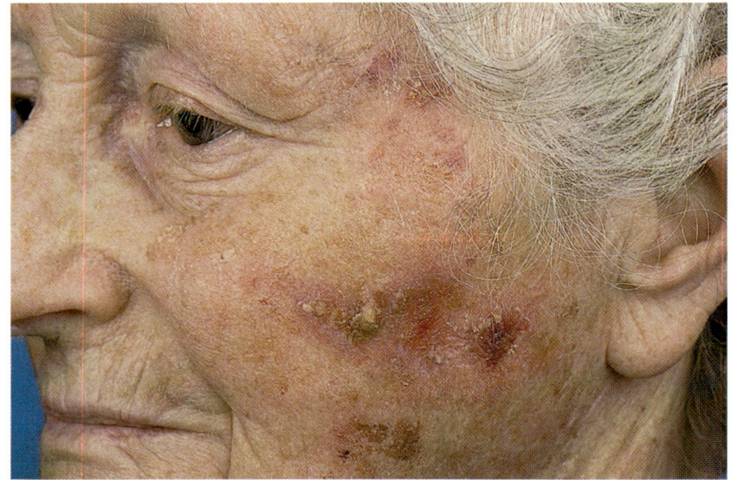

Figure 433 Actinic (solar) keratoses. Multiple, slightly raised, hyperkeratotic, partly crust-covered areas on the face.

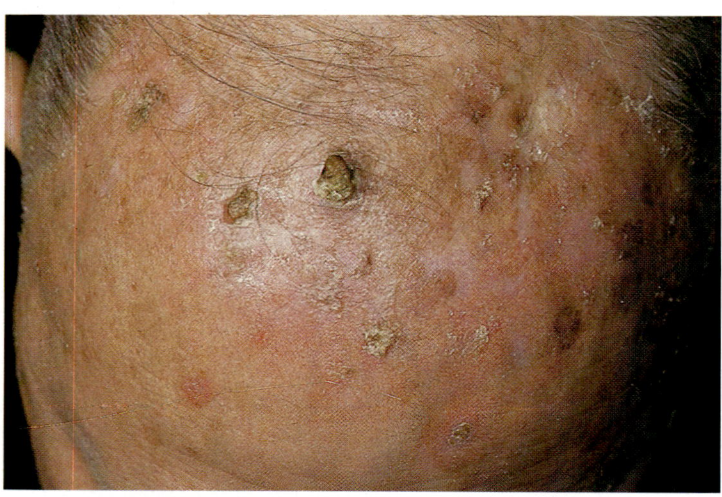

Figure 434 Actinic (solar) keratoses. Telangiectatic areas on the scalp with hyperkeratosis of varying degrees.

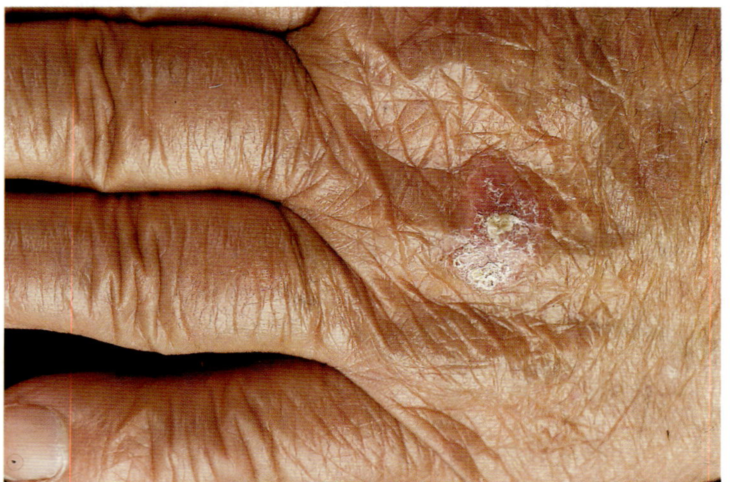

Figure 435 Actinic (solar) keratoses on light-exposed, atrophic skin.

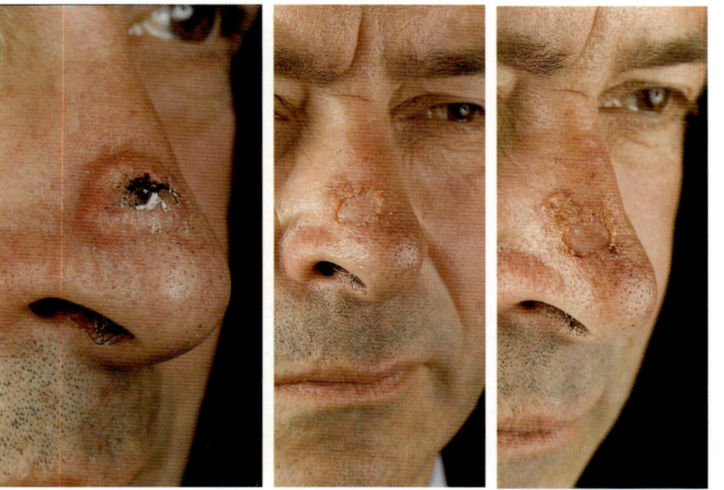

Figure 436 Keratoacanthoma. Left: Round tumor with central pitting which is filled with a cornified cone. Center: Partial spontaneous involution 3 months later. Right: Residual scar after two more months.

Actinic Keratoses, Keratoacanthoma

A. Actinic Keratoses

Actinic or solar or senile keratoses develop spontaneously as a consequence of prolonged exposure to ultraviolet radiation. They occur mainly in older people, particularly in individuals with outdoor occupations, such as farmers and sailors. Increasing exposure to UV-light from changing recreational habits and reduction of the protective ozone layer will gradually cause the incidence of these skin changes to increase, even in persons not exposed to sunlight through their occupations. Actinic keratoses must be taken seriously because they represent a precancerous lesion and may evolve into squamous cell carcinoma. This makes actinic keratoses more than just a cosmetic problem. Malignant transformation into invasive cancer does not occur very often and develops only after the actinic keratosis has existed for a long time. However, in patients with long-term suppression of the immune system, squamous cell carcinoma can develop within a few years.

Clinical Features

1. Initially, actinic keratoses are erythematous lesions of up to 1 cm in size. Their surface is covered with a crust of scales which gives it a slightly rough texture.
2. Some of the changes show increased pigmentation in some segments.
3. Occasionally, the lesions are covered with thick keratinic layers with the appearance of a cutaneous horn (cornu cutaneum).
4. Increased infiltration of the base and beginning ulceration are an indication for biopsy to rule out squamous cell carcinoma.

Therapy

1. In early cases, application of a fatty ointment **(R. 33a, b)** and a sunscreen (see below) is sufficient.
2. Topical corticosteroids, occasionally in combination with urea or salicylic acid **(R. 39b),** suppress the inflammatory reaction temporarily.
3. For topical treatment of advanced lesions, the cystostatic drug 5-fluorouracil is applied to the involved areas twice daily for 2 to 6 weeks until an erosive reaction occurs (it should not be applied to the eyes, the nasolabial fold or the oral region). The surrounding healthy skin must be covered with a zinc paste.
4. The patient must be followed regularly until the lesions are healed.
5. All lesions suspected of malignant transformation must be biopsied; excisional biopsy is recommended for smaller lesions.
6. The existing actinic damage cannot be reversed. The skin must be protected against sunlight to avoid damage from UV-exposure (hats with a broad rim, sunscreen ointment with a high lightprotective factor **(R. 45);** no excessive exposure to sunlight).

B. Keratoacanthoma

Keratoacanthoma, a so-called pseudo-carcinoma, occurs frequently and must be mentioned here. It is a solitary tumor that occurs in areas exposed to the sun, especially in fair-skinned individuals. The tumor develops without pre-existing changes within a few weeks and disappears spontaneously after several weeks or months. It usually leaves a shallow scar. Damage to the underlying bone or cartilage structures is visible occasionally.

Clinical Features

A firm, skin-colored to red nodule of up to 2 cm in size with a central crater filled with keratin that gradually increases in size is typical.

Therapy

The tumor usually runs a favorable course; observation of lesion with regular examinations is sufficient. Since the extent of scar formation cannot be predicted and the lesion is difficult to distinguish from squamous cell carcinoma, we recommend early excision and histologic examination.

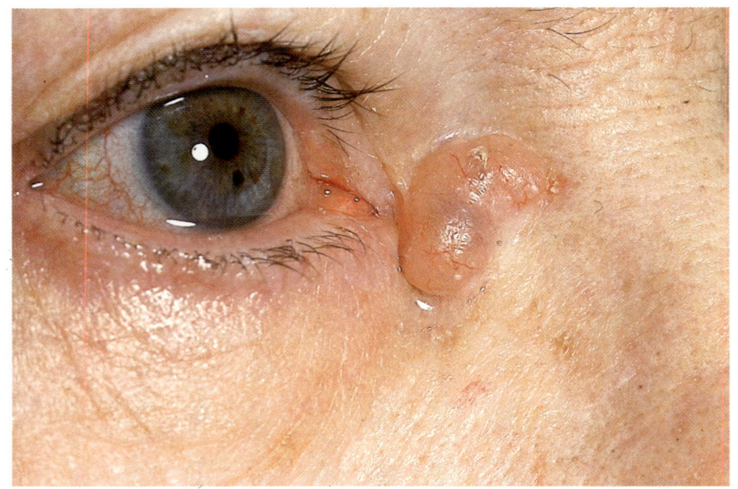

Figure 437 Basal cell carcinoma. Glassy appearance of tumor with ectatic blood vessels.

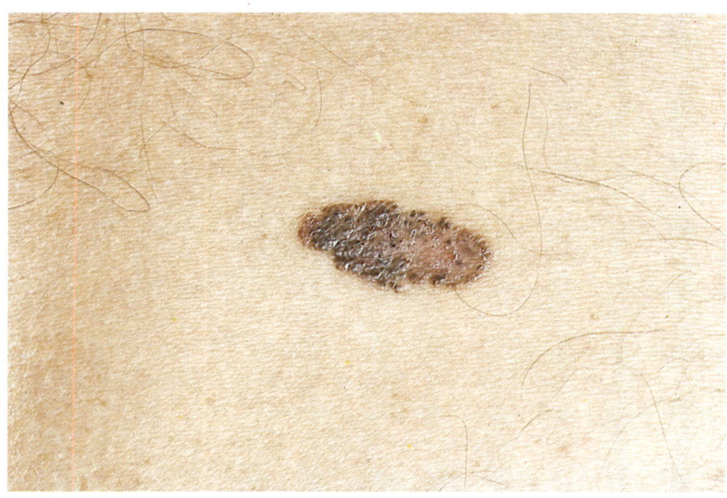

Figure 438 Pigmented basal cell carcinoma. Slightly raised tumor with marginal nodular seam and marked melanin pigmentation.

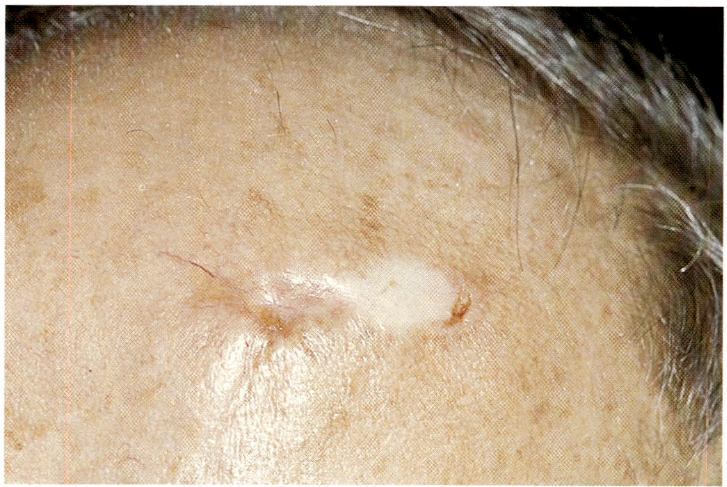

Figure 439 Basal cell carcinoma of the type basalioma planum et cicatricans. White indurated area adjacent to atrophic retracted region, similar to scar formation.

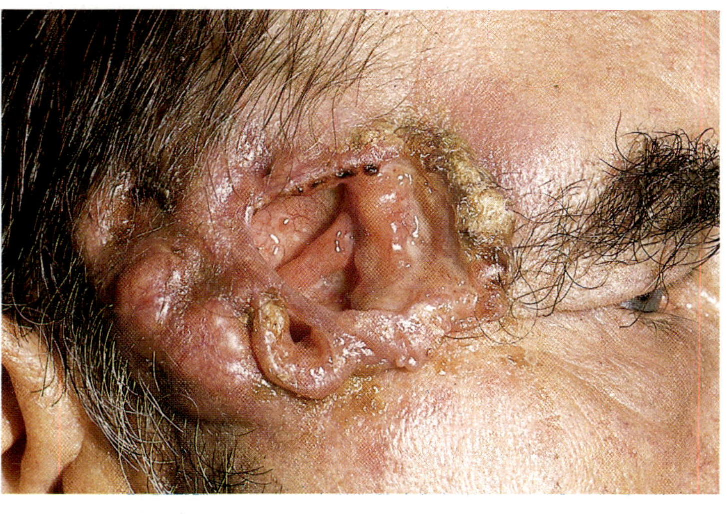

Figure 440 Basal cell carcinoma of the type ulcus terebrans. Extensive tumor in the temporal area with destructive growth and deep ulcer formation.

Basal Cell Carcinoma (BCC)

Basal cell carcinoma metastasizes extremely rarely, but must be taken seriously because of its aggressive destruction of skin, cartilage and bone. The fact that more than 80% of all basal cell carcinomas develop in the face, plus their frequent occurrence in fair-skinned individuals in sunny climes (Australia, the Southern states of the U.S.) indicate sunlight as an important causative factor. In addition, genetic factors and exposure to carcinogens, especially chronic exposure to arsenic (occupational and therapeutic exposure) may play a role. Increased occurrence of basal cell carcinoma is observed in patients with long-term suppression of the immune system (e.g., in patients with organ transplantation). In more than 40% of all patients, additional basal cell carcinomas develop later.

Clinical Features

Five different types of basal cell carcinoma can be distinguished on the basis of their morphology:

1. *Nodular basal cell carcinoma.* This is a skin-colored, or somewhat lighter, transparent, soft nodule with overlying tiny telangiectasias. It grows slowly and may develop into a rodent ulcer after a growth period of up to several years.
2. *Rodent ulcer.* With further growth, the blood supply to the central parts of the tumor becomes inadequate, and central ulceration develops with crust formation and occasional bleeding and weeping. The marginal nodules continue to grow and appear like a string of pearls covered by telangiectasias, the typical appearance of basal cell carcinoma.
3. *Ulcus terebrans.* Most ulcerated basal cell carcinomas remain restricted to the skin for a long time, but ulcus terebrans shows very aggressive growth that can lead to significant destruction in the face. The tumor can grow into the nose and into the orbital cavity, resulting in loss of eyesight. Life-threatening complications can occur when the skull is invaded (meningitis or massive hemorrhage caused by erosion of blood vessels).
4. Superficial, so-called *pagetoid basal cell carcinoma.* This tumor is found mainly on the trunk. It is a flat, scaling, slightly infiltrated, sharply delineated lesion that grows into the periphery over many years. Its margin shows nodular appearance, like a string of pearls, which is typical for basal cell carcinoma. Flat, atrophic scar formation appears in the center; superficial ulceration and crust formation is seen rarely. In exceptional cases, an aggressive tumor with infiltrating growth can develop in this basal cell carcinoma.
5. *Sclerodermiform basal cell carcinoma.* This tumor develops mainly on the face. Clinically, it has the appearance of a circumscribed, flat, occasionally slightly depressed lesion, like a scar. On close examination, it can be recognized as a basal cell epithelioma by the telangiectasias that are present in the tumor. These basal cell carcinomas are often mistaken for scars for many years and can grow to a significant size; they can then be difficult to manage.

All basal cell carcinomas show varying pigmentation irrespective of their biological behavior. This can make it difficult to distinguish this tumor from malignant melanoma. The tumors can be differentiated by their nodular margin which is typical for basal cell carcinoma. This does not signify a special entity of the tumor.

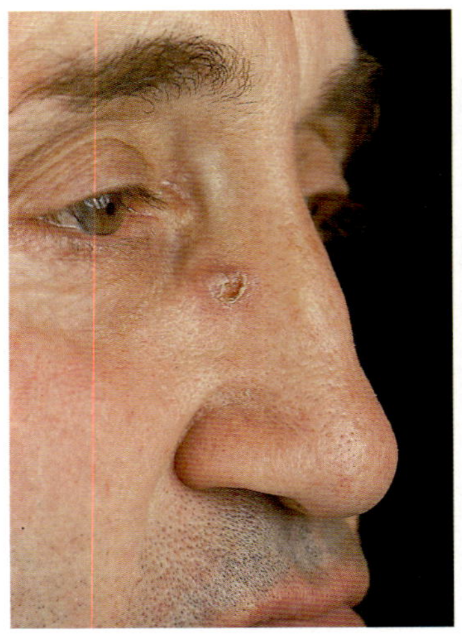
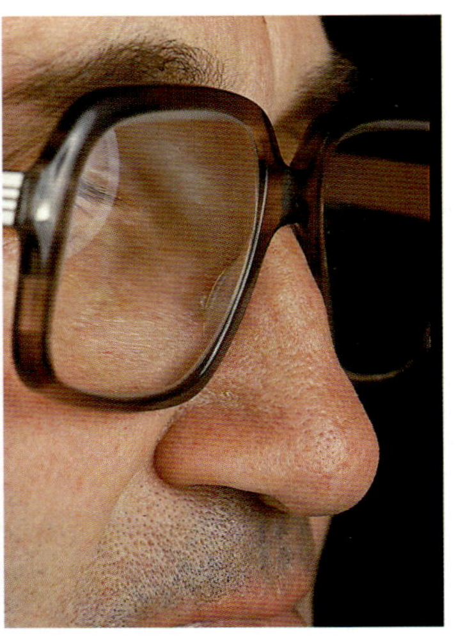

Figure 441 Basal cell carcinoma. Left: Centrally pitted tumor on the right side of the nose. Right: The lesion was covered by the eyeglasses and was mistaken for a skin irritation for a long time.

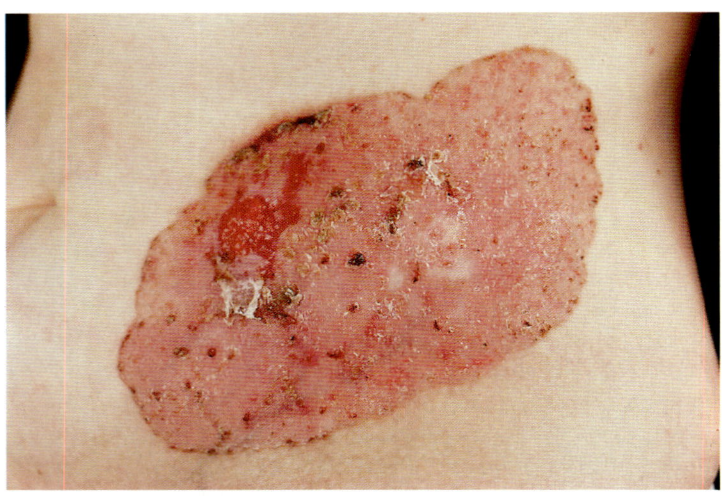

Figure 442 Basal cell carcinoma on the trunk. Sharply demarcated, slightly raised, reddened focus with a distinct margin which existed for many years.

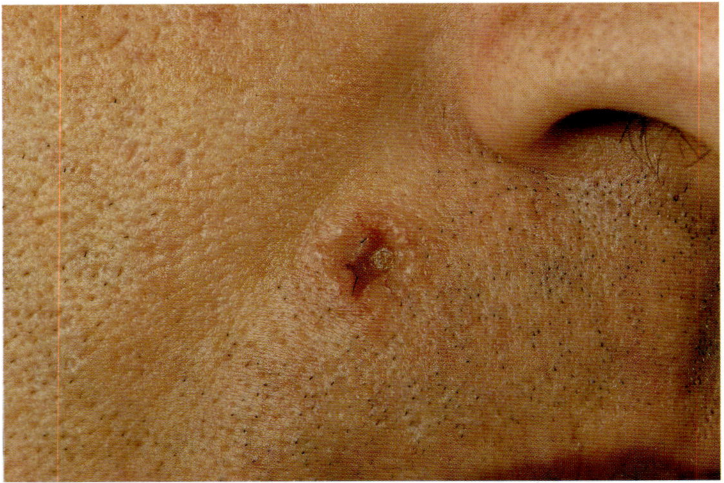

Figure 443 Basal cell carcinoma of the upper lip with glassy marginal wall and central ulceration.

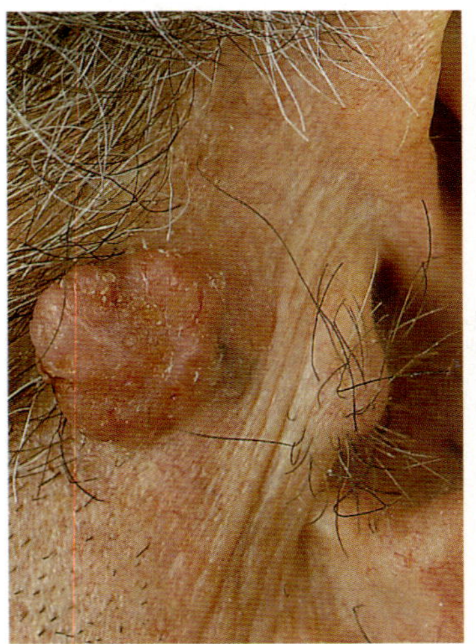
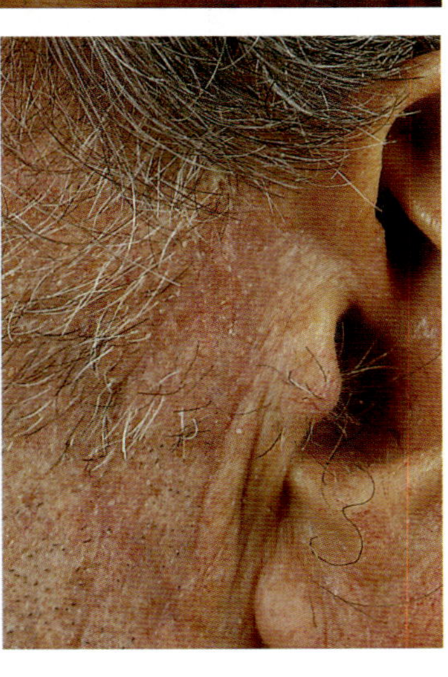

Figure 444 Basal cell carcinoma. Left: Nodular tumor in the left pre-auricular area. Right: Appearance one month after surgery.

Therapy

1. Excision of the tumor is the treatment of choice. Depending on the size of the tumor, a simple, spindle-shaped excision may be sufficient. Larger tumors may require a more extensive resection with subsequent plastic surgery to cover the defect. Three-dimensional histologic examination of the tissue surrounding the excised lesion is mandatory to confirm complete excision of the tumor. Basal cell carcinomas, even small ones, must be excised well into normal tissue, with a "safety margin" of at least 0.3 to 0.5 centimeters. On the face, even small tumors may require plastic surgery to cover the defect. Surgical treatment has the advantage that complete removal of the tumor can be confirmed histologically, and the resulting scars usually become less conspicuous with advancing years.
   Surgical procedures that result in complete tissue destruction, without the possibility of histologic examination, such as electrocurettage, cryosurgery of CO_2 laser are recommended only in exceptional cases for treatment of basal cell carcinomas.
2. Radiation therapy: In the hands of an experienced radiotherapist, the results of radiation treatment of basal cell carcinomas can be as good as those obtained with surgical procedures. The diagnosis must be confirmed by biopsy before radiation treatment is started. Today, radiation therapy is recommended for elderly patients (more than 70 years old) with extensive tumors who present with an increased operative risk.
   Ten to twenty radiation treatments are required; the treatments are followed by an inflammatory reaction that lasts several weeks. The cosmetic result is initially good, but deteriorates later. This treatment carries the risk of radiation-induced carcinoma 10 to 20 years later.
3. The patient must be seen at regular intervals (every 6 to 12 months) for follow-up examinations, and the affected areas checked for possible recurrences; the remainder of the skin must be examined for possible additional basal cell carcinomas, especially in the areas exposed to light.

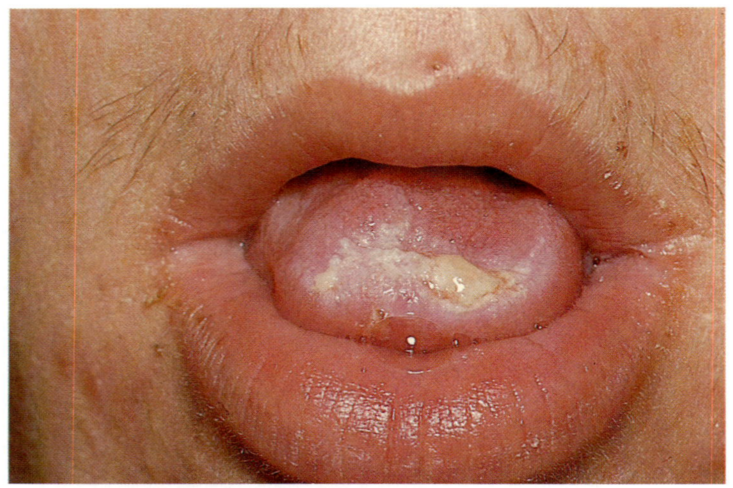

Figure 445 Leukoplakia. White hyperkeratosis of the tongue with poorly defined borders.

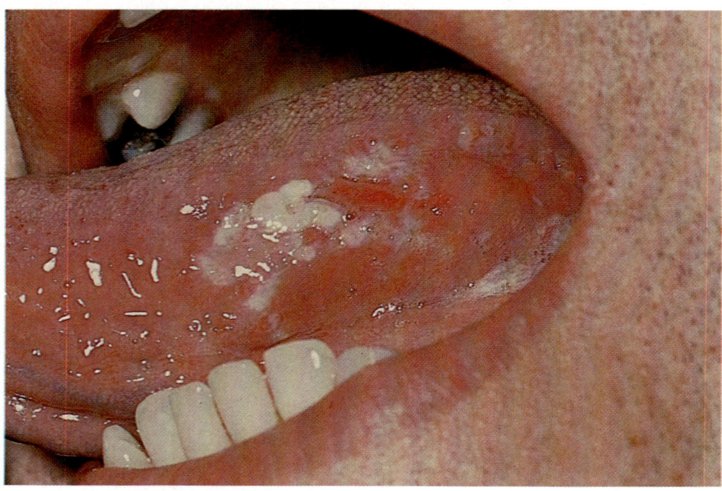

Figure 446 Leukoplakia-like Bowen's disease on the rim of the tongue. Partly erosive and partly leukoplakic, slightly raised tumor with irregular margins.

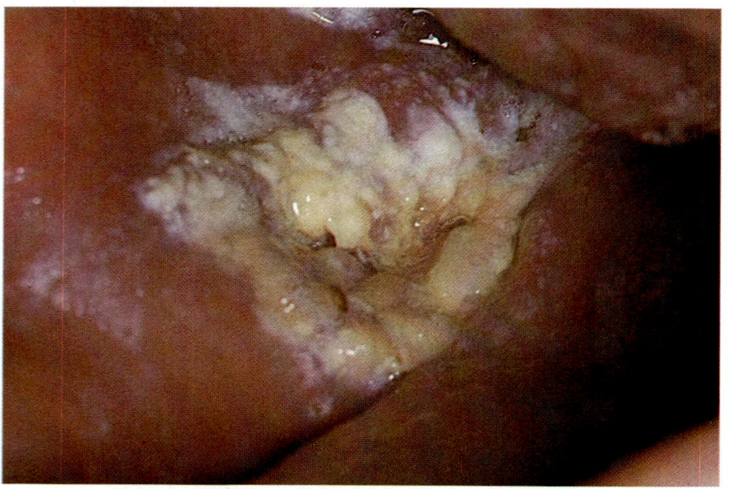

Fgure 447 Leukoplakia carcinoma on the buccal mucosa. Diffuse leukoplakia with indistinct irregular margins. A markedly hyperkeratotic infiltrating carcinoma is visible in the center of the lesion.

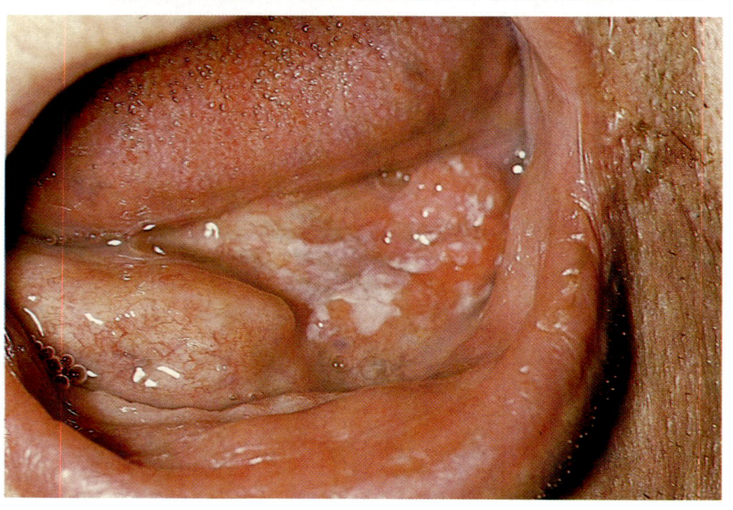

Figure 448 Leukoplakia-like Bowen's disease of the floor of the mouth. Diffuse, partly erosive, partly leukoplakia-like tumor with indistinct margins.

Leukoplakia

Leukoplakia is a plaque-like lesion on the red of the lips or the oral or genital mucosa. Ninety percent of these lesions are benign and do not require tumor-specific treatment. However, approximately 10% of all leukoplakias must be regarded as precancerous lesions that can mask a carcinoma in situ. Occasionally, one may find widespread carcinomatous changes in part of the leukoplakia (leukoplakia carcinoma). Furthermore, in some cases of mucosal carcinoma, leukoplakia may be present on the surface from the beginning, or it may develop later. Leukoplakia develops frequently as a result of mechanical irritation (defective teeth, poorly fitting dentures), from chemical irritation (smoking), or in hereditary or acquired diseases, such as viral papilloma, mucosal lichen planus (see page 93), white sponge nevus and congenital dyskeratosis. Consultation with a dermatologist or stomatologist who has experience with these conditions is recommended.

Clinical Features

1. A white patch or an indurated white plaque which is sharply delineated or sometimes has diffuse borders is characteristic. Occasionally erosions and a knobby, verrucous surface are seen.
2. The lesion is often located in the corners of the mouth, but the entire oral mucosa can be involved. Similar changes can be seen on the mucosa of the genitals.
3. Irregular, spotty leukoplakia lesions on an erythematous base, or lesions with erosions, ulcerations, and irregular, exophytic growth are always suspicious of carcinoma.

Therapy

1. Treatment is unnecessary if the cause of the mucosal irritation is known and can be eliminated. In these cases, the leukoplakia usually disappears with time after the irritation has been removed. Smoking should be stopped and dentures repaired. Follow-up examinations are necesssary until the lesion is healed.
2. Local application of vitamin A acid solution can occasionally effect healing.
3. When no cause can be found or when the leukoplakia does not heal within 4 to 6 weeks with the measures mentioned previously, or when carcinoma is suspected, the patient should be referred to an ENT specialist or an oral surgeon for excision of the entire lesion. Lesions that are too large for total excision can be treated with excision of the suspicious area. When histologic examination reveals malignancy, the tumor should be treated with a more radical procedure, such as wide excision, neck dissection or radiation therapy.

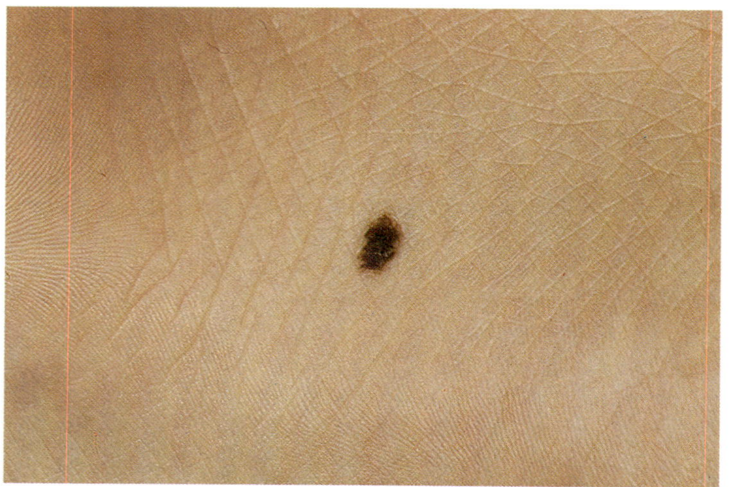

Figure 449 Nevomelanocytic nevus with signs of proliferation, clinically recognizable by the ragged, somewhat indistinct margin.

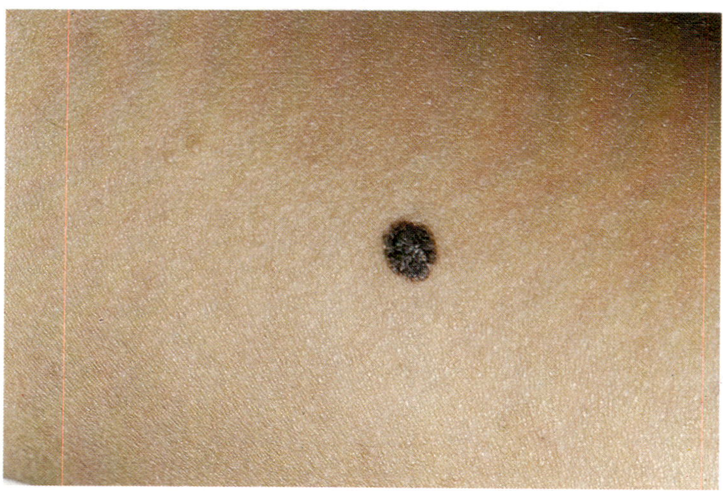

Figure 450 Nevomelanocytic nevus. Polycyclic margins and black-brown pigmentation as signs of increased proliferation.

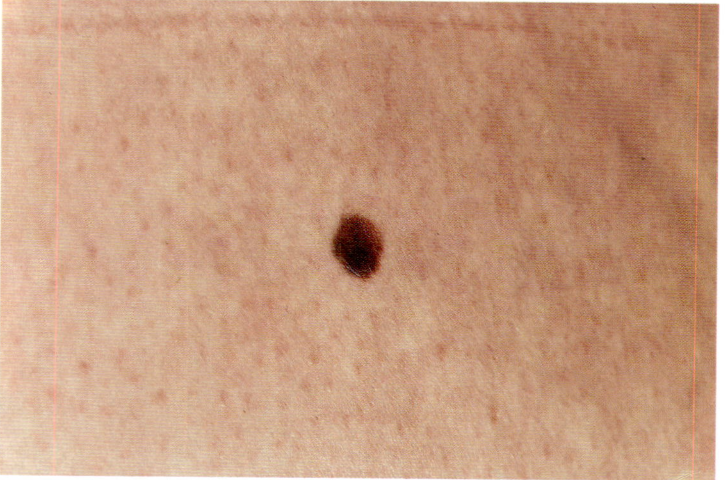

Figure 451 Superficial spreading melanoma. These early cases are often difficult to distinguish from a nevomelanocytic nevus by appearance alone.

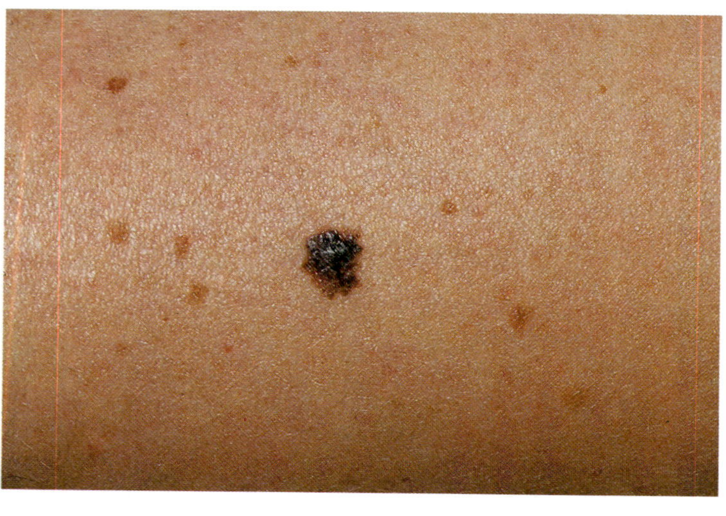

Figure 452 Early superficial spreading melanoma. Polycyclic margins, heterogenous pigmentation, slightly raised in the darker parts.

Malignant Melanoma

The incidence of this extremely malignant tumor has increased 10-fold in the last 40 years. In some patients, especially those with fair skin, excessive exposure to sunlight appears to be a factor. Patients with previous primary melanoma and those who have family members with malignant melanoma – by history or as a manifest finding – are especially prone to develop malignant melanoma.

It is extremely important to recognize the tumor as early as possible; the patient's chances of survival are much better with early treatment. The prognosis depends on the thickness of the tumor and its level of invasion. Superficially growing tumors have a more favorable prognosis when they are removed early. The attending physician must be familiar with the early signs of malignant melanoma and should refer the patient to a department of dermatology for evaluation (e. g., examination with the dermatoscope) and treatment.

A. Premalignant Changes and Early Types of Malignancy

In the early stage, as long as the tumor is only a few millimeters in size, it can be very difficult to differentiate a melanoma from a nevomelanocytic nevus. More than 80% of malignant melanomas occur on apparently normal skin. A few develop in benign nevomelanocytic nevi that have been present for some time, but these are exceptions. (For development of a malignant melanoma from a congenital nevomelanocytic nevus see page 203.)

Small pigmented tumors must be regarded as suspicious when the following criteria are present:

1. Rapid growth over a period of a few weeks or months.
2. Changes in pigmentation, especially darker discoloration, either of parts or of the whole lesion. Central hyper- or hypopigmentation. Grey, blue or red discoloration of the tumor.
3. Inflammatory, reddened margin.
4. Ragged borders.

Other very suspicious signs in small and also in larger tumors are:

5. Weeping, crust formation.
6. Bleeding, spontaneously or after minimal trauma.
7. Itching.

All these symptoms are only suspicious signs and can occur in traumatized or "active" nevomelanocytic nevi as well. Single or repeated trauma to a nevomelanocytic nevus does not induce development of a malignant melanoma. Lymphogenic cutaneous satellite tumors in the vicinity of the lesion are not just a suspicious sign, but confirm the presence of a malignant melanoma. The differential diagnosis, early forms included, should consider nevomelanocytic nevi and many other skin tumors, such as angiokeratoma, pigmented basal cell carcinoma, seborrheic keratosis, pyogenic granuloma, etc. Consultation with an experienced dermatologist and oncologist is essential.

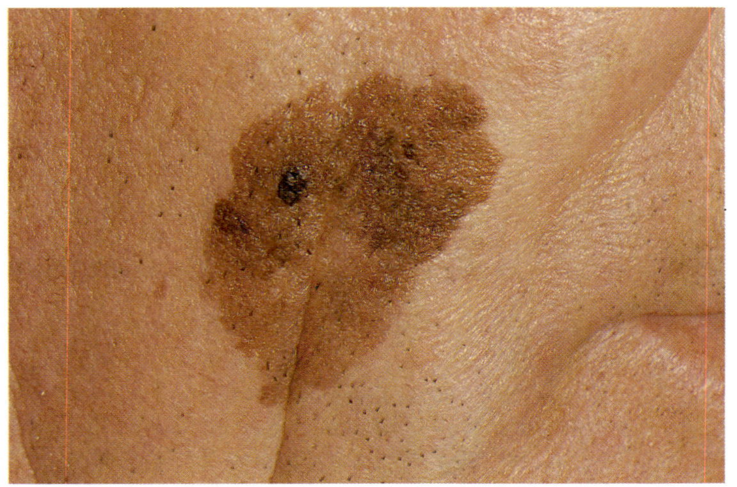

Figure 453 Lentigo maligna (melanosis circumscripta praeblastomatosa Dubreuilh). Well-defined, heterochromic pigmentation of the skin with notched borders.

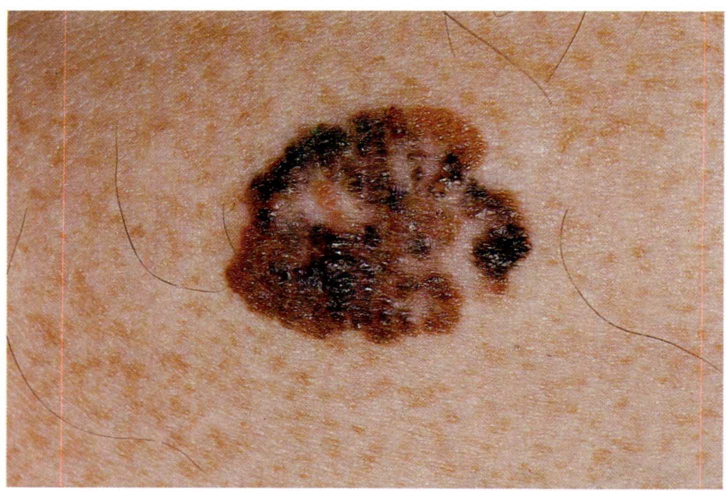

Figure 454 Superficial spreading melanoma. Slightly raised tumor with notched borders and mainly dark-brown pigmented nodules and depigmented areas of regression.

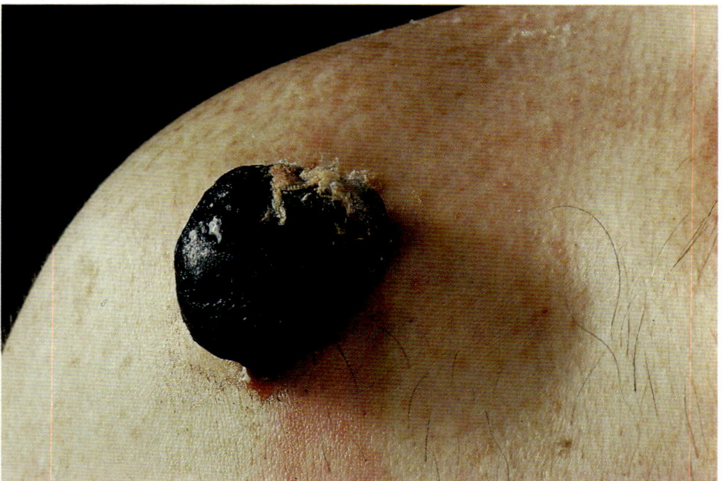

Figure 455 Nodular melanoma. Round, nodular, sharply delineated black tumor with easily traumatized surface.

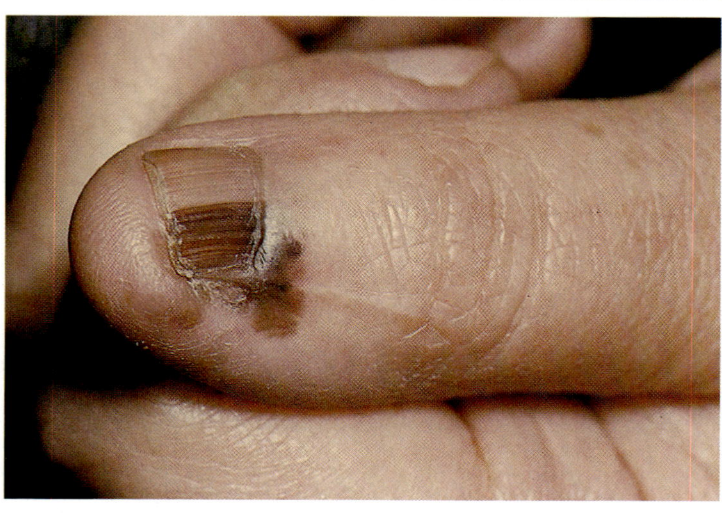

Figure 456 Acral lentiginous melanoma. Horizontal, not yet nodular growth phase. Irregular pigmentation adjacent to the nail, partly extending into the nail plate.

B. Clinical Types of Melanoma

Clinical Features

Four different morphological types of melanoma can be distinguished:

a) Superficial Spreading Melanoma (SSM) (approximately 70% of all melanomas).

The tumor presents itself in its superficial form for a few months to several years and grows at a moderate speed. Typically, it is a flat tumor with a notched border and usually consists of many tiny nodules. Individual central or marginal areas may show signs of regression and may be skin-colored or have a reddish or bluish color (from deep-seated remnants of pigment). Later, nodular or erosive changes occur in parts of the tumor, indicating a poorer prognosis (greater maximal thickness of the tumor). Superficial spreading melanomas are found mainly on the trunk and the extremities.

b) Nodular Melanoma (NM) (16% of all melanomas).

This is a dark-brown to black pigmented tumor that grows vertically and horizontally in a nodular fashion. Mild trauma often causes bleeding and weeping. The tumor metastasizes rapidly and has a poor prognosis. Amelanotic tumors are observed occasionally. Nodular melanomas occur mainly on the trunk and the extremities.

c) Lentigo Maligna Melanoma (LMM) (5% of all melanomas).

This tumor occurs almost exclusively on the face, usually in older people and on skin injured by excessive exposure to sunlight. It originates from lentigo maligna (Hutchinson's freckle), which can be seen as an in situ melanoma that is limited to the epidermis for a long time. Lentigo maligna is a sharply or poorly delineated lesion with irregular borders and variegation of pigmentation. After 3–15 years, one or more black nodules which represent invasive lentigo maligna melanoma may develop in the flat freckle.

d) Acral Lentiginous Melanoma (ALM) (5 to 10% of all melanomas).

This also is a tumor that grows horizontally for some time and presents as an enlarging brown patch. The typical location of this tumor is on the hands and feet, occasionally subungual or in the skin surrounding the nails.

e) *So-called Unclassifiable Melanomas (UCM).*

Approximately 3 to 4% of all melanomas do not fall into the above categories.

Local metastases into the surrounding skin and the regional lymph nodes as well as distant metastases characterize the later stages.

Therapy

All tumors suspicious of melanoma should be excised well into the healthy tissue with a safety margin of at least 3 millimeters, as long as no metastases are present (a diagnostic biopsy should be avoided!). Further treatment is determined by histologic criteria (depth of the tumor, maximal thickness). For a long time now, the discussion pertaining to the size of an adequate safety margin continues. According to current opinion, tumors of up to 0.75 millimeters maximal thickness should be excised with a safety margin of 1 cm. Deeper tumors should be excised with a safety margin of 2 to 3 cm. Deep fatty tissue should be removed down to the fascia. If the evaluation reveals involvement of the regional lymph nodes, these should be removed as well. The value of prophylactic removal of the regional lymph nodes is controversial. In advanced cases, polychemotherapy, also in combination with cytokines (interferon alpha, interleukin 2) can be tried. The effectiveness of these treatments, however, has not yet been proved. According to the present state of knowledge, interferon alpha-2 b, given as an adjuvant in high-risk patients, can prolong the life of these patients.
All patients with malignant melanoma should be seen regularly for clinical follow-up examinations, initially every three months, later at longer intervals. These follow-up examinations should extend over a period of at least 10 years.

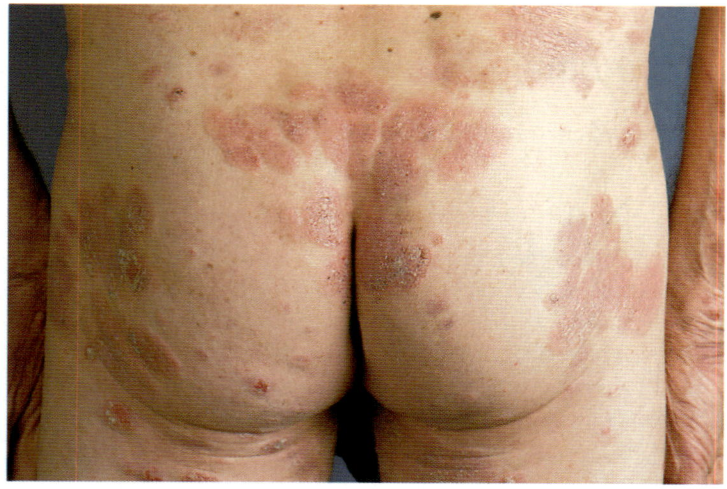

Figure 457 Cutaneous T-cell lymphoma. Mycosis fungoides. Multiple, sharply demarcated infiltrates.

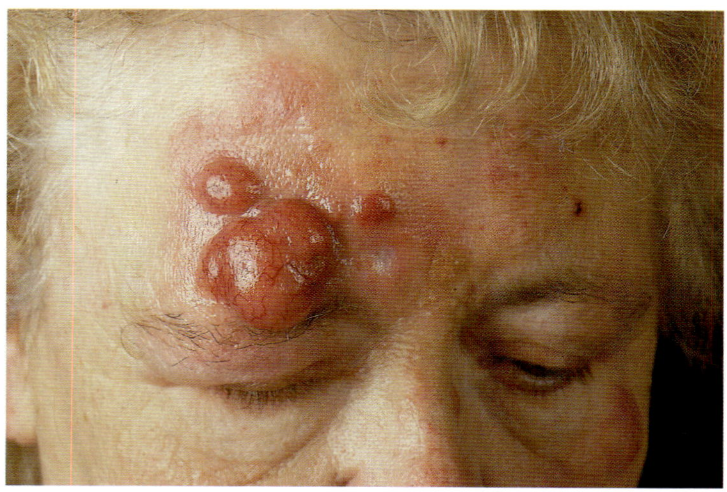

Figure 458 Cutaneous T-cell lymphoma. Tumors with nodular growth.

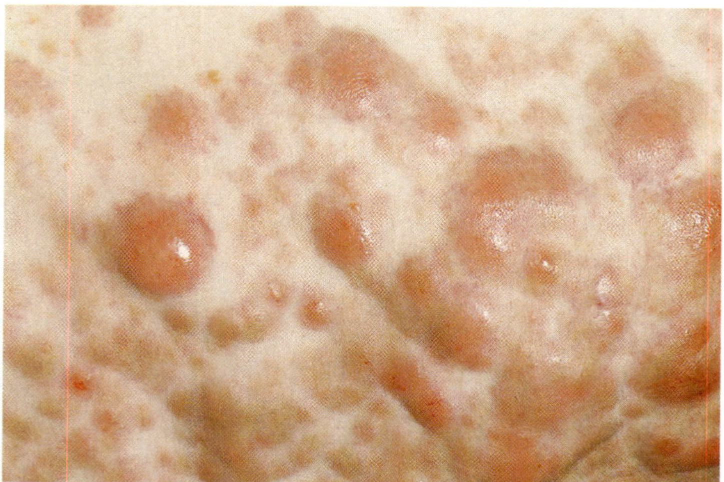

Figure 459 Malignant lymphoma (immunocytoma) of the skin. Densely arranged tumors in various stages of development.

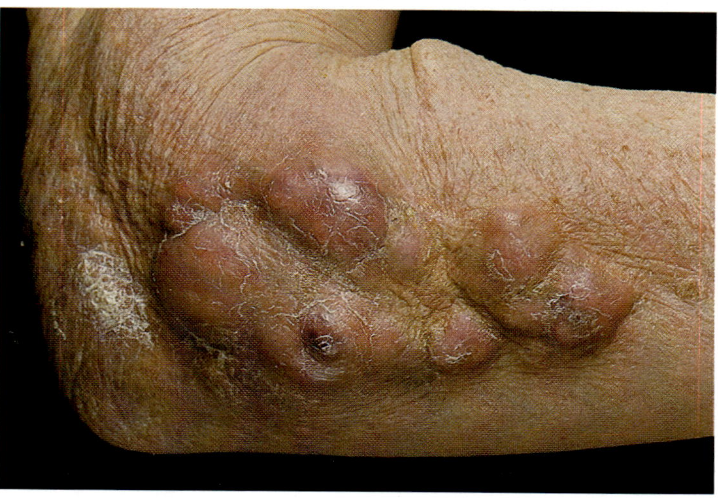

Figure 460 Centroblastic malignant lymphoma of the skin (retothelial sarcoma). Nodular, firm aggregate of tumors.

Mycosis Fungoides and Other Malignant Lymphomas

The term "malignant lymphomas" includes many diseases characterized by malignant proliferation of cells of the lymphatic system. A thorough knowledge of the early symptoms is important for the practicing physician. The first signs of the disease can be skin changes and generalized symptoms, such as fatigue, malaise and increasing weight loss which may lead to cachexia, as well as symptoms caused by the space-occupying growth of malignant lymphomas in lymph nodes, liver, spleen or bone marrow. The lymph nodes can be enlarged and palpable, as in chronic lymphatic leukemia. The disease can last for many months or years, depending on the degree of malignancy. Early diagnosis and treatment can often produce long-term remission or even cures.

Malignant lymphoma can affect the skin as a primary or secondary (metastatic) tumor. With primary skin involvement, the disease can often be limited to the skin for many years, especially with mycosis fungoides, a cutaneous T-cell lymphoma, but less often with other malignant lymphomas. Pseudolymphoma is a term used for lymphocytic inflammatory reactions due to a number of different causes (e.g., Borrelia infections, analgesics) that can resemble malignant lymphomas clinically and histologically. These tumors are benign and often regress completely with time (e.g., lymphocytoma; see page 59).

Clinical Features

a) Mycosis fungoides

The precursor stage consists of uncharacteristic itching and widespread eczematous plaques which may last for several years before it is followed by tumorous infiltrates and nodules in the skin. The disease generally develops slowly and may last for 5 to 10 years or even longer. Mycosis fungoides must be regarded as a malignant lymphoma of low malignancy.

b) Other malignant lymphomas

Individual or multiple, small or larger, often ulcerating nodules or nodular infiltrates of red to brown-red to blue-red color, are typical cutaneous lesions of this condition. The tumors can remain restricted to the skin for some time before internal organs become involved. Frequently, only a few nodules are present that can regress with treatment. The tumors usually recur after a remission of weeks, months or even years.

Among solitary or multiple malignant lymphomas, one distinguishes lymphomas of high- and low-grade malignancy. In rare cases, a malignant lymphoma appears early as disseminated multiple small lesions involving the entire skin. In these patients, the disease runs a rapid course with fatal outcome within a few months.

Therapy

Lasting cures are rare in patients with malignant lymphoma and cutaneous manifestations, but long-lasting remissions can occasionally be achieved with appropriate therapeutic measures. An exact classification based on histologic and immune-cytologic criteria should be attempted before treatment is started.

1. Malignant lymphomas of the skin are sensitive to radiation, especially low-voltage therapy and radiotherapy with fast electrons.
2. PUVA therapy can also produce long-lasting remission of mycosis fungoides, especially when it is combined with retinoids (so-called re-PUVA therapy).
3. Treatment with cytostatic drugs and corticosteroids should be carried out in a department of dermatology or in a department of hematology with experience in oncology. Chemotherapy is carried out with different combinations, depending on the degree of malignancy and the clinical stage of the disease.

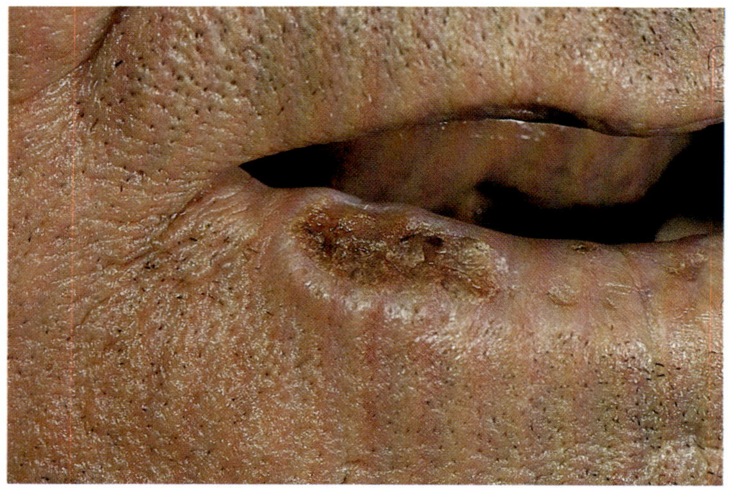

Figure 461 Squamous cell carcinoma of the lower lip. Centrally ulcerated tumor with a firm, raised margin.

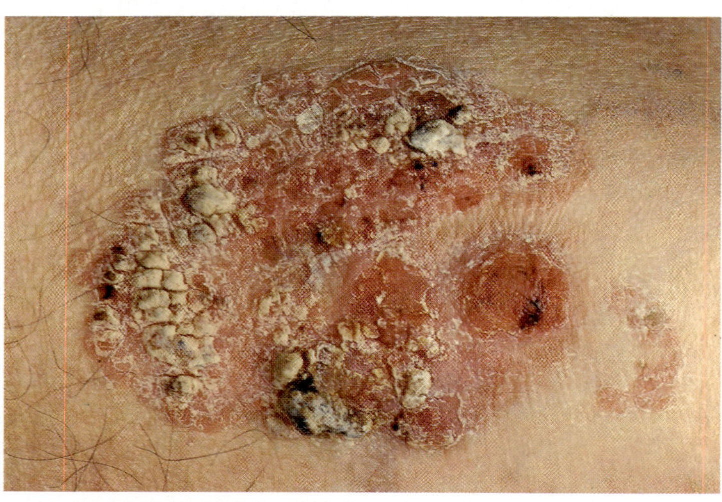

Figure 462 Bowen's disease. Flat, partly hyperkeratotic, partly erosive tumor, resembling psoriasis. The tumor developed over a period of several years.

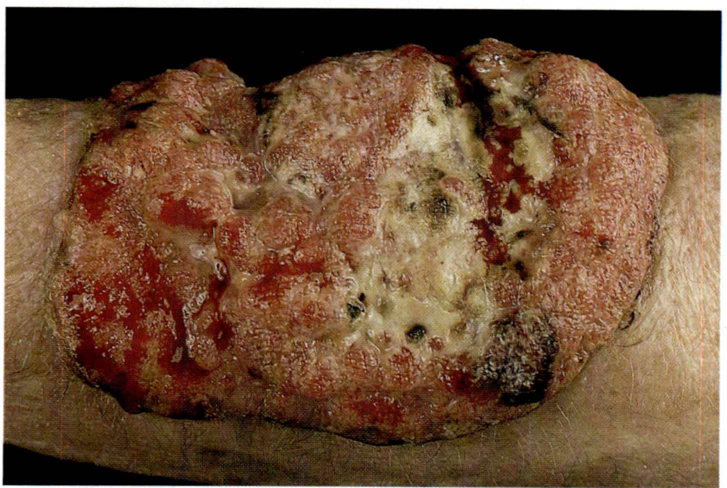

Figure 463 Squamous cell carcinoma of the forearm. Exophytic tumor with necrotic surface.

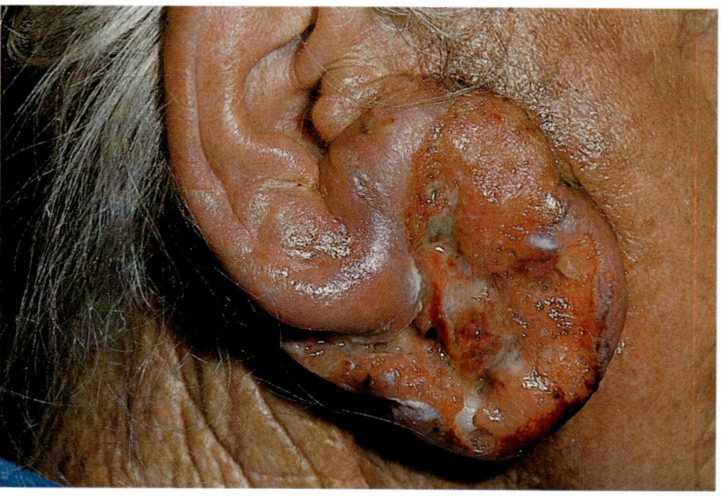

Figure 464 Squamous cell carcinoma of the ear. Ulcerating tumor, infiltrating the auricle.

Squamous Cell Carcinoma

Squamous cell carcinoma is the true carcinoma of the skin, caused by malignant proliferation of keratinocytes. Contrary to basal cell carcinomas, this tumor almost always occurs in precancerous alterations, or on skin damaged by chronic exposure to ionizing radiation (sunlight, x-rays) or by carcinogens (tar, arsenic). In rare cases, it develops on the basis of chronic inflammation (lupus vulgaris, chronic leg ulcer) or on contracted scars.

Chronic exposure to sunlight is by far the most frequent cause of squamous cell carcinoma of the skin. This tumor develops predominantly on areas of the skin exposed to light, such as the face, the scalp and the dorsum of the hand, and in individuals who work outdoors (farmers, sailors, etc.), especially in those with fair skin. The carcinogenic effect of sunlight depends on its content of short-wave UV radiation (UVB: wave lengths 280–320 nm) and is most pronounced in the mountains, at the sea (reflection), and when the sun is at its zenith. Because of the increasing exposure to UV light (vacation, sun lamps, shrinking ozone layer), a significant increase in the incidence of light-induced carcinoma must be expected in the upcoming decades.

Long-lasting suppression of the immune system also promotes the development of squamous cell carcinomas, as follow-up examinations of patients with organ transplants, especially patients with kidney transplants, have shown. Patients with an acquired defect of the immune system, such as individuals with HIV infection, are at greater risk of developing squamous cell carcinoma. The latency period between exposure to the carcinogen and development of the tumor can be as much as 25 to 30 years, as is known for arsenic and x-rays.

With prompt treatment, squamous cell carcinomas can often be cured. The cure rate for small squamous cell carcinomas (up to 3 cm) is more than 90%. Squamous cell carcinomas originating from precancerous lesions, such as actinic keratoses, grow very slowly and are often neglected for quite some time. Metastases are seen especially in neglected cases of carcinomas, or in carcinomas of the body's orifices, such as of the lips, vulva, anus or penis and in carcinomas of the oral cavity. Squamous cell carcinomas developing on skin damaged by light exposure have a relatively good prognosis. One must keep in mind, however, that these patients can later develop other carcinomas on their damaged skin.

Carcinoma of the oral mucosa often develops on premalignant changes, such as leukoplakia or erythroplakia, but also without these preexisting changes. The commonly seen carcinoma of the lower lip is usually caused by long-lasting exposure to UV light. Tobacco use is evident as the etiologic cause of carcinoma of the oral mucosa. Alcohol is another risk factor, but to a lesser degree. Many patients with intra-oral carcinoma are heavy consumers of tobacco and alcohol. Members of the Mormon Church, as well as Seventh-Day Adventists, who do not smoke or drink alcohol, practically never develop carcinoma of the oral mucosa. The prognosis of carcinoma of the oral mucosa is much less favorable than that of squamous cell carcinoma of the skin and the lower lip.

Poor hygiene of the foreskin is considered to be the most important cause for carcinoma of the penis. Cleanliness can be hindered by a phimosis, thus increasing the risk of developing a carcinoma of the penis. Carcinoma of the penis practically never develops in circumcised individuals. Long-term immunosuppression as in organ transplant patients also increases the risk of developing carcinoma of the penis.

Clinical Features

1. Initial changes appear as chronic eczema-like lesions with discrete, slowly increasing keratinization.
2. With a more endophytic growth, an ulcer develops with a firm wall and papillomatous changes; a more exophytic growth will lead to a raised papillary verrucous tumor with a thick horny surface, which occasionally has the appearance of a cutaneous horn. Long-standing squamous cell carcinomas occasionally have a friable, weeping or bleeding surface.
3. Necrotic changes in the tumor and bacterial infection can produce malodorous crusts.
4. Palpable and firmly enlarged regional lymph nodes are an indication that the cancer has already metastasized.

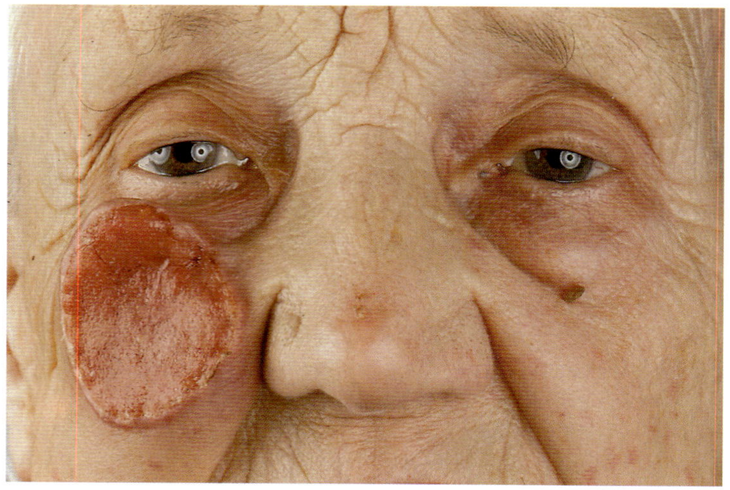

Figure 465 Squamous cell carcinoma on the right cheek. Round, centrally ulcerating tumor.

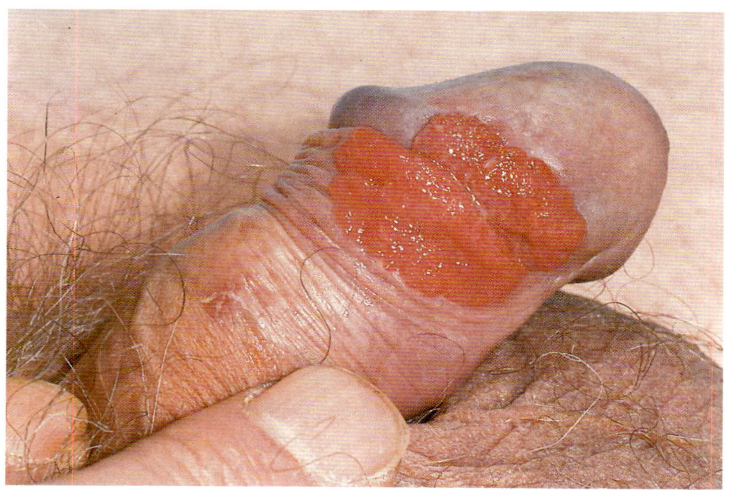

Figure 466 Carcinoma of the penis.

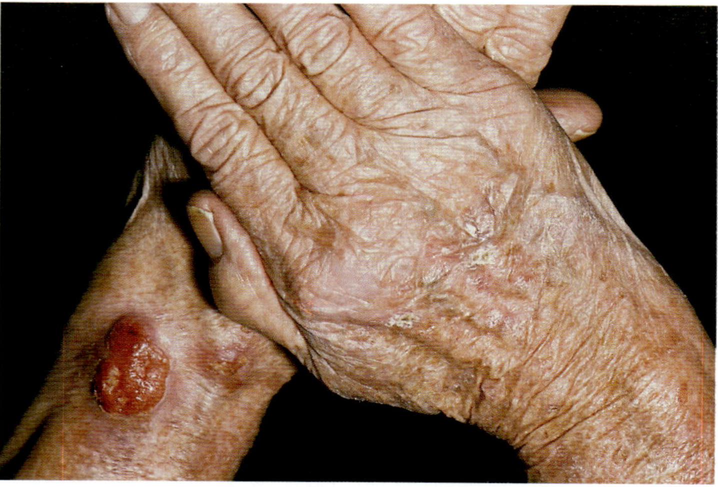

Figure 467 Squamous cell carcinoma on actinically damaged skin; dorsum of the left hand.

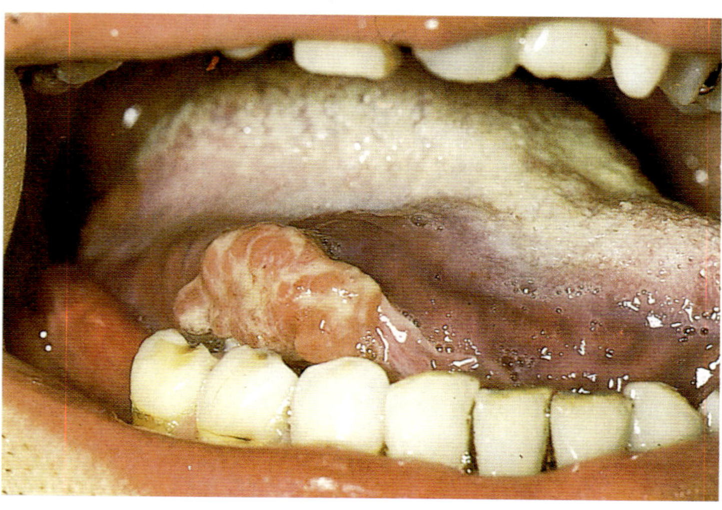

Figure 468 Squamous cell carcinoma on the floor of the mouth.

Precise information regarding these points tends to improve the therapeutic result and to reduce the cost of treatment.

3. Another important point is to prescribe an appropriate amount of the effective drug. Small amounts are relatively more expensive than larger quantities. For a circumscribed dermatosis which generally heals quickly (e.g., acute contact dermatitis), the prescription of a small tube can be quite economic. For chronic skin diseases, the prescribed amount should be sufficient to allow the patient to carry out adequate topical treatment until the next office visit. The following are rough estimates of the amounts necessary to treat certain areas of the skin. The amounts indicated are for ointments. For creams the amounts should be 10–30% more, for lotions the amounts should be doubled.

Table 1

Treated area	Amount for one treatment (gm)	Amount for 14 days for application twice daily (gm)
Hands, face	2	50
Anogenital area	2	50
One arm, chest or back	3	80
One leg	4	120
Entire body	25–40	approx. 1000

4. A thin application of a cream or an ointment is usually sufficient. Application of a thick layer does not increase the effectiveness of the active ingredient because its resorption is not dependent on the thickness of the applied layer. By "treating" the surroundings, this only increases the amount of the medication used. It is possible, however, to force penetration of the drug remnants that have remained on the surface by saturating the skin with fat. This can be done by applying an ointment containing the effective drug in the morning and a drug-free ointment in the evening.

5. With expensive corticosteroid preparations, a so-called interval therapy can be used. This alternates periods of therapy with preparations containing the drug and periods of therapy with drug-free preparations in intervals of 2–3 days. With this regimen, the effect can even be better, because cortisone tachyphylaxis can be avoided. Treatment is more cost effective and cortisone side effects occur less frequently.

6. Compounding medications can also be less expensive. Mixing standard (U.S.P.) bases with commercial preparations is not recommended, however. Commercial preparations are often complicated emulsions that can become unstable when mixed, and they usually become more expensive when processed further in a pharmacy. On the other hand, prescriptions with U.S.P. bases and active medications have the advantage that they are free of preservatives. It is preferable for the primary care physician to limit the use of these prescriptions to a few preparations with which experience can be gained.

Medications and Measures for External Treatment

A. Wet Dressings

They are anti-inflammatory, cooling and desiccating and are helpful for weeping, erosive and ulcerative lesions. They can be used to debride wounds by cleansing the skin of crusts and exudates and by helping to maintain drainage of affected sites. It should be remembered that prolonged use of disinfectant substances can have a cytotoxic effect and delay wound healing.
Application: Use several layers of gauze or pieces of linen (wick effect), renew every 20 minutes (caution: prolonged use can lead to maceration).

R. 1. Bland, anti-inflammatory:
Tap water,
Physiologic saline solution.

The addition of alcohol (isopropanol or ethanol 1:5 to 1:10) increases cooling, drying and degreasing (do not use on open wounds).

R. 2. Antibacterial:
Silver nitrate (1:1000), $KMnO_4$ (1:1000 to 1:10,000),
Zinc sulfate (1:1000 to 1:10,000).

B. Partial Baths (Hand Bath, Foot Bath, Sitz Bath) and Full Baths

Baths have anti-inflammatory, drying and antipruritic effects. Frequently used additions such as sulphur, ethereal oils and humic acid can help only a few dermatoses. Their irritating effects on the skin tend to aggravate the condition.

R. 3. Indifferent:
Add colloidal substances such as linit or oatmeal (Aveeno) or cornstarch. Add a handful of the substance to the running bath water.

R. 4. Disinfectant:
Add $KMnO_4$ until the bath water is a pale purple.

R. 5. Degreasing:
Acetone 1:20 or alcohol 1:10 is helpful for localized areas.
Seba-Nil, Ionax skin cleanser.

R. 6. Antiscaling:
Soft soap

R. 7. Regreasing:
Bath oils help prevent drying of the skin.
Alpha Keri
Ar-Ex
Domol
Lubrex
Surfol
Caution: Especially older patients must be warned that the tub will be slippery.

R. 8. **Toughening the skin:**
Powder with phenolsulfonic acid-phenolic urea methanal complex.

R. 9. **Antipruritic, anti-inflammatory:**
Tar preparations such as Balnetar (2.5%), Lavatar (33.5%), Polytar (25%), and Zetar emulsion (30%).

R. 10. **Shampoos:**
a) *Antiseborrheic:* preparations with salicylic acid or tars
b) *Antiseborrheic, antibacterial:* All Clear, Head and Shoulders
c) *Antiseborrheic, antimycotic:* preparations with ketoconazole

C. Powders

Powders have a drying effect and decrease friction. Thus they are very useful to keep skin folds such as in the groin, axillae and the submammary area dry. Active medications are released from powders to a lesser degree than from other vehicles.

R. 11. **Non-medicated (or inert):**
Talc, USP (talcum)
Cornstarch

Rx. Zinc oxide 25 gm
Talcum 25 gm

For wound cleaning:

Rx. Glucose 25 gm
Urea pure 25 gm

Debrisan powder

R. 12. **Anti-infectious:**
Powders with silver additives
Sure Shield
Bacitracin: Polysporin (with polymyxin B)

R. 13. **Antifungal:**
Tolnaftate: Aftate, Athlete's Foot Powder, Insulate Powder, Tinactin
Nystatin: Mycostatin, Nystop, Pedi-Dri (only effective against yeasts)
Miconazole: Lotrimin AF Athlete's Foot Powder, Micatin, Zeasorb-AF.

D. Solutions, Tinctures

Mixtures of pharmacologic agents with water (solutions) or alcohol (tinctures) or alcohol in conjunction with polyethylene glycol have a desiccating and defatting effect. After evaporation of the solvent, the effective substance remains on the skin. These are useful for the scalp, the interdigital areas of the foot and the skin folds. When prescribing dye solutions, the patient must be advised that their stains are difficult to remove from laundry and floors.

R. 14. **Antifungal, antibacterial:**

a) *Trimethylan dyes:*
– Brillant green 0.5% watery
– Castellani's paint
– Gentian (crystal, methyl) violet, 0.5% watery

b) *Tolnaftate:* Tinactin solution (effective against dermatophytes only)

c) Broad-spectrum antifungal agents
Miconazole: Micatin solution, Fungoid
Clotrimazole: Lotrimin, Mycelex OTC

d) *Clindamycin:* Cleocin T, Clinda-Derm
Erythromycin: Akne-mycin, Staticin
Tetracycline hydrochloride: Topicycline

R. 15. Antiviral:
Idoxuridine/dimethyl sulfoxide: Herpid
Idoxuridine (IdUr): Stoxil
Podophyllum resin: Podofin, Pod-Ben-25 (for treatment of condylomata acuminata)

R. 16. Anti-inflammatory, anti-infectious:

a) Solutions containing tar
Coal tar solution (liquor carbonis detergens; LCD).

b) Solution for the treatment of inflammation of the oral mucosa

Eucalyptus oil	0.1%
Oleum menthae	1.8%
Oleum thymi	0.2%
Tinct. myrrhae	5.0%
Tinct. salviae	2.0%
Glycerol (85%)	5.0%
Sorbitol 70% (non-crystal)	10.0%
Cremophor EL	12.0%
Saccharin-sodium	0.06%
Aqua purificata	63.9%

For mouth rinsing or gargling, a diluted solution is used (30 drops in one glass of water (circa 60 ml)). In severely ill patients, the mouth can be wiped with a cotton swab soaked with the undiluted solution.

R. 17. Disinfectants:
Disinfection of the skin for therapeutic reasons is rarely necessary. Repeated application of disinfectants to wounds leads to tissue toxic effects and delayed rather than accelerated wound healing. Most medications contain alcohol in high concentrations, which causes too much pain on large wounds. Topical medications containing mercury should be not used on large wounds, if at all, because of the risk of absorption.
Mercurochrome solution (caution: rare allergy to mercury possible, advantage: only minimal burning sensation upon application),
Merfen Orange (caution: allergy to mercury is possible),
Betadine solution (caution: allergy to iodine is possible),
Alcoholic iodine solution (caution: allergy to iodine is possible).

R. 18. Scalp tinctures (anti-inflammatory, containing corticosteroids):
Benecort topical solution (1–2 1/2% hydrocortisone)
Synalar solution (0.01% fluocinolone acetonide)
Lidex solution (0.5% fluocinonide)
Stiedex solution
Kenalog

R. 19. Antihidrotic:

Rx: Aluminum chloride (20.0–)30.0
Aqua dest. to make 100.0
Apply in the evening, leave on for 15 minutes, then rinse off.

E. Shake Mixtures

These are a combination of solid and liquid materials, i.e., "liquid powder". The effect is similar to that of powders: anti-inflammatory, desiccating, cooling, but better adherence, especially to large areas. Shake mixtures contain much water but little or no oil, thus they are not suitable for dry skin. As in powders, their effect is mainly through physical properties. There is little or no release of active medications.

R. 20. Indifferent:

a) *Desiccating:*
Non-alcoholic white shake lotion (Lotio alba aquosa):

Rx: Zinc oxide	20 gm
Talcum	20 gm
Glycerin	30 gm
Distilled water	30 ml

b) *Strong drying effect:*
Alcoholic white shake lotion:

Rx: Zinc oxide	20.0 gm
Talcum	20.0 gm
Glycerin	20.0 gm
Spirit dilut.	20.0 ml
Distilled water	20.0 ml

R. 21. Antipruritic:

Pramoxine hydrochloride: Prax lotion
Diphenhydramine: Benadryl suspension
(*Caution:* possible contact allergy).

R. 22. Strong anti-inflammatory effect through addition of corticosteroids:

Triamcinolone: Kenalog shake mixture.

R. 23. Antibacterial:

Vioform zinc shake mixture = Vioform 1% in Lotio alba aquosa or spirituosa (see **R. 20a, b).**

F. Gels

The base, usually propylene glycol with high liquid content (water or alcohol), has a cooling and antipruritic effect. Alcoholic gels have a drying effect and may cause skin irritation, especially when the skin is dry.

R. 24. Cooling, anesthetizing, antipruritic:

First generation antihistamines have a low topical anesthetizing and thus antipruritic effect. There is a risk of contact sensitization.
Tavist gel
Topical gel (contains menthol, camphor and benzyl alcohol).

R. 25. Acne medication:
Benzoyl peroxide has sebostatic, keratolytic and antibacterial effects (caution: contact allergy and irritation are possible).
3–5% for the face, 10% for the trunk.
Tretinoin (vitamin A acid) has keratolytic and sebostatic effects (caution: increased photosensitivity and skin irritation).

a) *Benzoyl peroxide:*
Acnegel, Benzagel: watery gel
Benzac, Clearasil BP Plus: watery gel
Panoxyl: alcoholic gel (greater defatting effect).
b) *Vitamin A acid:*
Retin-A gel
Aberela gel.

Gels are useful for sensitive skin, or slightly lubricating emulsions are possible **(R. 44).** Alternative treatment as short contact therapy of 10 minutes' duration.

R. 26. Antifungal:
Naftifine: Naftin gel

R. 27. Antiseborrheic, desquamatory effect:
Keralyt gel
PsoriGel scalp gel

R. 28. Antiparasitic:
Lindane and *benzyl benzoate:* Kwell, Scabene gel (see also **R. 40)**
Crotamiton: Eurax gel.

G. Pastes

These consist of powder components incorporated into a cream or ointment. They are indicated for acute inflammatory dermatoses where desiccation and a bland protective coating are desired. Pastes are not frequently used, and there are few that are commercially made.

R. 29. Bland, thick coating:
Zinc oxide paste (USP) (Lassar's):

Rx: Zinc oxide	25.0
Amyl. titric.	25.0
White vaseline	50.0.

R. 30. Moderate coating:
Soft zinc paste:

Rx: Zinc oxide	30.0
Olive oil	20.0
Lanolin	50.0

R. 31. Antifungal:
Nystatin:
In Germany there are numerous pastes (like Lassar's) containing nystatin (effective only against yeasts) available.

R. 32. Anti-inflammatory, anti-eczematous:

Tumenol zinc paste

Rx: Tumenol ammonium	5.0
Talcum	25.0
Zinc oxide	25.0
White vaseline to make	100.0

H. Emulsions: Lotions (Milk Type), Creams, Ointments

Lotions or creams are emulsions of the milk type (oil in water). Ointments are emulsions of either the butter type (water in oil) or are completely water-free and occasionally even water-repellant bases (vaseline, paraffin). A water-free base that can be easily washed off, for instance, is polyethylene glycol ointment, a so-called lipogel. These bases are often used in commercial preparations because of their good release of active medications. Preparations with a higher fat content irritate the skin more, and the occlusive effect increases. Lotions and creams are unstable and usually contain a significant amount of additives (preservatives, emulsifiers, stabilizers) that can occasionally cause intolerance reactions. On the other hand, patients usually find creams and lotions more pleasant than ointments because they are absorbed more quickly. It must be kept in mind that with increasing water content the quantity of topical medication also increases (see page 245).

R. 33. Preparations without active medication for interval therapy, for treatment of dry skin and for skin protection:

a) *Very strong lubricating effect, water-repellant:*
White vaseline USP
Unguentum molle (soft ointment)
Eucerin anhydric., mineral oil, liquid paraffin

b) *Strong lubricating effect:*
Hydrophilic petrolatum USP
Eucerin c. aqua

c) *Mild lubricating effect:*
Hydrophilic ointment
Unguentum emulsificans aquosum
Aquacare
Lubriderm
Purpose cream

d) *Cooling and mildly lubricating:*
Unguentum leniens

R. 34. Antibacterial:

Antibiotics are used much too often for topical therapy. Topical antibiotics are indicated only in rare cases. Their use may lead to the development of resistance and contact sensitization. Therefore, the following discussion does not cover preparations containing antibiotics that are indispensable for systemic treatment (e.g., gentamicin) or related drugs that can produce cross-resistance or contact allergies, e.g., neomycin.

Tetracycline hydrochloride: Achromycin ointment
Limited use because of frequent resistance of skin germs to tetracyclines.
Bacitracin: Bacitracin ointment
Fusidine acid: Fusidine ointment
PVP Iodine: Betadine ointment
Isodine ointment
possible resorptive effect
Tyrothricin: Sure Shield
Clioquinol: Vioform emulsion

R. 35. Antifungal:

a) *Miconazole:* Micatin
Econazole: Spectazole
Haloprogin: Halotex
Clotrimazole: Lotrimin
Mycelex
} Broad-spectrum antibiotics effective against yeasts and dermatophytes

b) *Tolnaftate:* Tinactin cream — selective against dermatophytes

c) *Nystatin:* Mycostatin or Nilstat — effective against yeasts only

d) *Amphotericin B:* Fungizone

R. 36. Antiviral:
Acyclovir: Zovirax ointment
Penciclovir: Denavir
Idoxuridine: Stoxil

R. 37. Antipsoriatic:
Anthralin (cignolin, dithranol): Anthralin causes dermatitis of the non-affected skin. Consequently, concentration of the active medication should be increased slowly until the optimal dose is reached (caution: irritation with excessive concentrations). The ointment should never be applied to the face. Oxidation products of this substance can cause permanent stains on clothing.
Lasan creams 0.1, 0.2, 0.4, 1%
Dithrolan ointment, Anthra-Derm ointment, Lasan Unguent
Prescriptions of anthralin should be compounded in graduated concentrations from 0.05 to 2%, preferably in white vaseline. Other antipsoriatic medications with limited indications (generally used for localized psoriasis) are:
Calcipotriene: Dovonex ointment

R. 38. Corticosteroids:
Corticosteroids are the most effective substances for topical anti-inflammatory therapy. To avoid undesirable side effects of cortisone, it is preferable to use short-term or interval treatment with stronger cortisone preparations, instead of using continuous long-term therapy with less potent preparations (attenuation of the cortisone effect by tachyphylaxis). The dispensation of commercial preparations diluted with an indifferent base is especially inexpedient in this regard. Long-term (more than 6 weeks, under occlusive dressings even earlier) use of topical corticosteroids can cause undesirable effects such as dermal atrophy, local hypertrichosis, development of telangiectasias, steroid rosacea of the face (see page 139), enhancement of infections and striae. All but the latter may be reversible. These adverse effects occur especially with prolonged application of

weak corticosteroid preparations to areas of thin skin (eyelids, face, genitals) or intertriginous areas such as axillae, groin, and the submammary region.

Some of the cortisone applied to the skin is resorbed and can produce systemic cortisone effects, especially with application of potent corticosteroids over large areas of the body (more than 25% of the body surface). Systemic side effects are more likely to occur with application of potent corticosteroids to areas of the skin with good absorption (in infants and children, intertriginous skin).

Penetration of the drug is enhanced by application under occlusive plastic gloves, shower cap, household plastic wrap, etc., or when affixed with tight-fitting clothing or tube gauze dressings. It must be considered that not only the desirable effects of cortisone, but also the undesirable effects are intensified by occlusive dressings, leading to folliculitis, for example.

The effect of corticosteroid preparations depends on the concentration as well as the selected drug. For practical purposes, corticosteroids can be classified in weak, medium and strong preparations. Weak preparations should be used for thin skin (face, small children) and in intertriginous areas. There are no differences in the effects of the different topical steroid preparations other than the varying potencies. The undesirable side effects can differ slightly in degree.

a) *Relatively weak cortisone preparations:*
   Hydrocortisone 1% cream and ointment: Generic
   Hytone
   Nutracort (lotion and cream)
   Dermacort cream
   Desonide 0.05% cream: Tridesilon

b) *Medium-strength cortisone preparations:*
   Triamcinolone 0.1% cream: Kenalog, Aristocort
   Desoximetasone 0.05% cream: Topicort-LP
   Hydrocortisone valerate cream 0.2%: Westcort,
   Fluocinolone
   Acetonide 0.025% cream: Synalar,
   Fluonid

c) *Strong cortisone preparations:*
   Betamethasone valerate 0.1% ointment: Valisone
   Amcinonide 0.1% ointment: Cyclocort
   Fluocinonide 0.05% cream: Lidex
   Desoximetasone 0.25% cream: Topicort
   Halcinonide 0.1% cream: Halog

d) *Very strong corticosteroids:*
   Clobetasol propionate 0.05% cream and ointment: Temovate
   Betametasone dipropionate ointment: Diprolene
   Diflorasone diacetate 0.05% ointment: Psorcon

e) *Steroids for application to mucous membranes:*
   Adhesive gel:

Rx: Betamethasone valerate		0.04
Polymethacrylic acid-sodium		1.0
Glycerol (85%)		4.0
Aqua purificata	to make	20.0

R. 39. Combined preparations containing corticosteroids:

Topical creams and ointments containing corticosteroids in combination with other medications are limited in the United States but are widely used in Europe, especially the combination with antibiotics and/or antifungal agents. These preparations are generally superfluous, and even worse, the physician may fail to perform adequate diagnostics when using them. Moreover, topical application of aminoglycoside antibiotics (such as gentamicin) can be hazardous because of the possible development of resistant organisms. Topical neomycin can cause contact allergy. The addition of disinfectants is acceptable.

a) *Iodochlorhydroxyquin and hydrocortisone:* Vioform hydrocortisone cream, ointment, lotion.

The combination of corticosteroids and urea or salicylic acid is useful to improve penetration and effectiveness.

b) *Hydrocortisone/urea:* Carmol HC, Alphaderm, Calmurid HC

Combinations of corticosteroids and coal tar have anti-inflammatory and antipruritic effects and are useful in chronic eczema. These combinations are not commercially available in the U.S.

R. 40. Antiparasitics:

The usual antiparasitic preparations are neurotoxic contact poisons. They are soluble in lipids and are easily resorbed, so that they may cause systemic toxic effects in infants and small children and during pregnancy. Package inserts provide directions for these patients. Lindane is accumulated in fatty tissue for a long time and may have potentially harmful effects on bone marrow, immune system and liver and can no longer be the first choice for the treatment of parasitoses.

Crotamiton: Eurax cream and lotion
Gamma benzene hexachloride (Lindane): Kwell (cream, lotion)
Scabene (cream, lotion)
5–10% Sulfur ointment (must be compounded)
Benzyl benzoate 20–25% lotion MSP (can be used during pregnancy)

R. 41. Antiphlogistic, antipruritic:

a) *Formulations with tar extracts*
for treatment of chronic eczematous conditions,
e.g., Wilkinson's ointment

Rx: Pix lithantracis	20.0
Sulfur praecip.	20.0
Sapo Kalin. med.	20.0
White vaseline, to make	100.0

b) Pure ichthyol 10-50% (e.g., Ichtholan 10, 20, 50%) is listed in the German text for enhancing the breakdown of abscesses in inflammation.
Caution: Coal tars are photosensitizing. Their content of aromatic hydrocarbons (carcinogenic) must be taken into account with long-term therapeutic application. With extensive application, damage to the kidneys is also possible. These undesired effects are not known for the tar products ichthyol and tumenol.

R. 42. Desquamatory:

a) *Salicylic vaseline:*
Rx: Salicylic acid 3.0-5.0 (-10%) in white vaseline to make 100.
Avoid prolonged total body use; systemic toxic effect from cutaneous absorption of salicylic acid is possible, especially in small children.

b) *Urea ointment:*

Rx: Urea	10.0
Aqua purif.	30.0
Unguentum cordes, to make	100.0

Commercial preparations with similar action:
Aquacare H.P. (10% urea cream)
Carmol 20 (20% urea cream)
Carmol 10 (10% urea lotion)

R. 43. Wound ointments, ulcer medications:
For this dermatological indication, there are a large number of different ointments that often contain many individual substances. Conclusive evidence for their effectiveness has been demonstrated for only a few individual components. Also, some of the more frequently used ingredients often cause contact allergies (Peru balsam, neomycin, benzocaine, sulfonamides). Local factors are more important for wound healing than topical medications. In poorly healing wounds (leg ulcers, decubitus ulcers, radiation ulcers) treatment of these local factors have first priority. In the absence of disturbing factors, a simple wound heals under a protective bandage that is permeable to air. Firmly adherent fibrin coatings and necroses can be easily softened by wet dressings. In addition, the bacteria which are present on all wounds contribute to the process with their fibrinolytic enzymes and collagenases.
Collagenase: Collagenase Santyl ointment
Dextranomer: Debrisan, Envisan Paste
Fibrinolysin and desoxyribonuclease: Elase ointment

R. 44. Acne medications:
Besides the primarily prescribed gels **(R. 25),** creams and the less oily emulsions are also useful, especially for sensitive skin; they can also be used for short intervals (5–10 minutes):

a) *Benzoyl peroxide:*
Clearasil cream

b) *Tretinoin, vitamin A acid:*
Retin-A cream

R. 45. Sunscreen preparations:
Most of the modern sunscreen preparations contain PABA (para-amino benzoic acid) or its esters or benzophenone derivatives. PABA protects the skin against ultraviolet light (wave lengths of 280 to 320 nm). Light of longer wave lengths and visible light penetrates PABA and causes tanning of the skin. PABA alone has a sun protective factor (SPF) of 4 to 10.
Benzophenone derivatives do not provide the same light protection as PABA. They filter a broader spectrum of UV rays, namely the wave lengths between 250 and 400 nm. PABA in combination with benzophenone derivatives provides a light protective factor of 10–15.

Other sunscreen preparations contain zinc oxide or titanium dioxide. They are completely impermeable for visible light and UV radiation, but as pastes they are cosmetically unsatisfactory. Since simple make-up (foundation) contains powder particles, it already provides a certain degree of light protection, depending on how thickly it is applied.

I. Corticosteroid Crystal Suspensions

R. 46. Intra- or sublesional injection of a corticosteroid crystal suspension with the Dermo-jet (principle of the inoculation pistol) or by intracutaneous injection represents an especially intensive form of local corticosteroid therapy. It is extremely important to avoid injecting the drug into the subcutaneous tissue (long-standing fat atrophy). Such injections should not be performed in the face due to the risk of a Hoigné syndrome.
Triamcinolone: Kenalog or Aristocort
Betamethasone: Celestone

Medications for Systemic Therapy

The following discussion includes commonly known medications also used for other indications, as well as drugs prescribed especially for the treatment of skin diseases.

A. Antibiotics

R. 47. Penicillins:
Oral: V-Cillin K
Pentids
Pen-Vee K
Parenteral: Bicillin
Wycillin
Dicloxacillin: Dynapen

R. 48. Broad-spectrum penicillins:
Amoxicillin, Ampicillin
Amoxicillin plus clavulanate potassium (Augmentin), effective against bacteria which form beta-lactamase.

R. 49. Tetracyclines:
Tetracycline: Achromycin, Sumycin
Oxytetracycline: Terramycin
Minocycline: Minocin
Doxycycline: Doxycline, Vibramycin (also available for i.v. injection)

R. 50. Cephalosporins:
Cefalexin: Keflex
Cefaclor: Ceclor
Cefixime: Suprax
Ceftriaxone: Rocephin
(Caution: Possible cross allergies with penicillin!)

R. 51. Erythromycin:
Erythromycin: Erythrocin, E-Mycin, Ilotycin
Clarithromycin: Biaxin

R. 52. Clindamycin:
Clindamycin should be reserved for difficult cases and not used routinely for acne therapy.
Cleocin

R. 53. Spectinomycin:
Trobicin, exclusively for treatment of gonorrhea

R. 54. Quinolones:
Norfloxacin: Chibroxin, Noroxin
Ofloxacin: Floxin
Ciprofloxacin: Cipro

B. Antimycotics

Systemic therapy is necessary for widespread or markedly inflammatory dermatomycoses that cannot be controlled with topical therapy, or when the hair is involved. Should mycoses of the nails require treatment, local therapy is often insufficient. Better resorption and higher effective levels of the medication can be achieved by administration with a fat-rich meal. The following medications are available for oral therapy:

R. 55. Griseofulvin:
The drug is effective selectively against dermatophytes and fungi. Undesirable effects are relatively rare. They include gastrointestinal disturbances, headaches, dizziness, insomnia, paresthesias, and very rarely leukopenia.
Commercial preparations:
Griseofulvin (micromized): Grifulvin V, Grisactin
Griseofulvin (ultramicromized): Gris-PEG, Grisactin Ultra, Fulvicin P/G
These drugs can be given in lower doses, since absorption is good.

R. 56. Ketoconazole:
This is a broad-spectrum antimycotic, effective against both dermatophytes and yeasts. Undesirable effects are rare (nausea, headaches, pruritus, gastrointestinal disturbances). However, there have been reported disturbances of liver function (some fatal) after prolonged use, so that the drug is no longer recommended for treatment of onychomycoses.
Commercial preparation: Nizoral tablets.

R. 57. Fluconazole:
Broad-spectrum antimycotic, also available for parenteral application. Its main indications are systemic mycoses, particularly with yeasts, as well as prophylactic treatment of HIV-infected patients and those receiving chemotherapy or radiation therapy.
Commercial preparation: Diflucan

R. 58. Itraconazole:
Broad-spectrum antimycotic for oral treatment of dermatomycoses, yeast mycoses and tropical mycoses. As with all imidazole preparations, interactions with other medications are possible due to interference with liver metabolism (cytochrome system). Regular check-ups are indicated when the drug is used for long periods (in dermatology especially for onychomycosis).
Commercial preparation: Sporanox

R. 59. Terbinafine:
In contrast to the above-mentioned imidazole derivatives, this medication is a so-called allylamine with fungistatic as well as fungicidal action on dermatophytes. This makes this drug especially effective for onychomycoses. Regular control examinations are recommended, especially during long-term treatment.
Commercial preparation: Lamisil

C. Virostatic Drugs

For systemic treatment of diseases caused by herpesvirus and varicella zoster virus, several virostatic drugs are available. Resistance can develop against these drugs, as has been shown, by unwarranted use of the medication. It is certainly not necessary to treat all recurrent herpes simplex conditions and every uncomplicated zoster with a systemic antiviral drug.

R. 60. Virostatic drugs:
Acyclovir: Zovirax tablets, Zovirax solution, i.v. therapy
Famciclovir: Famvir tablets
Valacyclovir: Valtrex tablets

Resorption of these drugs is poor, and i.v. administration is recommended for severe diseases. The effectiveness of prophylactic administration of acyclovir for recurrent herpes simplex infections is controversial, since the development of resistances is still unclear.

D. Antihistamines

For dermatologic therapy, mainly H_1-receptor blockers are used. They are most effective for acute urticaria and hayfever, but also helpful in the treatment of chronic urticaria. Their effectiveness, however, against pruritus of other etiologies is limited.
For practical purposes, antihistamines can be classified as those with and those without a sedative component. Although sedation can be helpful in the treatment of sleep disturbances caused by pruritus, it is not desirable in a day medication (responsiveness, traffic safety). Combinations of antihistamines with caffeine to reduce the sedative effect or with corticosteroids are not very meaningful because of their dissimilar pharmacokinetics.

R. 61. Antihistamines with little or no sedative effect:
Tripelennamine hydrochloride: PBZ
Cetirizine: Zyrtec
Loratadine: Claritin
Astemizole: Hismanal

R. 62. Antihistamines with sedative effect:
Promethazine: Phenergan
Hydroxyzine: Atarax, Vistaril
Chlorpheniramine: Chlor-Trimeton
Clemastine: Tavist
Cyproheptadine: Periactin
Dimetindene: Tritan, Fenistil

E. Corticosteroids

R. 63. Dermatologic indications for systemic corticosteroid therapy are severe and widespread diseases or acute problems that require a rapid therapeutic effect (adverse drug reactions, diseases of the pemphigus group), as well as skin disease with concomitant involvement of internal organs, such as lupus erythematosus. Undesirable effects and contraindications of corticosteroid therapy must be kept in mind, especially in chronic illnesses that require long-term therapy. These include Cushing's syndrome, hypertension, osteoporosis, a diabetogenic effect, edemas, peptic ulcers, glaucoma, cataracts, immunosuppression with increased incidence of infection, increased risk of thrombosis and induction of psychoses. For practical purposes, knowledge of a few selected corticosteroids and their effective strengths is sufficient.

Table 2

Drug	Cushing Threshold (mg)	Lowest Dose with anti-inflammatory Effect (mg)	Commercial Preparations
Hydrocortisone	40	40	Cortef tabs.
Prednisone	10	7	Deltasone tabs. Meticorten tabs.
Prednisolone	10	7	Prednisolone tabs.
Methyl-prednisolone	8	5	Medrol tabs.
Triamcinolone	8	5	Aristocort tabs.
Dexamethasone	2	1	Decadron tabs
Betamethasone tablets	2	1	Celestone tabs.

For long-term treatment, corticosteroids are administered according to the circadian rhythm of endogenous cortisone secretion: in the morning, or even better, every other morning (alternating administration), provided the status of the disease permits this. Systemic corticosteroid administration with i.m. injection of depot preparations does not allow adequate regulation of cortisone, as well as causing significant suppression of the adrenal cortex, so that it cannot be recommended. Combinations of corticosteroids with other active ingredients, especially antihistamines, can be ignored, at least in dermatologic practice.

Low-dose cortisone therapy, as discussed here, means administration of the drug in the lowest anti-inflammatory dose, if possible, below the Cushing level (see Table 2 above). A median dose would be equivalent to 30 to 50 mg of prednisone; a high dose would be equivalent to 100 mg or more of prednisone per day.

F. Retinoids

Retinoids, derivatives of vitamin A, have become very important in dermatological therapy in recent years. All retinoids are teratogenic, therefore treatment of women of childbearing age is not recommended (see respective package inserts).

Undesired effects include dry lips, loss of hair, and thinning of the skin, especially in the palmar and plantar areas. Elevation of the blood fats and of the hepatic enzymes is sometimes observed. These parameters must be checked at regular intervals during treatment with retinoids. Long-term therapy with retinoids can lead to alterations of bone (hyperostoses), which have been observed so far mainly in children.

Based on experience to date and with respect to economic principles when prescribing these expensive preparations, it is advisable to consult an experienced dermatologist before employing oral synthetic retinoids. At the present time, two preparations are available for systemic therapy: acitretin and isotretinoin.

R. 64. Acitretin (Neotigason):

Indications: Severe psoriasis, especially pustular psoriasis, psoriatic erythroderma, psoriatic arthritis, as well as several hereditary disorders of keratinization, and lichen planus. Other possible indications that are still experimental at the present time include chronic lupus erythematosus, cutaneous T-cell lymphoma and pre-invasive leukoplakia. The most significant limitation in the therapeutic use of acitretin is the drug's teratogenic effect. Treatment of women of childbearing age is not recommended (see package insert).

R. 65. Isotretinoin (Accutane/Roaccutane):

Indications: Severe forms of acne, especially acne conglobata, severe rosacea. For cutaneous T-cell lymphoma, a combination therapy with UV radiation, also in combination with a photosensitizing agent (Re-SUP or Re-PUVA), has been found successful. Treatment of women of childbearing age is not recommended because of the drug's teratogenic effect (see package insert).

G. Fumaric Acid

R. 66. Fumaric acid ester

A combination of several fumaric acid esters is available in Germany as Fumaderm for oral treatment of severe forms of psoriasis, however with varying success. The main undesirable effects are gastrointestinal problems, flush, leukopenia and an increase in creatinine. Regular laboratory tests before and during treatment are necessary.

Compression Bandages

For the general practitioner, a very important aid to prevent venous stasis is the compression bandage. Its effectiveness depends a great deal on the technique of application and the appropriate material for the respective indication.
Compression bandages or elastic stockings are prescribed prophylactically to prevent emboli and thromboses, especially in bed-ridden patients. Therapeutically, they are used for treatment of insufficiency of the leg veins or lymphedema. The only contraindication for compression bandages is arterial occlusive disease of stages III and IV.

If the condition of the skin requires frequent wound care (e.g., leg ulcers, stasis dermatitis), dressings and bandages are changed every day. The following chapter discusses in brief the materials available for these dressings.

Bandages with short tension tracts exert a strong working pressure and have a significant deep effect. They are used for compression therapy in ambulatory patients. Correct application of a compression bandage requires some practice.

Bandages with medium or long tension tracts have a higher resting pressure and are more suitable for the prophylaxis of thromboses in bed-ridden patients. They are more elastic and easier to apply.

Fixed bandages such as Unna's paste bandages or adhesive bandages are left in place for several days. They are usually applied by the physician and fit better.

If no special wound care is necessary, compression stockings are better for long-term treatment and are easier to apply. They should be custom-made and can be obtained as calf-sleeves, knee stockings, full-length stockings and pantyhose, depending on the extent of the venous insufficiency. Ready made support stockings are not appropriate for compression therapy.

Compression stockings are available for various indications in the following compression categories:
Compression category I: Ankle pressure 20 mmHg.
For mild varicosities (beginning varicosities of pregnancy).
Compression category II: Ankle pressure 30 mmHg.
For severe varicosities with occasional edema.
Compression category III: Ankle pressure 40 mmHg.
For sequelae of ulcus cruris (leg ulcer), postthrombotic syndrome.
Compression category IV: Ankle pressure 60 mmHg.
For lymphedema.

It must be kept in mind that the material becomes stiffer in the higher compression categories, and more strength is required to apply the stockings. This is especially important in older women who may not wear the stockings if they are too hard to put on. Since mild compression is better than no compression at all, it may be wise to prescribe a pair of stockings with less compression than is actually indicated. It may also be easier to apply two stockings of compression category II, thus providing the compression effect of Category III to IV.
A new pair of stockings must be prescribed every 6 months when continuous compression treatment is necessary and the stockings are worn regularly. Frequent washing prolongs the life of the stockings.

Index

A

Abscess 4, 132–133
Acid burn 156
Acne
  conglobata 2, 4–5, 133
  excoriée 3
  necroticans 86
  steroid-induced 20–21
  vulgaris 2–5
Acneiform eruption 21
Acrocyanosis 34
Acrodermatitis chronica atrophicans 59
Actinic keratosis 224–225
Addision's disease 108–109
AIDS 168–171
Allergic dermatitis 37
Alopecia 68–71
  androgenetic 70–71
  areata 68–69, 109
Angioedema 19, 153–155
Angioma
  senile 192–193
  venous 192–193
Angular cheilitis 99
Aphthae 10–11
Arterial disease, obstructive 28–29
Arteriosclerosis 28–29
Arthritis, psoriatic 127
Atheromas 184–185
Atopic dermatitis 40–45, 125, 133
Atrophie blanche 30–31
Atrophy, senile 7

B

Balanitis 73, 179
  simplex 178
Bandages, elastic 262
Basal cell carcinoma 226–229
Baths 246
Bedbug bites 80–81
Bee sting 78–79
Benign symmetric lipomatosis 196–197
Black hairy tongue 162–163
Blue nevus 204–205
Borrelia burgdorferi 59
Bowen's disease 230, 238
Bromhidrosis 77
Bullae 22–23
Bullous pemphigoid 22–25
Burn 158–159
  acid 156–157
  chemical 156–157

C

C1-Inhibitor deficiency 155
Café au lait macules 205
Callus 208–211
Candidiasis 47, 83, 99, 116–119
Carbuncle 132–133
Carcinoma
  basal cell 226–229
  oral mucosal 236–237
  squamous cell 9, 32, 54, 136, 225, 238–241
Cheilitis 98–99
  angular 171
  chronic actinic 8–9
Cherry angiomas 192
Chilblains 33, 64–65
Chloasma 110–111
Chondrodermatitis helicis 8–9
Clavi 208–209
Cold panniculitis 65
Comedones 2–6

Compression bandages 262
Condylomata
  acuminata 217–219
  lata 176
Contact dermatitis 36–39
Corn 208–209
Cornu cutaneum 8
Cradle cap 40
Creams 251–256
Creeping eruption 150–151
Crusta lactea 40
Culicosis bullosa 78
Cutis
  marmorata 35
  vagantium 90
Cysts, senile 7

D

Decubitus
  ulcer 26–27
Dermatitis 36–53
  artefacta 12–15
  atopic 40–45, 99, 125, 133
  contact 36–39
  herpetiformis 24–25
  phototoxic 94–95
  radiation 136–137
  solaris 94–95
Dermatofibroma 187
Dermatosclerosis 30–31
Dermographism, white 42–43
Diaper
  dermatitis 47–48
  rash 116
DLE 100–101
Dressings, wet 246
Drug eruption
  fixed 16, 19
  maculopapular 16–17
Dry skin 148–149

E

Eczema 36–53
  ear 50–51
  herpeticum 74–75
  hyperkeratotic, palmoplantar 46–47
  lichenified 52
  nummular 51–53
  occupational 37
  palmoplantar 44–45
  vesicular 44–45
Elastosis 7
Elephantiasis 102–103
Emulsions 251–256
Endangiitis obliterans 28
Ephelides 110–111
Epidermolysis bullosa 24–25
Eppinger stars 193
Erysipelas 56–57, 103
Erythema
  chronicum migrans 58–59
  multiforme 60–61, 73
  nodosum 62–63
Erythrasma 82–83
Erythroplakia 241
Exanthema, macular 17
Exfoliatio areata 161, 163

F

Fasciitis, necrotizing 57
Favre-Racouchot's disease 5–7
Fibroma 186–187
Fiddler's neck 209–211
Flea bites 80–81
Folliculitis 131
Freckles 110–111
Frostbite 54–55
Fuchs' syndrome 61
Fungal diseases 112–121
Furuncle 130–131
Furunculosis 131–132

G

Gangrene, diabetic 28
Gels 249–250
Geographic tongue 162–163
Giant nevus 203
Gingivitis 142
Gingivostomatitis, herpetic 11, 72
Glossitis, median rhomboid 164–165
Gluten-sensitive enteropathy 25
Gonorrhea 172–173

Granuloma
annulare 66–67
pyogenic 206–207
telangiectaticum 207
Grass dermatitis 94
Gumma 177

H

Hair loss 68–71
Halo nevomelanocytic nevus 203
Hemangioma 188–193
strawberry 188–189
Hematolymphangioma 102
Hematoma 7
Hemorrhage 7, 21
Henoch-Schönlein disease 21
Herald patch 122
Hereditary angioedema 154
Herpangina 142
Herpes
genital 178
keratitis 73
simplex 72–75
zoster 160–161
Herpetic gingivostomatitis 72–73
Hertoghe's sign 42–43
Hidradenitis, suppurative 133
Hirsuties papillaris penis 181
Hirsutism 70
Histiocytoma 186–187
HIV-infection 168–171
Hyperhidrosis 76–77, 121
Hyperpigmentation 109
Hypertrichosis 97

I

Ichthyosis vulgaris 148
Immunocytoma 236
Impetigo 133–135
Ingrown nail 106–107
Injury, self-inflicted 12–15
Insect bites 79
Intertrigo 82–83
Itching 85
Ixodes ricinus 58–59

K

Kaposi's sarcoma 168–171
Keloid 194–195
Keratoacanthoma 224–225
Keratolysis, pitted 76–77
Keratoma plantare sulcatum 76–77
Keratosis
actinic 6, 8, 224–225
seborrheic 212–213
solar 224–225
Knuckle pads 208
Koebner's phenomenon 92
Kraurosis
penis 178–179
vulvae 178–179

L

Larva migrans 150–151
Leg ulcer 29
Lentigines
senile 8
solar 110–111
Lentigo maligna 234–235
Leukoplakia 230–231, 241
oral hairy 168–171
Lice 88–91
Lichen
planus 92–93
simplex chronicus 52
Lichenification 42
Light reaction 94–97
Lingua
geographica 163
plicata 162–163
villosa nigra 163
Lip diseases 98–99
Lipoatrophy 20
Lipoma 196–197
Lipomatosis, benign symmetric 196–197
Livedo reticularis 34–35
Lotions 251–256
Lupus erythematosus 100–101
Lyell's syndrome 19
Lymphangiosarcoma 103
Lymphedema 15, 57, 102–103
Lymphocytoma 58–59
Lymphoma
cutaneous T-cell 236–237
malignant 236–237

M

Maculae caeruleae 90
Madelung's
 fat neck 196
 syndrome 197
Malum perforans 26
Mees' lines 106
Melanoma, malignant 232–235
Melasma 110–111
Milia 198–199
Miliaria 104–105
Molluscum contagiosum 168, 200–201
Morphea, generalized 32
Mosquito bites 79
Münchausen syndrome 13
Mycosis 112–121
 fungoides 237
Myiasis 151

N

Nail diseases 106–107
Necrobiosis lipoidica 66–67
Necrolysis, toxic epidermal 18–19, 61
Neurofibromatosis von Recklinghausen 205
Neurosyphilis 177
Nevomelanocytic nevi 202
Nevus
 araneus 193
 flammeus 189–191
 nevomelanocytic 202–205
 pigmented 202–205
 spilus 110, 204–205
 spindle cell 204–205
 Spitz 204–205
Nits 88
Nummular eczema 51–53

O

Ointments 251–256
Onychogryphosis 106
Onychomycosis 114–115
Onychophagia 13
Oral hairy leukoplakia 168–171

P

Painful piezogenic pedal papules (PPPP) 196
Panniculitis, cold 65
Paraffin granuloma 14
Paraphimosis 180–181
Paronychia 107, 118–119
Pastes 250–251
Pearly penile papules 180–181
Pediculosis 88–91
Pemphigus
 vegetans 22
 vulgaris 22–23
Perlèche 98–99, 171
Perniosis 64–65
Phimosis 180–181
Phlebitis 146
Photoallergic reaction 97
Phototoxic
 dermatitis 94
 reaction 18–19
Pigmentation 108–111
Pigmented nevi 203
Pilar cyst 185
Pitted keratolysis 77
Pityriasis
 alba 108–109
 rosea 122–123
 versicolor 119–121
Pompholyx 41, 44–45
Porphyria cutanea tarda 96–97
Port-wine stain 189
Postthrombotic syndrome 32
Powders 247
PPPP 196
Prurigo 124–125
Pruritus 84–87
Pseudocars 6–7
Pseudocysts 5–6
Pseudolymphoma 237
Psoriasis 126–129
Purpura 21
 senile 6–7
Pustular psoriasis 126–129
Pustules 130–131
Pyodermas 130–135
Pyogenic granuloma 206

Q

Quincke's edema 153

R

Radiation damage 136–137
Raynaud's phenomenon 34–35
Retention cyst 184–185
Reticuloid, actinic 97
Rhinophyma 138–139
Ritter's disease 134
Rosacea 138–139
Rosacea-like dermatitis 138–139

S

Sand flea bites 150–151
Scabies 140–141
Scalding 158–159
Sebaceous glands, heterotopic 181
Sebocystomatosis 184
Seborrhea 3
Seborrheic
  dermatitis 49–51
  keratosis 212–213
Self-inflicted skin lesions 12–15
Shake mixtures 249
Shingles 161
Shock 153
Skin tags 186–187
SLE 100–101
Solutions 247–249
Spider nevi 192–193
Spindle cell nevomelanocytic nevus 204–205
Spitz nevus 204–205
Squamous cell carcinoma 9, 32, 54, 136, 225, 238–241
Stasis
  dermatitis 31, 48–49
  purpura 31
Steal phenomenon 29
Steroid
  acne 20
  rosacea 139
Stevens-Johnson syndrome 61
Stewart-Treves syndrome 103
Stings 79
Stockings, elastic 262
Stomatitis 142–143
Strawberry hemangioma 188–189
Sun reactions 94–97
Sunburn 94–95
Suppurative hidradenitis 133
Sutton's nevus 202–203
Sweating, increased 77
Symplepharon 19
Syphilis 168, 174–177

T

Tattoo 144–145
Thrombocytopenia 21
Thrombophlebitis 146–147
  erysipelatoid 57
Thrush 83, 99, 116–119
Tick 58, 59
Tinctures 247–249
Tinea 112–115
Tongue
  black hairy 162–163
  fissured 162–163
  geographic 162–163
Toxic epidermal necrolysis 18, 61
Trichilemmal cyst 185
Trichomycosis 75
  palmellina 76–77
Trichotillomania 13, 70–71
Trombidiosis 80–81

U

Ulcer 26
Ulcus cruris 29
Unguis incarnatus 106–107
Urticaria 19, 152–154
UV-light reaction 94–97

V

Varices 30, 146
Varicosis 30
Venous
  disorders 29–33
  lake 192–193
Verrucae vulgares 214–215
Vesicles 22–23

Violinist's callus 209–211
Vitiligo 108–109
Vulvitis, herpetic 73–74
Vulvovaginitis 179
  herpetic 73

W

Warts
  common 214–219
  flat 216–217
  infectious 214–219
  plantar 216–217
Wasp stings 79
Wen 185
Wet dressings 246
Wickham's striae 92–93

X

Xanthelasma 220–221
Xanthoma 220–221
Xerosis 149

Z

Zoster 160–161